DATE DUE

NO 9 '95			
FE 12 '98			
NY 4 '99			
DE 6 05			

DEMCO 38-296

STANDARD OF CARE

ALSO BY THE AUTHOR

The Rights of Patients
Judging Medicine

Co-authored

Informed Consent to Human Experimentation:
The Subject's Dilemma
(with Leonard Glantz and Barbara Katz)

The Rights of Doctors, Nurses and Allied Health Professionals
(with Leonard Glantz and Barbara Katz)

Reproductive Genetics and the Law
(with Sherman Elias)

American Health Law
(with Sylvia Law, Rand Rosenblatt, and Ken Wing)

Co-edited

Genetics and the Law, Genetics and the Law II, and
Genetics and the Law III
(with Aubrey Milunsky)

The Nazi Doctors and the Nuremberg Code:
Human Rights in Human Experimentation
(with Michael Grodin)

Gene Mapping: Using Law and Ethics as Guides
(with Sherman Elias)

STANDARD OF CARE

The Law of American Bioethics

GEORGE J. ANNAS

New York   Oxford
OXFORD UNIVERSITY PRESS
1993

Oxford University Press

Oxford   New York   Toronto
Delhi   Bombay   Calcutta   Madras   Karachi
Kuala Lumpur   Singapore   Hong Kong   Tokyo
Nairobi   Dar es Salaam   Cape Town
Melbourne   Auckland   Madrid

and associated companies in
Berlin   Ibadan

Published by Oxford University Press, Inc.,
200 Madison Avenue, New York, New York 10016

Library of Congress Cataloging-in-Publication Data
Annas, George J.
Standard of care : the law of American bioethics /
George J. Annas.
p.   cm.   Includes bibliographical references and index.
ISBN 0-19-507247-2
1. Medical laws and legislation — United States.
2. Bioethics — United States.
I. Title.   [DNLM: 1. Bioethics.
2. Ethics, Medical.
3. Legislation, Medical — United States.
W 50 A613s]   KF3821.A95   1993
344.73′041 — dc20   [347.30441]
DNLM/DLC   for Library of Congress   92-18728

9 8 7 6 5 4 3 2 1

Printed in the United States of America
on acid-free paper

In Memory of My Father
George J. Annas, Sr.

Acknowledgments

As with virtually all of my writing, I owe enormous amounts of thanks to the conversations, commentaries, and criticisms of my wonderful colleagues at Boston University's Law, Medicine and Ethics Program: Leonard H. Glantz, Wendy K. Mariner, and Michael A. Grodin. Many of these chapters also benefited from the comments and questions of audiences of physicians, lawyers, judges, students, and the general public who heard them in their early forms as lectures. It is also a pleasure to once again acknowledge the unswerving support Norman A. Scotch, under whose leadership at Boston University's School of Public Health this book was written.

Major portions of Chapters 1, 4, and 13 have appeared in the *New England Journal of Medicine*; Chapters 2, 3, 6, 8, 12, 14, 18, and 19 in the *Hastings Center Report*, Chapters 5 and 7 in *Law, Medicine and Health Care*, Chapter 9 in the *American Journal of Public Health*; Chapter 10 in the *Villanova Law Review*; Chapter 11 in the *Emory Law Journal*; Chapter 15 in the *Western New England Law Review*, Chapter 17 in the *American Journal of Law and Medicine*; and the final chapter in the *Connecticut Law Review*.

Contents

III Public Sector Bioethics

STANDARD OF CARE

Introduction

The nation's leading bioethicists, meeting at the fall 1992 "Birth of Bioethics" conference in Seattle, were startled when keynoter Shana Alexander told them, "I trust my lawyer more than I trust my doctor." Even in the midst of an unrelenting lawyer-bashing Presidential campaign, the bioethicists should not have been surprised. American law, especially civil rights law, is dedicated to fostering individual rights, equality, and justice. Law sides with patients to oppose the arbitrary use of power whether by physicians or the government; the rubric is patient rights. This is why American law, not philosophy or medicine, is primarily responsible for the agenda, development and current state of American bioethics. It seems natural to Americans, for example, that the morality of abortion has been recast as the "right to abortion" and that the morality of medical treatment near the end of life is now called simply the "right to die." America is, after all, the most rights-centered society on earth, and our Constitution's Bill of Rights and Fourteenth Amendment naturally lend themselves to defining personal decisionmaking in terms of constitutional rights.

It seemed perfectly appropriate to me when *Roe v. Wade*[1] was seriously threatened in *Webster*[2] that Planned Parenthood asked me to write an amicus brief to the U.S. Supreme Court on behalf of American bioethicists. My colleagues Leonard Glantz, Wendy Mariner, and I filed this brief in March 1989 on behalf of an ad hoc group we called Bioethicists for Privacy composed of philosophers, theologians, attorneys, and physicians from twenty-one states who either taught medical ethics or who had a major professional interest in the subject.[3] This was the first bioethics brief ever filed with the U.S. Supreme Court. Then, after the Court issued its decision in *Cruzan*[4] on the right to die in 1990, a group of bioethicists, meeting at their annual retreat shortly after the decision was rendered, felt it appropriate to draft a bioethicists' statement on the decision to help guide physician reaction. It was published in the *New England Journal of Medicine.*[5]

Both the brief and the statement were not about what philosophers would term ethics; they were about the state of American law: what it is and what it should be. And in America the state of the law often depends on the U.S. Supreme Court's interpretation of the Constitution. This is because the Constitution restricts the power of the state and its officials to interfere with the rights of its citizens. Politics also determines law. This is why the election of President Bill Clinton produced a major shift in virtually all laws and federal policies affecting abortion.

The case-based common law approach to adjudication of conflicts is used in all former British colonies, and is the fundamental way judges make decisions (applying principles deduced from previously decided cases to decide current cases) in the English-speaking world. In this regard, applying accepted legal principles to decide a specific case is a substantially identical process to applying ethical principles to decide a specific case. And because lawyers are experts at procedures, lawyers tend to be seen as the experts at procedural decisionmaking, even in the "ethical arena." Many of the chapters in this book, for example, are based on specific cases that have been decided in U.S. courts — but the analysis these courts used is often the same one a group of ethicists would have applied.

"Standard of care" is a legal term denoting the level of conduct a physician or health care provider must meet in treating a patient so as not to be guilty of negligence, usually called malpractice. That standard is generally defined simply as what a reasonably prudent physician (or specialist) would do in the same or similar circumstances. This is a profession-centered standard, and encompasses a wide range of practices. When I began my own career in health law some twenty years ago, I spent most of my time with physicians telling them that they did not take the law seriously enough — that they were unfairly paternalistic and did not permit their patients to exercise basic human rights. Although I still believe that patients often (even usually) have great difficulty in actually exercising their rights in most hospitals and long-term care facilities, I now spend most of my time telling physicians and health care providers that they are taking the law too seriously — and are in danger of letting fear of liability replace reasoned judgment, and abdicating their responsibility to define "good medical care" and set the standard for such care.

For far too many physicians, the first question they ask is not "Is this the right thing to do?" but, rather, "Is this legal?" or, worse, "Can I get sued if I do this?" The answer to the latter question is always yes, and the question is virtually meaningless since in the United States anyone can sue anyone for almost anything. Asking the question in this context, however, has physicians stating explicitly that lawyers and judges, rather than physicians and their patients, should be responsible for setting the medical standard of care, and that protecting themselves from lawsuits is more important to physicians than treating their patients to the best of their ability.

This is where the term "defensive medicine" came from. It should be emphasized at the outset that *any* medical treatment done primarily to protect the physician from potential lawsuits (rather than to benefit the patient), although sometimes legal, is by definition unethical. And to the extent that exaggerated legal concerns, rather than patient-centered and sound professional practice concerns, determine treatment decisions, medicine both abuses patients and abdicates its responsibility to set the standard of care. One core thesis of this book is that while the standard of care in the United States is strongly influenced by the law, for this standard to be beneficial to both patients and the public it must be based much more on doing the "right thing" (which is practicing good medicine with the informed consent of the patient) than doing what is legally safest in terms of potential liability.

This book uses a case-based approach to explore fundamental value questions confronting society with a view toward stimulating thought and discussion that can help clarify which values deserve legal support in the U.S. Because it deals with fundamental human rights, however, it should also help clarify which values should underlie international human rights law. The realm of human rights law is necessarily somewhat removed from U.S. bioethics in the sense that America is constitutionally and culturally unique. On the other hand, because human rights are based on human characteristics, the universal is more important than the particular. The short term quest is to demonstrate how law shapes both ethical discourse and medical practice. The longer term quest is to use these examples to help articulate an international agenda for human rights in health.

Of course, as a lawyer I can easily be accused of having a jaundiced eye and of seeing legal issues where others see only ethical concerns. Can the proposition that American law is primarily responsible for the development of the current state of American bioethics be proven? The arguments and examples presented in this book, I believe, provide sufficient proof. It is nonetheless useful to begin our exploration of the world of law and bioethics with an example of the pervasiveness of law on bioethics in America. The development of a uniquely American invention, the bioethics committee (usually called simply the ethics committee) illustrates the point clearly, and in a variety of contexts.

ETHICS COMMITTEES

When I began to write a regular column on law for the bioethics journal, *The Hastings Center Report*, more than fifteen years ago, my first column was entitled "In re Quinlan: Legal Comfort for Doctors."[6] The subtitle referred to the New Jersey Supreme Court's suggestion that instead of bringing cases like *Quinlan*[7] to court, families and physicians should rely on a hospital ethics committee. The court based this recommendation on a suggestion of a Texas pediatrician, Karen Teel, that a committee "composed of physicians, social workers, attorneys and theologians" could help diffuse the "professional responsibility for decision." I was unenthusiastic about the New Jersey solution, noting that "The idea seems to be that all feel more (ethically?) 'comfortable' with decisions thus arrived at for which no one individual is seen as responsible and for which no individual can be held legally accountable."

Although the *Quinlan* case has been the touchstone for legal and ethical discussions of the right to refuse medical treatment for more than fifteen years, no other court has delegated immunity-granting authority to an ethics committee. On the other hand, the strategy of using ethics committees to provide "comfort" for physicians and others worried about either legal liability or public reaction has prospered. Ethics committees have grown from an anomalous entity to provide ethical comfort to a few, to an almost standard entity to provide ethical cover for many.

Without the threat of legal liability and community disapproval (which could lead to new laws), ethics committees would probably not have developed at all. As the cases explored in this book illustrate, law and ethics are distinct, though related, activities. The law is mandatory, setting standards that can only be breached at the risk of civil or criminal liability. Ethics is aspirational, setting forth universal goals that we should try to meet, but for which we suffer no temporal penalty when falling short. Ethicists often criticize the law as too blunt, as scaring people unnecessarily, as interfering, and as counterproductive. All of these criticisms are sometimes fair.

In the 1960s some states required that hospital review committees approve any abortion before it could be legally performed. And when kidney dialysis began, and there was a shortage of dialysis machines, some hospitals set up committees to decide which of the competing candidates would receive dialysis. *Roe v. Wade* (and its companion case, *Doe v. Bolton*[8]) ended the abortion committees, and both public reaction and the End Stage Renal Disease Act ended the dialysis patient selection committees. Public reaction was spurred by Shana Alexander's November 1962 *Life* article, "The God Committee." Although there have been periodic attempts to use similar "ethics committees" to make decisions for individual patients (for example, psychosurgery committees), prospective decisionmaking by committee for individual patients has never held wide support, either in the medical community or the public.

The Infant Care Review or "Baby Doe" committees were established in many neonatal intensive care units across the country as a direct response to the Reagan administration's Baby Doe regulations.[9] Under the threat of intrusive federal investigations, the American Academy of Pediatrics and others recommended an alternative: hospital-based committees that would be available to review contested decisions to withdraw treatment from handicapped newborns. Many of these committees have survived, even though the federal Baby Doe regulations did not.

Institutional Review Boards (IRBs)

The most longstanding "ethics"-type committee is the Institutional Review Board, or IRB. This committee was created by law, and specific federal regulations govern its conduct. In the 1960s, when such committees were rare, they were usually designated as human studies or human subjects

committees. In the 1970s their name was changed to "institutional" committees—and this has always seemed just right, because the primary function
of the committee is to protect the institution, and its membership is almost
exclusively made up of researchers (not potential subjects) from the particular institution. These committees have changed the face of research in the
United States, by requiring researchers to justify their research on humans
to a peer review group prior to recruiting subjects. But this does not mean
that they have made research universally more "ethical." In at least a few
spectacular instances, these committees provided ethical and legal cover
that enabled experiments to be performed that would otherwise not have
been performed because of their potentially devastating impact on human
subjects. The most dramatic examples are the experiments with the permanent artificial heart at the University of Utah and the Humana Heart Institute in Louisville, and xenograft experiments at Loma Linda, the University
of Pittsburgh, and Cedars-Sinai Medical Center, Los Angeles. The success
of IRBs can be traced primarily to their very specific mandate, their standards of decisionmaking (spelled out in federal regulations), and their support by the medical and research-funding communities.[10] Their failures can
generally be traced to an overidentification with the perceived needs and
interests of the institution and with the lack of expertise in particularly
novel or complex research.

Institutional Ethics Committees (IECs)

Unlike IRBs, IECs have no standard mission and operate under no governing regulations. Since they have no standard mission, and vary widely in
terms of purpose, composition, authority, and resources, they are also
impossible to evaluate. Insofar as their primary mission is to protect the
institution by providing an alternative forum to litigation or unwanted
publicity, the term ethics is inappropriate, and the committee should be
called a risk management committee or a liability control committee.

Like all of the previous committees that could be labeled ethics committees, their primary preoccupation has been to respond to legal changes and
challenges, rather than to do anything a philosopher might label "ethics."
Many such committees, for example, have drafted their institution's policy
on such issues as brain death, the withdrawal of life support, and the
implementation of required request laws. Other ethics committees see their
primary function as staff education. This is entirely laudable, and ultimately it may be the most effective method of behavior modification.

A few of these committees consult in individual cases that are brought to
them. They are least suited for this role. Consultations are almost always
better when performed one on one, and this is probably why the ethics
consultant is replacing the ethics committee in this role.[11] If they are to
provide a forum for dispute resolution, the committees must follow some
basic due process guidelines. Once these are provided, however, the committee becomes like an administrative agency (of the kind envisioned by the
Quinlan court), and both its procedures and the substantive rules it applies

are likely (and appropriately) to be much more legal in nature than ethical. This helps explain why law consistently dominates ethics in the institutional setting, and why IECs can seldom aspire to anything higher than the lowest common denominator the law allows. On the other hand, ethics committees can function well as simply a neutral forum for discussion to attempt to resolve disputes—but in this case the ethics label seems misleading.

Professional Organizations and Ethics Committees

Ethics committees have become an integral part of many professional medical organizations. The American Academy of Pediatrics was the moving force behind the Baby Doe ethics committees and has its own ethics committee as well. Both the American College of Obstetricians and Gynecologists (ACOG) and the American Fertility Society (AFS) also have their own ethics committees. These two organizations formed a cosponsored national ethics committee in 1991 to, among other things, suggest guidelines for human embryo research. Since the federal government abandoned its support for the Ethics Advisory Board in 1980, there has certainly been a need for such a group. Whether ACOG and AFS are the proper organizations to sponsor it, however, is a more difficult question. In seeking an answer, it is useful to review how these organizations have used their own ethics committees in the recent past.

The AFS set up its ethics committee, composed almost exclusively of its own members, to make recommendations about the new reproductive technologies that its members use. The committee was well aware that the central and most contested subject for recommendations was the status of the extracorporeal human embryo and what could and could not ethically be done to it. Rather than build on previous studies, like those of the Ethics Advisory Board, England's Warnock Commission, and Australia's Waller Commission, the AFS ethics committee opted to "solve" their members' problem by redefinition. The committee decided that extracorporeal human embryos were not really embryos at all, but were "preembryos," an invented term for what had previously been called preimplantation embryos. The committee's definition of this neologism is "a living, genetically unique entity with a statistical potential to implant, if exposed to a receptive uterus, and to be delivered as a newborn infant." The embryo, on the other hand, is described as "far more complex" and giving rise to "the rapidly growing and maturing fetus."[12] All this would seem unimportant wordplay, except that redefining the preimplantation embryo as a nonembryo permitted the committee to advise its members that anything goes with these now nonembryos:

> Currently, the responsibility for establishing policies on the transfer or nontransfer of preembryos lies with the programs that offer medical assistance in reproduction. Each program should develop and announce to candidate couples explicit policies on the options of transfer, donation, preembryo research, storage, and discard.

This basic recommendation is repeated in the sections on cryopreservation of embryos and research on embryos.

ACOG's ethics committee meets more regularly than AFS's, and it develops much shorter policy opinions, usually three pages long, for its members. A typical opinion is on "Multifetal Pregnancy Reduction and Selective Fetal Termination."[13] Like embryo research, this topic is highly controversial, and one in which national policy guidelines would be highly desirable. ACOG's very able, but primarily physician-composed, committee worked on this policy for years, and it did its homework. The committee properly distinguished multifetal pregnancy reductions (usually the by-product of fertility drugs) from selective fetal termination (when one of two or more fetuses is diagnosed as having an abnormality). Nonetheless, when it came to the ethical bottom line, it was the same as the AFS's bottom line: its member practitioners could "ethically" do whatever they and their patients decided in each case. For multiple pregnancy reduction, "the issue of patient choice and physician participation and consultation will need to be analyzed individually." And for selective fetal termination:

> Any decisions to select among fetuses will be considered ethically questionable by some persons. But for others, the benefits in selecting among fetuses ought to be carefully balanced against the potential risks and losses involved. Ethical justification for the use of selective termination in individual instances will rest on this balance.

Both the AFS and ACOG committees probably did the best they could. But both wound up not with ethical statements at all, but with practice platitudes that supported their members' business practices by saying that they should continue to do whatever they thought right. They provide virtually no guidance as to either how ethical decisions should be made or what ethical principles should govern them. In other words, there are no right or ethical answers; there is no better or best way to practice; there is only the lowest common practice denominator, which will be supported by the organization's ethics committee (and this support should provide ethical cover for existing business practices).

The ACOG-AFS joint venture may be a genuine attempt to move from a professional support group function to an effort to grapple with the multitude of ethical issues involved in the new reproductive technologies and embryo research. But historians of bioethics can be forgiven for expecting little more than an attempt to continue business as usual under the "ethical cover" of a high-profile committee.

ETHICS AT THE GOVERNMENTAL LEVEL

At the federal level, the Human Genome Project's pledge to use 3–5 percent of its budget to fund legal and ethical studies is the first national research effort to take law and ethics seriously from the outset. This is certainly good news and could provide a useful model for all public funding of research. Nonetheless, it must be recognized that such direct funding runs the risk of coopting ethics for expedience, and of having politics dictate the appropriate subjects for ethical discourse. It has already become routine, for example, for scientist speakers at Human Genome Project-sponsored conferences to insist both that ethics is being "taken care of" by this funding and that the project itself is not stopable. In other words, the one ethical question that has never been open for debate is whether the Human Genome Project should continue at this time. Oversimplified to be sure, the message is: leave us alone to do our science, and we'll cut you ethicists in (a bit) on the action.

The scientists may, of course, be correct. But they have not yet made a convincing case that the Human Genome Project is the highest priority in either medicine or molecular biology, that it deserves a privileged status, and that it is not fair game for ethicists who question either its current pace or the potential problems with the application of its likely products. Bioethicists can be flattered that the program's sponsors are running for ethical cover without being coopted into providing such cover before the ethical analysis is performed.

When the case of Nancy Cruzan, a case substantially identical to the Karen Quinlan case, was reviewed by seventeen judges (including those on the U.S. Supreme Court) in 1989 and 1990, not one even mentioned ethics committees. It is good that ethics committees are no longer considered as legal agents by judges, and it would be better if lawyers (and legal considerations) were removed from them altogether. In rethinking the proper role of ethics committees, it may be useful to return to the 1970s and Alexander Solzhenitsyn's 1978 commencement address at Harvard University. Solzhenitsyn insisted that although a society without an objective legal scale is "terrible," one with no other scale "but the legal one is not quite worthy of man either":

> A society that is based on the letter of the law and never reaches any higher is taking small advantage of the high level of human possibilities. The letter of the law is too cold and formal to have a beneficial influence on society. Whenever the tissue of life is woven of legalistic relations, there is an atmosphere of mediocrity, paralyzing man's noblest impulses.[14]

Setting up an additional bureaucratic entity called an ethics committee to make legal pronouncements can only make medicine more legalistic and impersonal. Moreover, encouraging a group of lay people to attempt to practice law makes no more sense than encouraging a group of lawyers to attempt to perform surgery. What we might try instead is to engage in a real effort to see if multidisciplinary committees can "do ethics" and encourage real change in our hospitals and medical care facilities to go beyond the law and risk management to "do the right thing." Good ethics (and a good ethics committee) begins where the law ends.

WHERE THE LAW ENDS

The reconstituted Reagan-Bush U.S. Supreme Court seems to have taken as its project increasing in the power of the government to control the personal lives of its citizens. We now have a Supreme Court that sees it as reasonable and responsible to take rights *away* from its citizens. This is perhaps most notable in the area of abortion, enhancing the authority of police and the power of prison officials, limiting freedom of religion, and increasing the authority of the executive branch to limit the constitutional rights of recipients of federal funds.

These issues are explored in Part I of this book, "The U.S. Constitution and Bioethics." The book opens with perhaps the most discouraging opinion by the Court in modern times, *Rust v. Sullivan*,[15] which upholds government limits on free speech in the doctor–patient relationship. The effect of the war on drugs on our constitutional liberties is then examined. Finally, the excruciating case of Angela Carder shows how balancing the rights of citizens and the power of the state can directly affect both the way citizens are born and the way they die in American hospitals. The next two sections explore constitutional rights at the beginning and end of life. The first deals with abortion, surrogate motherhood, the status of the extracorporeal human embryo, and the role of genes in defining motherhood; the second deals with the "right to die" from constitutional, judicial, and legislative perspectives. The implicit message of Part I is that we can no longer rely on the U.S. Constitution to protect us from government intrusion into the doctor–patient relationship and into personal decisionmaking regarding reproduction, birth, treatment refusals, and death. We *do* need more than law here, and perhaps with the death of constitutional law as we have come to know it may come the birth of a new bioethics as a new countervailing force capable of providing some protection for individual liberties now under governmental and bureaucratic assault.

Part II, "Private Sector Bioethics," deals explicitly with areas in which the Constitution has never played a major role, either because they have been dominated by private players or because the Constitution provides strong authority for government dominance. Here the major concern is more often money and markets than government power, and the increasing shift from medical ethics to business ethics. The AIDS epidemic and our response to it are used to examine the legal (and ethical) obligations of physicians to care for patients with AIDS; and the desperation fueled by the epidemic (and the quest for profits) is used to focus a discussion on the appropriateness of drug regulation in the face of patient demands for experimental interventions. The second section in this part explores the legal and ethical issues entangled with our fascination with biotechnology; the Human Genome Project and commerce in human cell lines are emphasized.

Part III, "Public Sector Bioethics," addresses issues that have not been dealt with by the law from a primarily constitutional perspective. Special attention is given to organ transplants, resource allocation, and killing. The first section explores the power politics of fetal tissue transplantation, our concept of death and its link to organ transplantation, and informed consent to artificial heart experimentation. The second section is relatively brief, although it can be argued that resource allocation should be *the* central issue in contemporary bioethics. Nonetheless, the law has had little to say about resource allocation. Thus it is a central area in which ethics could (and should) take a leadership role. Both chapters in this section deal with rationing. The first explores the meaning of this term in the current debate on controlling the cost of health care while increasing access and quality; the second is a hypothetical U.S. Supreme Court opinion set in the year 2020 that explores some of the constitutional and ethical issues involved in explicit medical care rationing schemes. The final section is provocatively labeled simply "killing" and is designed to catalyze thought. The contexts chosen are purposefully unusual, with the goal of emphasizing the limits of legal solutions. This section examines decisionmaking in choosing which of two Siamese twins should be given the chance to survive and discusses whether the method used to kill a person (sometimes a patient) matters and, if so, why.

Finally, the book concludes with an examination of the growth of the field of health law over the past three decades, its relationship to bioethics, and a suggestion for shaping its development in the current decade. The last paragraph of the book contains an assertion by mythologist Joseph Campbell that also provides a fitting conclusion to this introduction: In America, a pluralistic, multicultural society, "lawyers and law are what hold us together. There is no ethos."[16]

THE U.S. CONSTITUTION
AND BIOETHICS

1

Brave New Medicine: Restricting Doctor–Patient Conversations

The century opened with George Bernard Shaw's 1905 play about British physicians, *The Doctor's Dilemma*. The dilemma then was to decide which of two patients to treat. In 1991 the U.S. Supreme Court created an end-of-the-century dilemma by forcing U.S. physicians working in federally subsidized family planning clinics to choose between accepting federal funding and remaining silent about abortion or providing full information to their women patients and forgoing such funding. This dilemma is unprecedented in the United States, and by its decision, the U.S. Supreme Court radically departed from past precedents and almost enthusiastically rewrote basic legal and ethical rules implicit in the doctor–patient relationship. Understanding the legal justification for restricting physician conversations in federally funded clinics is formidable and involves a mixture of abortion politics, government-funded medical services, and our view of society's obligations to the poor. Because this case portends a new rigidity and statism in the Supreme Court that may (contrary to current trends) make medical ethics much more important than medical law, it is fitting to use it to open our exploration of constitutional rights and bioethics at the millennium.[1]

THE CASE OF *RUST v. SULLIVAN*

In 1988 the Department of Health and Human Services (HHS) announced radically revised regulations governing the 4,000 family planning clinics that had been receiving federal funding under Title X of the Public Health

Service Act since 1970. These clinics serve approximately 4 million poor women. The announced purpose of the regulations was to redefine what Congress meant in 1970 by section 1008 of the act: "None of the funds appropriated under this title [Title X] shall be used in programs where abortion is a method of family planning."[2] Title X does not fund abortion, and Title X clinics do not perform abortions. But the Reagan administration also wanted to prohibit these clinics from referring clients for abortion and discussing abortion with them as well. Neither promotion nor encouragement of abortion by family planning clinics was alleged, but HHS said that a 1982 audit of fourteen such clinics had revealed practice variations. Specifically, one clinic counseled about abortion alone if the woman said she had already decided on an abortion; four clinics provided women with brochures prepared by abortion clinics; and at two clinics women seeking an abortion were allowed to use the phone to make an appointment for it.

The 1988 revisions state, among other things, that "a Title X project may not provide counseling concerning the use of abortion as a method of family planning or provide referral for abortion as a method of family planning." As an example of this provision, usually called the "gag rule," the regulations state that if a pregnant woman herself requests information on abortion, it is permissible to "tell her that the project does not consider abortion an appropriate method of family planning and therefore does not counsel or refer for abortion." The program is required to refer the pregnant patient "for appropriate prenatal and/or social services by furnishing a list of available providers that promote the welfare of the mother and unborn child."

The regulations were almost immediately declared unconstitutional by two U.S. Circuit Courts of Appeal.[3] Another Circuit Court, however, found them constitutionally acceptable,[4] and in May 1991 the U.S. Supreme Court, in the 5 to 4 decision in *Rust v. Sullivan*, agreed.[5] The case presented a facial challenge, a claim that the regulations were invalid as written, rather than as actually applied. Two basic questions were presented to the U.S. Supreme Court: Did the regulations reflect a plausible construction of congressional intent? and Were the regulations constitutional?

THE MAJORITY OPINION

Writing for the five-Justice majority, Chief Justice William Rehnquist made the case look straightforward. As to statutory interpretation, he noted that the language of section 1008 is very broad and thus provides HHS with almost unlimited authority to construe its meaning. Further he found (as other courts did) that the legislative history is "ambiguous and fails to shed light on relevant [1970] congressional intent." In such circumstances, the Court usually defers to the agency's expertise. Even though the 1988 revisions marked a drastic departure from past HHS interpretation of the 1970 act, the Court concluded that the agency's "reasoned analysis" (based in large part on the 1982 audit) provided a sufficient justification for its change of policy.

The constitutional issues were treated as equally straightforward. The Court had previously held that the government may not erect a "barrier" to prevent citizens from exercising their constitutional rights. On the other hand, the government may fund one constitutionally protected activity (such as childbirth) and not fund another constitutionally protected activity (such as abortion).[6] In *Rust*, Justice Rehnquist used an inept analogy — the constitutional authority of Congress to establish a National Endowment for Democracy to encourage other countries to adopt democratic principles without having to fund a program to encourage communism and fascism. One would have thought that democracies would be less likely than dictatorships to require single ideologically based messages and to restrict conversation among its citizens. The real analogy is whether workers at the studio could be prohibited from using the word "communism" in private conversations. When can a democratic government restrict conversations in the context of a doctor–patient relationship on the basis that the relationship is partially subsidized by the government?

The Court conceded that it is possible that the doctor–patient relationship in general might be a "traditional relationship" that "should enjoy protection under the First Amendment from government regulation, even when subsidized by the Government." But the Court decided that it need not determine the constitutional status of the doctor–patient relationship in this case because other doctors are available who are not legally constrained in what they can tell patients, and

> . . . because the Title X program regulations *do not significantly impinge* upon the doctor–patient relationship. Nothing in them *requires* a doctor to represent as his own any opinion that he does not in fact hold. Nor is the doctor–patient relationship established by the Title X program *sufficiently all-encompassing* so as to justify an *expectation* on the part of the patient of comprehensive medical advice. The program does not provide post-conception medical care, and therefore a doctor's silence with regard to abortion cannot reasonably be thought to mislead a client into thinking that the doctor does not consider abortion an appropriate option for her. (emphasis added)

In the Court's view of the limited doctor–patient relationship in the Title X clinic, "the general rule that the Government may choose not to subsidize speech applies with full force." According to the Court, if poor women may in fact not be able to get full medical information elsewhere, this is because of their poverty, not because of any obstacle raised by the government's Title X regulations. Poor women remain in the same position of ignorance regarding options they would have been in had the government not funded Title X clinics at all.

THE DISSENTS

Four Justices dissented, all agreeing that there was no need to reach the constitutional issues because section 1008 could reasonably be interpreted simply to prohibit using federal funds to perform abortions, rather than also to prohibit talking about them. Justice Harry Blackmun, in an opinion joined by Justices Thurgood Marshall and John Paul Stevens, also argued that the majority was wrong on the constitutional issues. In his view, the regulations are "the type of intrusive, ideologically based regulation of speech" that violate the First Amendment and cannot be justified simply by funding. In addition, the regulations violate the pregnant woman's Fifth Amendment rights to make decisions about her pregnancy free from affirmative government interference by both forbidding speech about abortion and simultaneously requiring referral for prenatal care. Thereby, "the Government places formidable obstacles in the path of Title X clients' freedom of choice." Justice Blackmun would also constitutionally protect the doctor–patient relationship on the basis that it "embodies a unique relationship of trust," in which doctors provide patients with "guidance, professional judgment, and emotional support," involving not only their health, but "often their very lives."

THE SCOPE OF *RUST*

This case is part of the continuing political debate on the government's role in limiting the ability of physicians and their pregnant patients to decide about abortion. It could thus be comforting to think that this case only applies to doctor–patient conversations about abortion. Unfortunately, legal decisions cannot be so easily confined, and the case provides precedent giving Congress and the executive constitutional authority to limit what doctors can say to their patients in all relationships that are partially federally funded. Therefore Americans should be more concerned about the Court's current views on poverty in the United States and the nature of the doctor–patient relationship than about the Court's view on abortion (a subject that is discussed in Part II of this book).

We have come to accept, as a matter of both law and medical ethics, that open and honest discussion is crucial to the doctor–patient relationship. We accordingly deplore the practice in Plato's Greece whereby, for slaves, "verbal communication between healer and patient was reduced to a minimum."[7] But restricting conversation between doctor and patient was a matter of Reagan-Bush policy, as was distinguishing patients according to economic class.

It is true that poverty (unlike race) does not define a "suspect class," and thus laws that affect only the poor have never been subjected to a high degree of scrutiny by the Court. On the other hand, as Justice Marshall has argued passionately and persuasively in the past, the Court cannot legitimately use this low standard of review to completely ignore what is happening in the real world. In his words: "It is perfectly proper for judges to disagree about what the Constitution requires. But it is disgraceful for an interpretation of the Constitution to be premised upon unfounded assumptions about how people live."[8] The *Rust* opinion, based as it is largely on the assumption that poor women have access to helpful physicians outside the family planning clinics, is untenable in its real world application. In this sense it provides strong judicial support for the perpetuation of a two-tiered health care system in which poor people and minorities are disproportionately represented in the lower tier. The fact that such a system is not unconstitutional is no excuse to ignore its existence by pretending that this Court decision does not directly affect the constitutionally protected choices of poor women, mostly of color.

The Court's description of the doctor–patient relationship, quoted above in part, is equally abstract and unrealistic. Physicians see their patients one by one in the real world, and all are unique. What does it mean to tell physicians that they cannot convey medically relevant information to their patients, but that this restriction does not "significantly impinge" on their relationship with their patient? And whose "expectation of comprehensive medical advice" is the Court talking about? The regulations themselves were adopted because pregnant patients were coming to Title X clinics inquiring about abortion; it was certainly their expectation that they would be given the appropriate information. Moreover, physicians can mislead patients as much by silence as by direct advice. In the doctor–patient context a half truth is the same as a lie, and it violates both medical ethics and the doctrine of informed consent. By legally approving inherently unethical behavior, *Rust* is a direct attack on medical ethics in the doctor–patient relationship.[9] It is in this regard that physicians must endorse the medical ethics of informed consent as their guiding principle, rather than the legal restrictions of *Rust*.

IMPLICATIONS OF *RUST*

It cannot be overemphasized that *Rust* is not primarily about abortion, but about poverty and the practice of medicine. Some of the major constitutional issues it raises are the following: How much control over doctor–patient conversations can the federal government now claim for care it funds through Medicare and Medicaid? Could HHS limit the amount of information physicians could give such patients about alternative treatments that are not paid for by Medicare or Medicaid to help control health care expenditures? Under a system of national health insurance, could we have "state medicine" with the doctor–patient dialogue prescribed by federal regulations, at least as long as some "private" physicians were available for those who could pay for them? And how could such regulations be enforced? Could videotapes of all doctor–patient contacts be required for compliance monitoring? Could the government use agents posing as patients to check on what a physician actually says?

Although *Rust* would permit affirmative answers to all of these questions, I think even the five Justices in the majority would try to answer all of them in the negative. This is because *Rust* differs from these other scenarios in that it applies only to poor people. If these new Title X regulations applied to white, middle-class Americans, they would have been seen as intolerable not only by the Congress and the Court, but by the President as well. The underlying philosophy is that the poor should be grateful that the government spends any money on them at all. In this sense the Court seems to view Title X funding as a charitable act rather than a government obligation. Recipients are free to take it or leave it, but they cannot expect to have any right to either determine what is given or to know what is left out. A portion of Wallace Shawn's monologue on the poor would not be out of place in the Court's opinion: "And so we'll teach the poor that yes, yes, we're going to give them things, but *we* will decide how much we'll give, *and* when, . . .".[10]

The Title X regulations thus seem to be viewed by the Court's majority not as rules that regulate doctors, but as rules that regulate the poor. Since physicians can't practice medicine without patients, however, the final message of *Rust* is that the Court devalues not only poor people, but also physicians who care for them. Doctors can have no higher constitutional status than their patients. Neither the bar nor organized medicine was fooled. Both the American Medical Association and the American Bar Association Houses of Delegates voted unanimously to condemn *Rust*.

The current American tragedy is that so many Americans have no health insurance and little access to care. Only Congress and the President can change that, and, after *Rust*, only Congress and the President can restore free speech rights for physicians who care for the poor in Title X clinics. Congress did its part in October 1991 by passing a statute restoring free speech rights to physicians in federally funded family planning clinics. President George Bush, however, vetoed the measure, and the House of Representatives was ten votes short of the two-thirds majority needed to override the veto. Thus even though overwhelming majorities of both the House and Senate said that Congress did not and does not intend to grant authority to issue these regulations, the Court and the President together were able to adopt them on the now-untenable basis that they are simply fulfilling the will of Congress.

Even more chilling was President Bush's veto message, reiterating his support of Title X regulations while at the same time insisting "there is no 'gag rule' to interfere with the doctor/patient relationship. I have directed that in implementing these regulations, nothing prevents a woman from receiving complete medical information about her condition from a physician."[11] This, of course, purposely (and politically) misses the point: a pregnant woman *can* be told all about pregnancy; the question is whether she can be told about abortion as one option to continuing her pregnancy.

In March 1992 HHS sent a letter to all Title X clinics saying that the gag rule did not apply to physicians. But agencies cannot change federal regulations by letter. That is why a federal appeals court properly enjoined enforcement of the gag rule in November 1992, until proper regulation amendment procedures, including an opportunity for public comment, were followed.[12] The election of President Clinton, who almost immediately renewed his campaign pledge to rescind the gag rule by executive order, sounded the death knell to this bizarre chapter in American legal history. However, to prevent any future President and five members of the Supreme Court from being able to require a two-thirds majority of both the House and Senate to preserve free speech rights for physicians and their patients, *all* health care appropriations must include language in which Congress specifically bars HHS and other agencies from restricting speech in the doctor–patient relationship.

Shaw's Colenso Ridgeon ultimately solved his patient-selection dilemma by fantasizing that if he rejected Louis Dubedat as a patient, and he died, his widow Jennifer would marry him. Concluding that *Rust* applies only to Title X clinics would be just as destructive a fantasy. Shaw's solution for the inherent conflict-of-interest problems in British medicine was a national health service. At the end of the century, the current Supreme Court majority notwithstanding, we can no longer tolerate second-class medicine for the poor and second-class rights for the physicians who care for them. Our modern dilemma is not whether all Americans should have access to quality medical care, and physicians who can freely and honestly talk to them, but how to make this goal a reality.

2

Trend Surfing:
The War on Drugs and Prisoners

To a large extent the interpretation of the Constitution is an exercise in creating and defining America. There is a constant tension between government power and the rights of individual citizens in most areas involving bioethics, especially at the beginning and end of life. The Court often speaks to major social movements by recasting the Constitution in ways the Justices believe are good for the country. This is well illustrated in two cases decided in 1989 involving the use of illegal drugs and in a 1990 case involving the rights of prisoners.

All three of these cases demonstrate how the Court's view on drug use and abuse can influence its interpretation of the Constitution, and the "war on drugs" is likely to insure that the United States will remain far ahead of all other countries in the world in terms of the share of its population (455 per 100,000) in prisons.[1] Our incarceration rates, for example, are more than ten times those of Japan and Sweden, and we have, percentagewise, five times more black males in our prisons than does South Africa.[2] When crime and drug use is widely viewed as out of control, longstanding constitutional safeguards for those accused of crime and drug abuse become almost as much a target as criminal activity itself.

CRACK, SYMBOLISM, AND THE CONSTITUTION[3]

Ever since the use of illegal drugs, especially crack, was labeled the country's number one public health and safety issue by President George Bush, we have seen more and more repressive ways proposed to attack the problem. As long as the use of illegal drugs was largely confined to America's underclass, and as long as the violence drug dealing produced was limited largely to the inner city, use of these drugs was not seen as a central societal issue. But times have changed. What was commonplace drug use in the 1960s is now a disqualification for positions in law enforcement, and even for the post of Justice of the Supreme Court of the United States. Much of the reaction to drug taking is sanctimonious, hysterical, and hypocritical.

Nonetheless, both legal and illegal drugs can impair job performance, and employers have legitimate concerns about their employees taking drugs on the job in particular settings. How far should employers be able to go in testing and screening their employees for drug use? The U.S. Supreme Court decided its first two cases on this question in March 1989. Although the cases left much to be decided and debated, they began the process of greatly expanding the limits of government-mandated drug testing.

The Railroad Rules

The first case involved regulations promulgated by the Secretary of Transportation under the Federal Railroad Safety Act of 1970.[4] These regulations, promulgated in 1985, were based in part on a 1979 study that concluded that 23 percent of railroad operating personnel were "problem drinkers" and in part on statistics that showed that from 1975 through 1983 there were forty-five train accidents involving "errors of alcohol and drug-impaired employees" resulting in thirty-four deaths and sixty-six injuries. The regulations required the collection of blood and urine samples for toxicological testing of specified railroad employees following any accident resulting in a fatality, release of hazardous materials or railroad property damage of $500,000; any collision resulting in a reportable injury or damage to railroad property of $50,000; and any incident involving a fatality of a railroad employee. After such an event, all crew members must be sent to an independent medical facility where both blood and urine samples will be obtained from them in an attempt to determine the cause of the incident. Employees who refuse testing may not perform their job for nine months. Under another provision, the railroad *may* perform breath and urine tests on individuals it has "reasonable suspicion" are under the influence of drugs or alcohol while on the job.

The Customs Service Rules[5]

In 1986 the Commissioner of Customs announced the implementation of a drug-testing program for certain customs officials, finding that although "Customs is largely drug-free . . . unfortunately no segment of society is immune from the threat of illegal drug use." Drug testing was made a condition of placement or employment for positions that meet one of three criteria: have direct involvement in drug interdiction or enforcement of drug laws; require the carrying of firearms; or require handling classified material. After an employee qualifies for a position covered by the rule, the employee is notified by letter that final selection is contingent upon successful completion of drug screening. An independent drug testing company contacts the employee and makes arrangements for the urine test. The employee is required to remove outer garments and personal belongings, but may produce the sample behind a partition or in the privacy of a bathroom stall. A monitor of the same sex, however, is required to remain close at hand "to listen for the normal sounds of urination," and dye is added to the toilet water to prevent adulteration of the sample. The sample is then tested for the presence of marijuana, cocaine, opiates, amphetamines, and phencyclidine. Confirmed positive results are transmitted to the medical review officer of the agency and can result in dismissal from the Customs Service. Test results, however, may not be turned over to any other agency, including criminal prosecutors, without the employees' written consent.

The Fourth Amendment's Protection

The Fourth Amendment provides:

> The right of the people to be secure in their persons, houses, papers, and effects, against unreasonable searches and seizures, shall not be violated, and no Warrants shall issue, but upon probable cause, supported by Oath or affirmation, and particularly describing the place to be searched, and the person or things to be seized.

Constitutional protections only apply to acts of the government, and not to acts of private employers. The Court, however, had no trouble concluding that the railroad was acting as an instrument of the government. Of course, tests carried out on Customs Service employees, done pursuant to government rule, are covered by the Constitution.

The Court, in opinions written by Justice Anthony Kennedy, also easily found that blood and urine tests are "searches" under the Fourth Amendment. As to the taking of a blood sample, the Court noted: "This physical intrusion, penetrating beneath the skin, infringes an expectation of privacy that society is prepared to recognize as reasonable." Moreover, the chemical analysis of the blood "is a further invasion of the tested employee's privacy interests." Breath tests, the Court found, implicated "similar concerns about bodily integrity and . . . should also be deemed a search." And although urine tests do not entail a surgical intrusion, "analysis of urine, like that of blood, can reveal a host of private medical facts about an employee, including whether she is epileptic, pregnant, or diabetic." The collection of urine also intrudes upon the reasonable expectation of privacy, especially when accompanied by a visual or aural monitor. The Court amazingly, and perhaps prudishly, seems to think that having one's urination monitored is a greater violation of privacy than having a needle penetrate one's skin and having blood removed through it. The Court quoted with approval the description by the Fifth Circuit Court of Appeals:

There are few activities in our society more personal or private than the passing of urine. Most people describe it by euphemisms if they talk about it at all. It is a function traditionally performed without public observation; indeed, its performance in public is generally prohibited by law as well as social custom.

A "Reasonable" Search?

Is this the type of search that requires a warrant, and, if not, is this type of search "reasonable"? The Court concluded that no warrant is required for two primary reasons: (1) there are virtually no facts for a neutral magistrate to evaluate (because both the circumstances justifying the search and the limits of the search are "defined narrowly and specified in the regulations that authorize them") and (2) the delay needed to procure a warrant might result in the destruction of valuable evidence as the drugs and/or alcohol metabolize in the employee. Warrantless searches have traditionally required at least some showing of "individualized suspicion"; but the Court made it clear that "a search may be reasonable despite the absence of such suspicion" at least if the interference is "minimal" and it takes place in the employment context. This is because "ordinarily, an employee consents to significant restrictions on his freedom of movement where necessary for his employment, and few are free to come and go as they please during working hours."

Blood tests are not unreasonable because they are usually "taken by physician . . . according to accepted medical practice" and are "safe, painless, and commonplace." Breath tests, although not done by medical personnel, involve no piercing of the skin and can be done "with a minimum of inconvenience or embarrassment." Urine testing was seen as the most difficult, because it involves "an excretory function traditionally shielded by great privacy." However, the railroad regulations do not require direct observation, and the test is done in a medical environment "by personnel unrelated to the railroad employer, and is thus not unlike similar procedures encountered often in the context of a regular physician examination."

More important, however, seems to have been the Court's view of the "diminished" expectation of privacy employees have when they enter certain occupations. The railroad industry was described as "regulated pervasively to ensure safety." The Court notes that an "idle locomotive" is harmless, but "it becomes lethal when operated negligently by persons who are under the influence of alcohol or drugs." Customs employees are involved in drug interdiction and so "reasonably should expect effective inquiry into their fitness and probity." This is especially true, the Court opined, because:

Drug abuse is one of the most serious problems confronting society today [and] the almost unique mission of the Service gives the Government a compelling interest in ensuring that many of these covered employees do not use drugs even off-duty, for such use creates risks of bribery and blackmail against which the Government is entitled to guard.

Unlike the railroad case, however, there was virtually no evidence that drug use is a problem in the Customs Service. Only five of 3,600 employees who had been tested under the program were found positive for drug use. The Court, however, termed this finding a "mere circumstance," concluding that the Customs program was designed to prevent the promotion of drug users to sensitive positions, as well as to detect such employees. In the Court's words:

> The Government's compelling interests in preventing the promotion of drug users to positions where they might endanger the integrity of our Nation's borders or the life of the citizenry outweigh the privacy interests of those who seek promotion to these positions, who enjoy a *diminished expectation of privacy by virtue of the special, and obvious, physical and ethical demands of those positions.* (emphasis added)

Nonetheless, the Court did send back the section of the rules that dealt with individuals who had access to "classified" material for further proceedings because the list of positions covered (which ran from attorney to messenger) seemed overly broad to meet the goals of the rule.

The Dissents

The railroad decision was a 7 to 2 opinion with Justice Marshall writing a strong dissent because he saw the opinion as gutting the Fourth Amendment. He agreed that "declaring a war on illegal drugs is good public policy," but concluded that "the first, and worst, casualty of war will be the precious liberties of our citizens." He was especially critical of the Court's reading into the Fourth Amendment an exception to the probable cause requirement when "special needs" of nonlaw enforcement agencies make either warrants or probable cause inconvenient requirements. The Court did this, he noted, by equating past cases that dealt with minimal searches of a person's possessions with a search of the person's body itself, thereby widening the "special needs" exception without requiring *any* evidence of wrongdoing on the part of the person. Justice Marshall concluded that the Fourth Amendment has basically been found inapplicable to certain areas by the Court without any more justification than the vague notion of waging an efficient "war on drugs."

The most powerful and surprising dissenting voice, however, was raised by Justice Antonin Scalia in the 5 to 4 Customs case. Like the railroad case, the Customs case was driven by the "war on drugs" and "the Government's compelling interests in safety and in the integrity of our borders." As Justice Scalia argued, however, whereas there was evidence of drug and alcohol abuse resulting in accidents and injury in the railroad case, in the Customs case "neither frequency of use nor connection to harm is demonstrated or even likely." He concluded therefore that the "Customs Service rules are a kind of immolation of privacy and human dignity in symbolic opposition to drug use." Justice Scalia noted, for example, that the record disclosed not even one incident of the speculated harms actually occurring, nor even one incident "in which the cause of bribe-taking, or of poor aim, or of unsympathetic law enforcement . . . was drug use." Instead, the evidence was that the Customs Service is "largely drug free." The regulations thus expose "vast numbers of public employees to the "needless indignity" of urine screening simply so the Customs Service can "set an important example" in the country's fight against drugs. Justice Scalia properly concluded that such a solely symbolic justification is "unacceptable" when the Fourth Amendment is violated:

> The impairment of individual liberties cannot be the means of making a point. . . . Symbolism, even symbolism for so worthy a cause as the abolition of unlawful drugs, cannot validate an otherwise unreasonable search. . . . Those who lose . . . are not just the Customs Service employees, whose dignity is thus offended, but all of us—who suffer a coarsening of our national manners that ultimately give the Fourth Amendment its content, and who become subject to the administration of federal officials whose respect for our privacy can hardly be greater than the small respect they have been taught to have for their own.

The Age of Screening

Justices Marshall and Scalia are correct. The Fourth Amendment now affords citizens far less protection against government searchers, and the lessening of protection cannot end with illicit drugs but will inevitably result in a lessening of respect for the bodily integrity of all citizens. It is also disturbing that the Court saw it as reasonable to use military requirements and border searches as analogous to government-mandated civilian workplace searches. Nor is rehabilitation sought in these cases, only punishment and deterrence.

Justice Scalia quite correctly noted that these opinions cannot be confined to railroad workers and Customs Service employees. They can immediately be extended to all employees who carry firearms and, from there, to all employees whose jobs, if performed under the influence of drugs, could harm the public, including: "automobile drivers, operators of potentially dangerous equipment, construction workers, school crossing guards." Moreover, as Justice Scalia argued, "a law requiring similar testing of private citizens who use dangerous instruments, such as guns or cars . . . would also be constitutional."

The war on drugs, of course, has special application to physicians. They, as much as Customs officials, might be chosen by the government as a "model" for other citizens. Since physicians have direct access to drugs and write prescriptions for them, the government could require drug screening as a condition of licensure on this basis. And if it could be shown that physicians, nurses, and other health care professionals have a serious drug and alcohol problem, which could seriously harm citizens, this would permit states and the federal government to pass laws requiring drug screening for employment or the granting of hospital staff privileges. Of course, private employers can adopt such rules themselves now and are not subject to the provisions of the Fourth Amendment. Some state constitutions, however, are more protective than the federal Constitution, and in those states, state and local government employees may be protected from mandatory screening in the absence of probable cause.

These cases left open a number of questions. Perhaps the most important was whether the government can require *random* drug screening, not related to a specific incident, to reason to suspect drug use, or to hiring or promotion. On the basis of these cases, it is reasonable to conclude that Justice Kennedy and the majority of the Court would find nothing constitutionally infirm in a random drug screening to further the "war on drugs." The cases also raise a generic issue of screening. If the government can compel screening to determine if an individual is using a substance whose use is forbidden by the criminal law, is there anything for which the government cannot mandate screening to protect the public? For example, what would prevent the government from requiring genetic screening for susceptibility to various diseases if and when such screening becomes available, assuming the screening for disease rendered the individual "less qualified" for the job, or potentially dangerous on the job? And what would prevent mandatory screening of health care employees and prospective employees for HIV infection under this rationale? The Court seems almost eager to view any screening test done by a physician as routine medical practice as de facto reasonable, without any real analysis of how intrusive such testing can be.

As the "age of screening" dawns, there will be more airport searches, more highway road blocks for sobriety testing, more intense border searches, and more screening tests for hiring, promotion, licensing, and continued employment. It is all part of our penchant to focus on individual citizens instead of systemic social problems. We seem to think that by treating citizens like grapes from Chile to be screened for cyanide, or apples to be screened for Alar, we can solve our societal problems of poverty, racism, and violence. It is the impulse that led us to concentrate on the captain's drinking when the Exxon Valdez ran aground and spilled its environmentally lethal cargo in Alaska's Prince William Sound.[6] Instead of reexamining the activities and planning of the oil industry to prevent and contain oil spills, we will likely see more drug and alcohol screening of tanker crews as the solution to oil spills. We like the easy way out, and mandatory drug screening seems cheap; it only costs us our Fourth Amendment security.

MANDATORY DRUG USE IN PRISON[7]

Almost immediately after endorsing constitutionally questionable steps to discourage drug use, the Court decided that antipsychotic drugs could be forcibly administered to competent prisoners in the name of prison discipline, even if the result might be death or permanent disability. How could our highest Court endorse such a prototypical totalitarian measure at this juncture of our history when totalitarianism is crumbling around the world, and drug use and abuse is so discouraged by our own government?

The Case of Walter Harper[8]

Walter Harper was convicted of robbery in 1976 and sentenced to the Washington State Penitentiary in Walla Walla. He was confined primarily to the mental health unit there from 1976 to 1980, where he voluntarily underwent antipsychotic drug therapy. In 1980 he was paroled on condition that he continue in treatment. He did, but in 1981 his parole was revoked after he assaulted two nurses at an inpatient facility. Upon his return to prison he was sent to the Special Offenders Center (SOC), a 144-bed facility operated by the Department of Corrections in Monroe. While there he voluntarily took medications until November 1982; after that and until June 1985 he was medicated by antipsychotic drugs against his will for all but one month because he was thought to be a danger to others.

The forced medication was administered consistent with SOC policy. The SOC policy provided that a prisoner could be subjected to involuntary drug treatment by a psychiatrist in a nonemergency situation only if the prisoner (1) suffers from a "mental disorder" and (2) is "gravely disabled" or poses a likelihood of serious harm "to himself, others, or their property." If the prisoner refuses medication, he is entitled to a hearing before a special committee consisting of a psychiatrist, a psychologist, and the associate administrator of the SOC, none of whom may be, at the time of the hearing, involved in the prisoner's treatment or diagnosis. The prisoner must be given twenty-four hours notice of the hearing (during which time he cannot be medicated), and he has the right to attend the hearing, to present evidence, to cross-examine witnesses, and to have a lay adviser help him. The prisoner may appeal a decision against him to the superintendent of the SOC and may later seek judicial review. After seven days of forced treatment, a committee composed in the same manner as the original committee must review the case. If the committee approves forced treatment again, it can continue indefinitely, provided a report by the treating psychiatrist is sent to the medical director of the Department of Corrections every fourteen days.

Harper had his hearing and was unsuccessful in his appeal to the superintendent. His forced treatment was periodically reviewed according to the policy. In February 1985 he filed suit, alleging that he had a constitutional right not to be medicated against his will without a judicial hearing. In March 1987 the trial court ruled that the SOC policy provided him with all that the U.S. Constitution required. On appeal, however, the Washington Supreme Court unanimously reversed the decision.[9]

The Washington Supreme Court was unimpressed by the SOC's antipsychotic medication policy and found it constitutionally defective as a matter of both substantive and procedural due process. Substantively, the Washington court found that Harper had a protected liberty interest to refuse antipsychotic drugs that was of the same importance as his liberty interest in being able to refuse electroconvulsive therapy (ECT). The court determined that this liberty interest could be overridden only if the state could prove "(1) a compelling state interest to administer antipsychotic drugs; and (2) that the administration of the drugs is both necessary and effective for furthering that interest."

As a procedural matter, the court held that these determinations must be made by a court after a hearing, which must also make a determination based either on the expressed desires of the patient or on substituted judgment. Representation by counsel was also required by the opinion, and any court order for forced treatment must be supported by "clear, cogent, and convincing" evidence. This opinion was unanimous (9 to 0).

The U.S. Supreme Court Decision

Justice Anthony Kennedy authored the 6 to 3 opinion of the U.S. Supreme Court, holding that the Washington court overstated both the substantive and procedural rights guaranteed to prisoners by the U.S. Constitution, and reversing their decision.

In terms of substantive rights, the Court agreed that prisoners do have a right "to avoid the unwanted administration of antipsychotic drugs." Nonetheless, this right must yield if the state can demonstrate that forcing treatment is "reasonably related to legitimate penological interests." Such interests do not include the use of drugs as punishment, but do include the use of drugs for treatment and to maintain order in the prison environment. This latter interest in "prison safety and security," the Court noted, is especially important because prisons are "by definition" made up of "persons with a demonstrated proclivity for antisocial criminal, and often violent, conduct."

In deciding whether a forced drug treatment regulation meets the "reasonably related to a legitimate penological interest" standard, a reviewing court should examine three factors: (1) the connection between the regulation and the state interest it is meant to foster; (2) the impact accommodating the asserted right will have on other prisoners, the guards, "and on the allocation of prison resources generally"; and (3) the absence of ready alternatives. Using these factors, the Court concluded that the SOC regulation is constitutional as a matter of substantive due process. Problems of potential abuse are avoided because:

> The fact that the medication must first be prescribed by a psychiatrist ensures that the treatment in question will be ordered only if it is in the prison's medical interests, given the legitimate needs of his institutional confinement.

As to procedural due process, the Court concluded that no judicial review is needed because "an inmate's interests are adequately protected, and perhaps better served, by allowing the decision to medicate to be made by medical professionals rather than a judge." Such professionals, the Court noted, are bound by the Hippocratic Oath, are in the best position to assess the risks of antipsychotic medication, and are best able to make medical judgments. Nor need the prisoner be provided with legal counsel at the hearing. In the Court's words: "It is less than crystal clear why *lawyers* must be available to identify possible errors in *medical* judgment."

The Dissent

Justice John Paul Stevens wrote the dissent, which was joined by Justices William Brennan and Thurgood Marshall. His major point was that the majority significantly undervalued Harper's substantive liberty interest and permitted an "institutionally biased" tribunal to substitute for due process of law.

Stevens characterized an individual's liberty interest in avoiding the forced administration of antipsychotic drugs as having both physical and intellectual dimensions, and he found forced treatment "degrading" when "it overrides a competent person's choice to reject a specific form of medical treatment." Forcibly using drugs "to alter the will and the mind of the subject," he argued, constitutes a "deprivation of liberty in the most literal and fundamental sense." Harper himself recognized the power of these drugs, stating he would rather die than take medication. At the time of this statement he was being forcibly medicated with prolixin, which acts "on all levels of the central nervous system as well as on multiple organ systems." The record indicated that prolixin

> can induce catatonic-like states, alter electroencephalographic tracings, and cause swelling of the brain. Adverse reactions include drowsiness, excitement, restlessness, bizarre dreams, hypertension, nausea, vomiting, loss of appetite, salivation, dry mouth, perspiration, headache, constipation, blurred vision, impotency, eczema, jaundice, tremors, and muscle spasms. . . . [It] may also cause tardive dyskinesia, an often irreversible syndrome of uncontrolled movements . . . and neuroleptic malignant syndrome, which is 30% fatal.

Harper had already been exhibiting dystonia (acute muscle spasms) and akathesia (physical-emotional agitation) by 1982. Stevens concluded that because of these potential adverse side effects, the Supreme Court of Washington properly equated such drug treatment with ECT, which could be refused in Washington by a competent prisoner.

Justice Stevens further noted that although the majority tried to interpret the SOC regulations to require a finding of potential medical benefit to the prisoner prior to medication, the regulations themselves contain no such requirement and permit "forced administration of psychotropic drugs on a mentally ill inmate based purely on the impact that his disorder has on the security of the prison environment," including a threat to property alone.

There is, in fact, no requirement in the SOC policy that the treatment be in the prisoner's best interest or be medically indicated. Instead, the prisoner's right to refuse treatment is directly subordinated to the institution's interest in order, and medication can be used simply as a chemical restraint. Of course, if an emergency exists, Justice Stevens agreed with other courts that medication may be given if the mental patient or prisoner "is suffering from a mental disorder and as a result presents an *imminent* likelihood of *serious harm* to himself or others." (emphasis added)

An emergency provision was also part of the SOC policy and was not challenged. What was at issue in this case is the power to drug a prisoner in the sole interest of prison security and management, without any serious discussion or consideration of alternatives (such as permitting those few inmates who actually refuse medications to do so, and isolating or physically restraining them). The minority concluded that by failing to adequately divorce the twin justifications of beneficial treatment and prison order, and by equating the state's interest in responding to emergencies with the state's interest in orderly prison administration, the majority had eviscerated the individual's substantive liberty interest "in the integrity of his body and mind" for institutional convenience.

The minority also found the procedural requirements of the SOC policy constitutionally deficient. Their main point was that the decisionmakers are inherently biased. The fact that two of them were physicians did not transform an otherwise unacceptable arrangement into an acceptable one. This is because the psychiatrists have a bias because they are reviewing the performance of their in-house colleagues (who, in turn, will be asked to review their performance). Moreover, since the panel members are all on the regular staff of the institution, they will be concerned not only with the inmate's welfare, "but also with the most convenient means of controlling the mentally disturbed inmate." As the minority noted, "The mere fact that a decision is made by a doctor does not make it certain that professional judgment in fact was exercised." In fact, institutional interests are likely to almost always take precedence over any concern with the medical indications for forced medication. This is because two of the three members of the reviewing committee are neither trained nor licensed to prescribe psychotropic drugs, one has no medical expertise at all, and all appeals are solely to the SOC superintendent.

There is, in fact, evidence of such institutional bias in Harper's case. For example, one drug, Taractan, was added to his medications in 1982 with the stated goal of "sedat[ing] him at night and reliev[ing] the residents and evening [staff] . . . alike of the burden of supervising him as intensely." Institutional control is also preserved by discontinuing medication only twenty-four hours prior to the hearing (when single doses of some drugs are designed to be effective for a month) and having the SOC itself appoint the prisoner's adviser. The minority accordingly concluded that "institutional control infects the decisionmakers and the entire procedure."

In Whose "Best Interests"?

What we should do about competent mentally ill persons who refuse drug treatment is an extremely difficult and contentious question. In the free world, however, we continue to give the individual patient, who is presumed to be competent, the legal right to refuse medication, even if the result is the unsatisfactory one of continued confinement to a mental institution (guardians are generally appointed to make decisions for those adjudged incompetent.)[10] This general rule now has an exception: competent mentally ill prisoners who are a danger to themselves, others, or property may be forcibly medicated. The psychiatric profession has generally hailed this decision as a victory for themselves and their patients. But their celebration is premature. This decision will likely serve only to make the public in general, and prisoners in particular, more suspicious of psychiatrists who will be seen as agents of an oppressive state rather than as independent physicians pledged to act in the best interests of their patients.

Psychiatrists must decide if they want to be agents of the state, just as other physicians have had to decide if they want to deliver lethal injections for capital punishment. Psychiatrists should take seriously the likelihood that even if they see forced medication as treatment, others will see it simply as a substitute for bars, straitjackets, and more guards. This case permits "treatment" solely for prison management. Although the holding is limited to prisoners, who have already been deprived of their basic right to liberty, the Court's general message cannot be so easily confined. For example, while the flagrant use of lobotomy as punishment, so well captured by Ken Kesey in *One Flew Over the Cuckoo's Nest*, seems constitutionally forbidden by the opinion, the use of ECT for prison management may be permissible.

On at least four occasions in the opinion, the majority states that the treatment Harper was forced to endure was "medically appropriate." This is a core problem. What are we to make of a psychiatric profession that believes forced medication with more than a half-dozen different major antipsycotic medications over a three-year period is "medically appropriate"? Should society ever permit physicians to inflict their own views of "appropriate treatment" on competent adults who disagree with their assessments? Since World War II at least we should be able to recognize the extremes that governments can go to with the assistance of physicians who believe in the government's policy. As historian Robert Proctor has noted: "Crudely put, you can do things with doctors that it would be very much harder to do without them."[11]

Finally, there is a sharp irony in this opinion. At a time when the U.S. Supreme Court has openly allied itself with President George Bush in his war on drugs, putting its weight behind the efforts to stop competent, free-living citizens from taking psychotropic drugs voluntarily, and at a time when prisons across the country are filling up with those involved in the sale and distribution of mind-altering drugs—at this time the Court decides that it is constitutional for the same government to force its incarcerated citizens to take drugs they don't want. Three years after these opinions it is clear that they have had little impact on the "war on drugs" in the United States.[12] Their primary impact has been to decrease the constitutional rights of U.S. citizens.

In Aldous Huxley's *Brave New World* citizens were conditioned to love their station in life, and society ran smoothly by making psychotropic drugs freely available to the population. Our government is now constitutionally free to pursue a different strategy—albeit one that has been tried and found ultimately ineffective by totalitarian governments: the forced medication of prisoners for the convenience of prison staff and the intimidation of the public. Unlike the rest of us, prisoners must "just say yes."

3

She's Going to Die:
The Tragedy of Angela Carder

In his short story, "The Use of Force," William Carlos Williams relates how a doctor (probably Williams himself) used extreme physical force to pry open the mouth of a recalcitrant child who, he suspected, had diphtheria that could only be diagnosed by viewing her throat.[1] The little girl resists his coaxing, and when, with her father's help, the doctor finally manages to jam the wooden tongue depressor between her teeth, the child opens her mouth just enough to crunch down on the blade to "reduce it to splinters." The doctor becomes furious with the child, whose mouth is now bleeding and who is "screaming in wild hysterical shrieks." But he knows he must see her throat for her own good, and it actually becomes "a pleasure to attack her. . . . The damned little brat must be protected against her own idiocy." Using a metal spoon and all his strength, he overpowers the child "in a final unreasoning assault." He learns her secret: she has diphtheria. We can agree that the doctor lost control and brutalized his child patient, yet still sympathize with him. Diphtheria was a life-threatening disease, and the child could not make a competent decision to refuse to have the doctor look at her throat. Moreover, her parents were present and consented to the entire procedure. It was the method, rather than the rationale, that was wrong.

The use of brute force has little, if any, role in the practice of medicine, although sometimes some force may seem necessary to treat children and mentally incompetent patients. The 1980s, a decade not known for its compassion, saw some physicians and judges moving beyond children and mentally incompetent persons to encompass pregnant women in the group of patients for whom force was sometimes seen as justifiable. The rationale was not that pregnant women were incompetent to make their own decisions, but, rather, that some of the decisions they made might take inadequate account of the possible consequences of those decisions on the soon-to-be-born child.

Although there have been dozens of lower court opinions involving attempts to force treatment, usually cesarean sections, on pregnant women, only two have reached appeals courts. The first was at the beginning of the 1980s.[2] The second opened the 1990s on an entirely different note and is the most important case to be decided in this area to date: the case of Angela Carder, known simply as *In re: A.C.* It provides a remarkable and dramatic example of how courts, at different levels, view patient and physician autonomy at the beginning and the end of life.[3]

ANGELA CARDER

Angela Carder was a 28-year-old, terminally ill, married woman who, on June 16, 1987, was approximately 26 weeks pregnant. She had suffered from cancer since she was 13 years old but had been in remission for approximately two years before she became pregnant. The pregnancy was planned, and she very much looked forward to the birth. Her health seemed reasonably good until about a week prior to this, when she was admitted to George Washington University Hospital in Washington, D.C., and a massive tumor was found in her lung. Various treatment options were considered, but none acted on. Within a few days the physicians determined that her condition was terminal and she would die within a short time. She was informed of this, and she agreed with a plan to deliver the child at 28 weeks, but insisted that her own care and comfort be primary. At approximately 4:00 p.m. on June 15, she was told that she might die much sooner.

Her husband, her mother, and her physicians agreed that keeping her comfortable while she died was what she wanted, and that her wishes should be honored. On the morning of June 16, this information was communicated to hospital administration. Legal counsel was consulted, who decided to consult the university's outside counsel. Outside counsel asked a judge to come to the hospital to decide what to do.

The Hearing[4]

Judge Emmett Sullivan of the D.C. Superior Court summoned lawyers, and with a police escort, rushed to the hospital where he set up "court." Legal counsel was, of course, present for the hospital. In addition, lawyers were appointed to represent both Ms. Carder and her fetus, and the judge invited the District of Columbia Corporation Counsel to participate as well. The lawyer for the hospital opened the proceeding:

> The apparent desire of the patient and her family is that if the patient is to die, that no intervention be done on behalf of the fetus. . . . The hospital is seeking declaratory relief from the Court to direct the hospital as to what it should do in terms of the fetus, whether to intervene and save its life.

The lawyer for the fetus expressed the view the fetus was "a probably viable fetus, presumptively viable fetus, age 26 weeks," and that the court's job was to "balance" the interests of the fetus "with whatever life is left for the fetus's mother." Ms. Carder's lawyer argued simply that his client opposed surgical intervention to remove the fetus. Her attending physician, Louis Hamner, had been her primary physician for approximately eleven weeks. He testified that Ms. Carder had agreed to have the child delivered at 28 weeks, but that because the odds of a major handicap were much higher at 26 weeks gestation, she did not want the fetus delivered earlier. He said Ms. Carder was heavily sedated and would likely die within twenty-four hours.

The chairman of the obstetrics department, Alan Weingold, recommended that the wishes of the patient and her family be honored. A neonatologist, Maureen Edwards, testified hypothetically, since she "had no direct involvement with the mother or with the family." She offered strong support for intervention on the basis that for any individual fetus, survival and morbidity are "very difficult to predict." When pressed, she put the likelihood of fetal viability at 50 to 60 percent, and the risk of serious handicap at less than 20 percent. The director of oncology, Lawrence Lession, testified that no treatment for her cancer would be useful.

The patient's mother testified that the previous day, after her daughter had been informed that her condition was terminal, she said, "I only want to die, just give me something to get me out of this pain." Ms. Carder's husband declined to testify, but did indicate that neither his mother-in-law nor he could handle raising a baby. No other witnesses testified.

Hospital counsel then asked the court to decide "what medical care, if any, should be performed for the benefit of the fetus of [Ms. Carder]." The lawyers' arguments to the judge focused not on what Ms. Carder wanted, or even on her best interests, but on the best interests of the fetus and on Ms. Carder's terminal condition. The lawyer for the fetus, for example, argued that it was not a choice between life for the mother or life for the fetus because, "sadly, the life of the mother is lost to us no matter what decision is made at this point." She urged that the cesarean be done. The lawyer for the District of Columbia argued that Ms. Carder's interests need not concern the court because of the "sad fact" that "the mother will die regardless of what we do." Ms. Carder's lawyer stated the case directly in an exchange that captures the essence of the hearing:

MR. SYLVESTER: As I see this, as I understand the medical testimony, if we were to do a C-section on this woman in a very weakened medical state, we would in effect be terminating her life, and I can't —

THE COURT: She's going to die, Mr. Sylvester.

The lawyer for the fetus concluded that: "all we are arguing is the state's obligation to rescue a potential life from a dying mother." The judge took a short recess and then issued his opinion orally. The centerpiece was Ms.

Carder's terminal condition. In the judge's words: "The uncontroverted medical testimony is that Angela will probably die within the next 24 to 48 hours." He did "not clearly know what Angela's present views are" respecting the cesarean section, but found that the fetus had a 50 to 60 percent chance to survive and less than a 20 percent chance for serious handicap. The judge concluded: "It's not an easy decision to make, but given the choices, the Court is of the view the fetus should be given an opportunity to live." He cited only one case, *In re Mayden* (discussed later in this chapter), an unreported 1986 opinion from a D.C. Superior Court (the only case anyone present had a copy of) that itself was wrongly decided.

After the Hearing

The court recessed at 4:15 p.m., but reconvened shortly thereafter when informed that Ms. Carder was awake and communicating. The first indication was that when Hamner informed her of the court's decision, she agreed to it (she was on a ventilator, and so mouthed her response). Shortly thereafter, Alan Weingold reported a more recent discussion with the patient in which she "clearly communicated" and, after being informed that Louis Hamner would only do the cesarean section if she herself consented to it, and understanding that, "very clearly mouthed words several times, I don't want it done. I don't want it done." Hamner confirmed this exchange. Weingold concluded:

> I think she's in contact with reality, clearly understood who Dr. Hamner was. Because of her attachment to him wanted him to perform the surgery. Understood he would not unless she consented and did not consent. This is, in my mind, very clear evidence that she is responding, understanding, and is capable of making such decisions.

The judge indicated that he was still not sure what her intent was. Counsel for the District of Columbia then suggested that it didn't matter what Ms. Carder wanted because the entire proceeding had been premised on the belief that she was refusing to consent. Therefore, her current refusal did not change anything. In his words: "I don't think we would be here if she had said she wants it." The judge concurred and reaffirmed his original order.

The Telephone Appeal

Less than an hour later, over the telephone, three judges heard a request for a stay so that arguments could be heard. Ms. Carder's lawyer told the judges that the cesarean section had been scheduled for 6:30 p.m., which gave them approximately sixteen minutes to hear arguments and make a decision. He argued that the cesarean section would likely end Ms. Carder's life and that it was unconstitutional to favor the life of the fetus over that of the mother without the mother's consent. The lawyer for the fetus argued that Ms. Carder had no important interests in this decision because she was dying; "unintended adverse consequences on the mother" are "insignificant in respect to the mother's very short life expectancy." The state's interest, she said, "overrides any interest in the mother's continued very short life, which is under heavy medication and very short duration."

A discussion ensued about the possibility of the fetus surviving, which the chief judge cut short by asking: "Let me ask you this, if it's relevant at all. Obviously the fetus has a better chance than the mother?" The lawyer for the fetus responded: "Obviously. Right." A few minutes later, the court denied the request for a stay, reserving the right to file an opinion at a later date. The proceeding was concluded at 6:40 p.m.

A Forced Abortion?

The cesarean section was performed, and the nonviable fetus died approximately two hours later. Ms. Carder herself, now confronted with both recovery from major surgery and the knowledge of her child's death, herself died approximately two days later. Five months later, the Court of Appeals issued its written opinion.[5] The opinion reads more like a Hallmark sympathy card than a judicial pronouncement. Its first paragraph, for example, ends with the following sentence: "Condolences are extended to those who lost the mother and child." The court acknowledges that its opinion might "reasonably" be seen as "self-justifying" and then goes on to rationalize the denial of the stay.

The opinion rests on a number of false assumptions. The most serious error is the statement that "as a matter of law, the right of a woman to an abortion is different and distinct from her obligations to the fetus once she has decided not to timely terminate her pregnancy." This is incorrect as both a factual and a legal matter. Ms. Carder never "decided not to timely terminate her pregnancy," and because of her fetus's affect on her health, under *Roe v. Wade* (discussed in Chapter 4) she could have authorized her pregnancy to be terminated (to protect her health) at any time prior to her death regardless of more restrictive legislation. By making the assumption that the logic of *Roe v. Wade* can require a woman to put her own life or health in jeopardy to protect her fetus, even her viable fetus, the court tells us that it simply has not read, or does not understand, the decision. And since the fetus itself was not viable, what actually happened is that the court forced Ms. Carder to have an abortion prior to her death, doing so on the false premise that a terminal diagnosis strips a pregnant woman of her constitutional rights.

The second basis on which the opinion rests is that a parent cannot refuse treatment necessary to save the life of a child (true), and therefore a pregnant woman cannot refuse treatment necessary to save the life of her fetus (false). The child must be treated because parents have obligations to act in the "best interests" of their children (as defined by child neglect laws), and treatment in no way compromises the bodily integrity of the parents. Fetuses, however, are not independent persons and cannot be treated without invading the mother's body. There are no "fetal neglect" statutes, and it is unlikely that any could withstand constitutional scrutiny.

Treating the fetus against the will of the mother requires us to degrade and dehumanize the mother and treat her as an inert container. This *is* acceptable once the mother is dead, but it is never acceptable when the mother is alive. The court seems to understand this and thus ultimately justified its opinion on the basis that Ms. Carder was as good as dead and had no "good health" to be "sacrificed": "The cesarean section would not significantly affect A.C.'s condition because she had, at best, two days of sedated life." But this reasoning will not do. It would, for example, permit the involuntary removal of vital organs prior to death when they were needed to "save a life." However, if the child had already been born, no court (even this one, I take it) would require its mother to undergo major surgery for its sake (for example, a kidney "donation"), no matter how dire the potential consequences of refusal to the child. And certainly no court would ever require the father of a child to undergo surgery, even to save the child's life. The ultimate rationale may be purely sexist: this situation will never apply to males like these judges; they are unable to identify with the pregnant woman and thus need not concern themselves about the future application of their decision to themselves.

What Went Wrong?

This cavalierly lawless and unprincipled opinion posed the question not whether the patient was competent, but whether the lawyers and judges were competent. What went wrong with the judicial process? At last three things: (1) the emergency nature of the hearing; (2) the refusal to recognize the patient as a person with rights; and (3) the self-justifying nature of the appeals court's opinion.

This case illustrates the general rule that judges should never go to the hospital to make emergency treatment decisions. First, judges know nothing about treatment decisions, and it is inappropriate for self-serving hospital lawyers to ask judges to make them, as well as unwise of judges to accept their invitation. Judges can render an opinion about the lawfulness of a proposed course of treatment or nontreatment (although even this is seldom called for). But to ask judges to make the treatment decision to protect the hospital from some speculative potential liability simply invites them to play doctor — something they might enjoy, but something about which judges possess no more competence than the average person on the street. Rushed to an unfamiliar environment, asked to make a decision under great stress, and having no time either for reflection or to study existing law and precedents, a judge cannot act judiciously. Facts cannot be properly developed, and the law cannot be accurately determined or fairly applied to the facts. The "emergency hearing" scenario is an invitation to arbitrariness and the exercise of raw force.

The only reason a judge should ever want to go to a hospital is to determine the competence of a patient. This *is* a proper judicial task. Thus it is astonishing that, although there was testimony about Ms. Carder's contemporaneous statements and her wishes, the judge never even bothered to go the short distance to her hospital room to talk directly to Ms. Carder. The reason, of course, is that because he viewed her as simply an inanimate container, he didn't care what the container's wishes were—and this is what makes the case so offensive. Angela Carder was competent and did not consent to the surgical intervention; surgery was ultimately performed over her express objection. She was totally dehumanized; her wishes and best interests ignored. This could only be done by assuming she was already dead—and this assumption could only survive as long as the judge refused to see the patient herself.

Finally, the appeals court did not act like an appeals court. It initially heard brief arguments over the phone and made a snap decision. Thereafter it did not wait for the "trial" judge to write a more formal opinion before issuing its own; it did not hear or invite arguments from the parties; and ultimately it wrote a "self-justifying" opinion, instead of a neutral and fair rendering of the law. The judges treated a live woman as though she was already dead, forced her to undergo an abortion, and then justified their brutal and unprincipled opinion on the basis that because she was almost dead, her fetus's interests in life outweighed any interest she might have in her own life or health. This is what happens when judges (and hospital lawyers who call them) forget what judging is all about and combine rescue fantasy with dehumanization of the dying.

This was *not* a hard case. Ms. Carder should have been asked to name a proxy to make decisions for her (when she was unable to communicate herself) shortly after her admission to the hospital. And if there really were facts in dispute, a case conference involving the patient, family, and all attending health care personnel (and even a *knowledgeable* health lawyer or ethicist) could have been held to assess them. Direct communication with the patient or the patient's proxy is almost always the most useful and constructive response to "problems" like those presented by this case. Calling a judge was a pathetic, unnecessary, and counterproductive panic reaction.

RIGHTING A WRONG

Most wrongly decided cases stay on the books. In a very unusual move, however, the D.C. Court of Appeals vacated this opinion in the spring of 1988.[6] Two years later it firmly reversed the original decision (7 to 1) and set forth the legal principles that should govern all doctor–patient relationships with pregnant patients: "We hold that in virtually all cases the question of what is to be done is to be decided by the patient—the pregnant woman—on behalf of herself and the fetus. If the patient is incompetent . . . her decision must be ascertained through . . . substituted judgment."[7]

The appeals court ruled that it was improper for the lower court judge to balance the mother's interests against the state's interest in the fetus in order to decide what to do. Instead, the appeals court concluded that the proper procedure would have been for the judge first to determine if Ms. Carder were competent (a step that would at least have required the judge to see her) and if she were competent then to permit her to make the decision herself. The appeals court reached this conclusion because it could find no persuasive rationale to justify depriving women of their constitutional and common law rights as citizens because they become pregnant, carry a fetus to viability, or continue pregnancy with a terminal illness.

If the pregnant patient is incompetent, the trial judge is to apply the substituted judgment doctrine to determine what she would decide if she could decide. To make this determination, the judge is to examine previous statements by the patient, the patient's value system, and what family members and loved ones, and even treating physicians, think the patient would want.

Appeals courts cannot find facts, and the appeals court accordingly did not determine what Ms. Carder wanted. On the other hand, the court did make it clear that judges are to do what patients in situations like this want done, and it could think of no "extremely rare and truly exceptional" case in which the state might have an interest sufficiently compelling to override the patient's wishes. The court also concluded unequivocally that the state had no interest sufficiently compelling to force surgery in the *A.C.* case itself.

All of this is solid and reasonable, and essentially follows the opinion of the American College of Obstetricians and Gynecologists' Ethics Committee, which was issued in August 1987. ACOG's committee concluded that when disagreements occur the physician should "convey the reasons for the current recommendation to the pregnant women, encouraging responsible behavior through education and counseling" and that "resort to the court is almost never justified." Law and medicine are on the same track here, and, in honoring the pregnant patient's decision as outcome-determinative, both are on the right track.

The Footnotes

One potential for misunderstanding and underestimating the importance and strength of this opinion are some of its twenty-three footnotes. Footnotes in legal opinions are an old problem. It is often stated, for example, that "footnotes are for losers." This implies that the judge writing the majority opinion will put material in footnotes at the request of other judges who will join the opinion only if the judge does. This material is thus meaningless. On the other hand, footnotes that set forth authorities or expand on the logic for the conclusions stated in the body of an opinion are often foundational. Some of the footnotes in *A.C.*, read separately from the opinion, could easily be taken out of context to present a misleading view of the opinion itself.

The opinion holds that in "virtually all" cases the pregnant woman herself, or through substituted judgment, should make the final decision. Footnote 2, however, seems to suggest a separate "tribunal" of some sort be formed to make the final decision on unspecified grounds: "Because judgment in such a case involves complex medical and ethical issues as well as the application of legal principles, we would urge the establishment — through legislation or otherwise — of another tribunal to make these decisions, with limited opportunity for judicial review." Of course, there are no "complex medical and ethical issues" to resolve if the only relevant issue is what the woman wants done.

This suggestion should not be taken any more seriously than legislatures and others have taken suggestions of a string of courts since the Karen Ann Quinlan case (discussed in Chapter 7) that have suggested establishing quasi-administrative agencies to resolve conflicts that should have been resolved in the doctor–patient relationship. The central idea in *A.C.* is not that an alternate decisionmaking tribunal or committee should be established; rather, it is that judges should never be called to hospitals to make emergency decisions. The judge in the hospital in an emergency situation will ultimately act arbitrarily, and the exercise will become one simply of using crude force. The court has now made the law crystal clear: it is now the obligation of physicians, hospitals, and hospital lawyers to follow it.

Prior Decisions

Footnotes 7 and 23 try to distinguish this case from the only other appeals court decision in this area, *Jefferson v. Griffin Spalding County Hospital Authority*,[8] and from a previously decided lower court opinion in the District of Columbia, *In re Mayden*.[9] In both of these cases the pregnant woman was "unquestionably competent," and both women refused to submit to cesarean sections based on religions objections. Even though the court refused to either directly challenge *Jefferson* or to directly overrule *Mayden*, it should be emphasized that neither decision can any longer be considered good law in the District of Columbia. In *Jefferson* the court relied completely on the testimony of one physician that, because of placenta previa, without a cesarean section there was a 99 percent chance that the soon-to-be-child would die and a 50 percent chance that the mother would die. Legally, the *Jefferson* court wrongly equated an almost child *before* birth with an actual child after birth. Reliance on medical "evidence" also proved misplaced. The child was ultimately delivered vaginally, without any surgical intervention, and both mother and child did fine.

The *Mayden* case is more important because it is a District of Columbia case, and the trial judge in *A.C.* relied on it. In footnote 23 the appeals court says it is neither "approving or disapproving" *Mayden*; nonetheless, its opinion effectively overrules it. In *Mayden* a woman had been in active

labor for almost sixty hours. The resident at the public hospital wanted
to do a cesarean section, but the woman, a Muslim who was specifically
determined to be competent, refused and her husband agreed with her. The
stated basis of the physician's wish to do a cesarean was that an infection
could begin at any time, and the infection could kill the baby or cause
brain damage. The likelihood of an infection increased every hour and was
between 50 and 75 percent without cesarean section. On this basis alone the
court ordered the cesarean. A healthy child was born, with no evidence of
infection. As in *Jefferson*, the competent refusal of a pregnant woman was
overridden because a physician disagreed with her decision. The *Mayden*
decision also contains two revealing statements: "All that stood between
the Mayden fetus and its independent existence, separate from its mother
was, put simply, a doctor's scalpel"; and "Neither parent . . . is a trained
physician." In short, *Mayden* seems to hold that if a doctor believes a
surgical procedure is necessary, and has the means to perform it, he should
be able to perform it even if the woman competently refuses, a result
precisely opposite to that in the final *A.C.* opinion.

Moreover, in *A.C.* the pregnant woman was dying, and the judge believed that the *only* chance for the fetus to live was an immediate cesarean.
In *Mayden* there was *no evidence* of medical problems to either the mother
or the soon-to-be-child, and all that seems to have been at issue is the
impatience of an obstetrics resident with a patient at a public hospital who
was a member of a religion he could not identify with. It appears that the
majority of the court decided to discuss *Mayden* only because the lone
dissenting judge appended the text of this previously unreported decision
to his dissent. Rather than ignore it altogether, the majority apparently
decided to add a final footnote to their already finished written opinion.

Two other footnotes are relevant. The first is note 17, in which we learn
for the first time in the court proceedings the views of Ms. Carder's personal
physician, who had been treating her for cancer for years. The court tells
us that he was not notified by the hospital about the hearing, but if he had
been notified, "he would have come to the hospital immediately and would
have testified that a cesarean section was medically inadvisable *both for
A.C. and for the fetus*." (emphasis in original) The court says this shows
that the record was deficient, but it shows much more. It shows that emergency hearings in hospitals are inherently unfair and arbitrary because it is
impossible to adequately prepare for them and to even assemble, much less
consider, the relevant facts and individuals.

The Use of Force

In footnote 3 the court notes that even though Angela Carder's attending
physicians refused to perform the cesarean, and another doctor who was
willing had to be found, "no physician was ordered to perform surgery or
to provide any treatment against his or her will." Likewise, the trial judge
in this case indicated that he didn't believe he had the authority to order a

physician to operate against his will. Everyone at the original hearing seemed to concur. Nonetheless, none of the judges to date has commented on the radical asymmetry: forcing invasive surgery on a competent adult (until this last opinion) seemed perfectly acceptable; forcing a physician to perform such surgery was always unthinkable. Both should be unthinkable. Even the lone dissenting appeals judge, who would have affirmed the decision and who defined "the viable unborn child" as "literally captive in its mother's body" (transforming the mother–fetus relationship into a warden–prisoner relationship), would draw the line at the use of physical force to perform surgery on an unwilling pregnant woman.

The dissenting judge, just as the trial judge in *A.C.*, apparently thinks that because it must be done by a trained physician, a major surgical procedure such as a cesarean section is not the use of force, whereas holding someone's hands down is. This is probably because judges are very familiar with restraining a person's physical liberty, but have no familiarity at all with medical procedures. It may also, of course, be simply that because judges are predominantly male and cesarean sections will never be performed on them, it is a surgical intervention they cannot see as offensive.

The use of force argument, if taken seriously, would lead to the repulsive conclusion that it is acceptable to force unwanted procedures on the defenseless, such as the anesthetized or quadriplegic, but not on those who can physically fight back. This is just one reason why the ultimate justification for surgical intervention must be the consent of the patient, not the patient's ability to fight the doctor. William Carlos Williams' language in "The Use of Force" is again helpful: force fouls the doctor–patient relationship subverting it into an assailant–victim relationship. He asks his small patient: "Will you open it [her mouth] now by yourself or shall we have to open it for you?" Without her agreement, their relationship rapidly deteriorates to a point where medical "treatment" can only be termed "unreasoning assault." It is thus not surprising that all the judges in *A.C.* find the use of force unacceptable.

The *A.C.* opinion and the ACOG standards come as close to saying that the decision of a pregnant woman, even one in labor, should *never* be overridden as any court or medical professional association can come. It is also impossible to think of any case where a competent pregnant woman's decision might be appropriately overruled by a judge that would be consistent with the *A.C.* opinion that force should never be used to physically restrain a competent woman. Not only surgery, but blood transfusions, injections, and even forcing a pill down a woman's throat, are prohibited.

The conclusion seems inescapable: the use of the judiciary to force pregnant women to undergo medical treatments against their will is not only counterproductive, unprincipled, sexist, and repressive—it is also lawless. Instead of trying to develop better procedures to force "treatment" on a few unwilling pregnant women, we should be trying to improve consensual prenatal and perinatal care for everyone. The law in this case correctly returns us to ethics.

Williams opens another of his *Doctor Stories* with the words, "That which is possible is inevitable."[10] Forcing pregnant women and those in labor to undergo surgery and other interventions against their will is certainly possible, as we have seen. If the decision in *A.C.* and the guidelines of ACOG are taken seriously, however, the use of force in the delivery room will no longer be inevitable.[11]

4

The Supreme Court, Privacy, and Abortion

Feelings, beliefs and opinions are strong and divided on the 1973 U.S. Supreme Court decision in *Roe v. Wade*, the Court's 1989 decision in *Webster* that signaled a retreat from *Roe*, and the Court's 1992 compromise decision in *Casey*.[1] Opinion polls on abortion since 1973 show that Americans are deeply ambivalent on the issue. A consistent majority believe abortion is immoral in most cases. Nonetheless, overwhelming majorities believe abortion should be available in cases of rape, incest, and severe genetic handicap, and more than two-thirds consistently say even though they believe abortion is either "wrong" or "immoral" the ultimate decision should be made by a woman and her physician rather than by government decree.[2]

Physician opinions seem to mirror those of society generally. For example, a 1985 surgery of 1,300 members of the American College of Obstetricians and Gynecologists found that 90 percent believed fetal abnormalities were a legitimate reason for first-trimester abortions (84 percent for second-trimester abortions); this was followed by agreeing to abortions because of a woman's physical health (75 percent), rape or incest (68 percent), a woman's mental health (56 percent), economic difficulties (36 percent), and personal choice (36 percent). Only about 25 percent of the public and 35 percent of obstetrician/gynecologists support "elective" abortions for whatever reason the woman might have.[3]

President George Bush, asked in 1989 whether he would wait for the U.S. Supreme Court to reconsider *Roe v. Wade* before taking presidential initiatives on abortion replied: "Wait. I think probably wait. . . . But I'd like to see the Supreme Court decision as soon as possible.[4] Then Attorney General Richard Thornburgh also wanted *Roe* overruled saying: "My guess is that [the U.S. Supreme Court] will return the regulations of abortions, like many health and safety questions, to the states. . . . The decisions will be made by state legislators and state governors and not by the federal government."[5]

Neither the President nor his Attorney General was ever willing or able to discuss the core issue involved in *Roe v. Wade* in public. The President, for example, said in the 1988 presidential debates that he hadn't thought through the penalties. Later he said the women were covictims, implying that only the physicians who perform abortions should be considered criminals. And the Attorney General is simply wrong: The shift in decisionmaking will not be from the federal government to state legislatures, but, rather, from decisions made by individual women and their physicians to decisions made by state legislatures. The core issue is what role the government should play in using the criminal law to restrict access to abortions that are sought by women and agreed to by their physicians.

ROE v. WADE

In *Roe v. Wade*,[6] and in all of the abortion cases that followed it (other than the financing cases), the Court has been faced with a *criminal* statute designed to limit access to abortion. In *Roe*, the Texas statute it was reviewing made it a crime to perform or to attempt an abortion, except to save the life of the mother. Justice Harry Blackmun, formerly legal counsel to the Mayo Clinic, wrote the opinion of the Court. One of his major goals was to prevent the government from interfering with the practice of medicine and in the doctor–patient relationship.[7]

The decision was 7 to 2, with Justices William Rehnquist and Byron White dissenting. Building on a series of cases, including a leading one dealing with contraception, that had described a "right to personal privacy, or a guarantee of certain areas or zones of privacy," the Court determined that a fundamental "right to privacy" existed "in the Fourteenth Amendment's concept of personal liberty and restrictions upon state action." The Court went on to hold that this fundamental right "is broad enough to encompass a woman's decision whether or not to terminate her pregnancy":

> The detriment that the state would impose upon the pregnant woman by denying this choice altogether is apparent. Specific and direct harm medically diagnosable even in early pregnancy may be involved. Maternity, or additional offspring, may force upon the woman a distressful life and future. Psychological harm may be imminent. Mental and physical health may be taxed by child care. . . . All these are factors the woman and her responsible physician necessarily will consider in consultation.

Although granting the abortion decision a very high degree of constitutional protection, the Court stopped short of declaring that a woman's right to an abortion was absolute, that she had a right to "abortion on demand." Instead, the Court recognized that the state also has interests that may at times be "compelling" enough to limit abortion. The Court identified two such interests: the protection of maternal health and the protection of fetal life. The protection of maternal health has always been a legitimate state interest. In the case of abortion, however, the Court ruled that this interest could never be so "compelling" as to prohibit abortion prior to the stage in pregnancy when it is less dangerous for the woman to carry the fetus to term than to have an abortion (about the end of the first trimester in 1973). The Court decided that during the first trimester the state could only regulate abortions to protect the woman's health by requiring that they be performed by a physician. Thereafter it could only regulate to protect women in ways reasonably calculated to enhance the woman's personal health, rather than in ways really designed to protect the fetus or to simply discourage abortions.

The second state interest the Court identified was the interest in "protecting the potentiality of human life." The Supreme Court did not decide that the fetus is not human, but only that a fetus is not a "person" as that term is used in the Fourteenth Amendment. The Court also properly noted that "the pregnant woman cannot be isolated in her privacy"; her interests in privacy must be weighed against the state's interest in the life of the fetus. The question is: When does the state's interest become so "compelling" that the state can justifiably interfere with the woman's constitutional right to have an abortion? No satisfactory answer to this question can be garnered from science, and any line of demarcation during pregnancy is inherently arbitrary. The Court decided to choose fetal viability, the interim point between conception and birth, at which the fetus "is potentially able to live outside the mother's womb, albeit with artificial aid," apparently because at this point the fetus is biologically identical to a premature infant.

After viability, which continues to occur near the end of the second trimester, but whose actual determination is a function of medical technology and skill, the state "may, if it chooses, regulate, and even proscribe, abortion except where it is necessary, in appropriate medical judgment, for the preservation of the life or health of the mother." Although states can regulate abortions after fetal viability (or, more accurately, restrict premature birth inductions), by 1990 only thirteen states had enacted post-*Roe* laws that attempt to restrict such abortions.[8]

EFFORTS TO MODIFY *ROE*

Efforts to amend the U.S. Constitution to change or overturn the decision were unsuccessful and have been all but abandoned. A parallel strategy is ongoing: the passage of state abortion statutes that are as restrictive as possible under the *Roe v. Wade* framework in the hope that the Supreme Court will permit some state restrictions and ultimately modify or abandon *Roe* altogether.

In this exercise, the states of Missouri and Pennsylvania have always been leaders. Missouri's post-*Roe* restrictive abortion statute, for example, was the first to reach the U.S. Supreme Court. In 1976 the Court declared most of its provisions unconstitutional, holding *inter alia* that a state *may not* outlaw a method of abortion that is safer than carrying a child to term, require the consent of a husband prior to an abortion, or require the consent of a minor's parent prior to an abortion.[9] In the years prior to *Casey*, the Court had struck down state statutory provisions that restrict abortion access by requiring any of the following: detailed "informed" consent provisions; second trimester hospitalization; a twenty-four-hour waiting period; the physician to personally obtain consent; record keeping not related to maternal health; reporting the basis for determining that a fetus is not viable; and the balance of maternal health versus fetal life when physicians perform a postviable abortion. Regulations that had been approved, on the other hand, include requiring a pathologic examination of fetal tissue, record keeping related to maternal health, general informed consent requirements, and the mandatory presence of a second physician at postviability abortions (provided there is an exception for emergencies).

Leonard Glantz derived six "not necessarily independent tests" that the Court has used in various combinations to invalidate or uphold regulations on abortions:

1. Has the state placed an obstacle in front of the woman or otherwise significantly burdened the pregnant woman's ability to choose an abortion?
2. Is abortion treated differently than similar medical or surgical procedures?
3. Does the regulation interfere with the exercise of professional judgment by the attending physician?
4. Does the regulation conflict with, or is it stricter than, accepted medical and scientific standards?
5. Is the regulation reasonably designed to protect maternal health in an area where no less restrictive or less expensive regulation will do?
6. Does the regulation, if a postviability rule, protect the fetus without putting the mother in jeopardy?[10]

The four approved restrictions all produce a positive answer to one of the last two questions and a negative answer to all of the first four questions. A similar, converse, observation can be made of the restrictions the Court has struck down: all produce a negative answer to one or both of the last two questions and a positive answer to at least one of the first four questions. It also appears that the more "yes" answers to the first four questions, the more likely the regulation will be struck down. It is "quite remarkable how consistent the Court has been in protecting a woman's right to obtain an abortion and a physician's right to perform one."[11]

Perhaps because the U.S. Supreme Court had been so consistent in upholding and expanding the rights recognized in *Roe*, opposition to *Roe* continued. One's position on abortion rights became a "litmus test" for judicial appointments. Under President Reagan, who personally said he considered abortion "murder," judges were appointed to the U.S. Supreme Court who were openly opposed to the *Roe v. Wade* decision. By 1989, with the addition of three Reagan appointees to the Court (Justices Sandra Day O'Connor, Antonin Scalia, and Anthony Kennedy) who joined the two original dissenters in *Roe* who were still on the Court, there first developed a possibility that a five-Justice majority might retreat from *Roe v. Wade* or overrule it entirely. This is why both sides in the abortion rights debate were so hopeful and fearful of the Court's decision in *Webster*, and why more friend of the court briefs were filed in that case than in any other case in the history of the United States.

CHALLENGING ANOTHER MISSOURI STATUTE

In 1986 Missouri enacted a statute that, among other things, provided that "The life of each human being begins at conception" [when a sperm of a man is united with an egg of a woman]; "Unborn children [from conception] have protectable interests in life, health, and well-being"; the attending physician must obtain the woman's informed consent personally and so certify; she must be informed by the physician "whether she is or is not pregnant"; all abortions performed after 16 weeks gestation must be done in a hospital; a detailed examination to determine viability is required after 20 weeks gestation; and the use of public funds, public employees, and public facilities "to perform or assist an abortion not necessary to save the life of the mother or for the purpose of encouraging or counseling a woman to have an abortion not necessary to save her life" are prohibited. A federal trial court declared all of these provisions unconstitutional and permanently enjoined Missouri officials from enforcing them.[12] The 8th Circuit Court of Appeals affirmed as to all but one provision.[13]

THE U.S. SUPREME COURT OPINION IN *WEBSTER*[14]

Because of the way it was argued, only three of the statute's provisions were actually ruled on by the Court. The Court ruled that Missouri *could* constitutionally prohibit state-employed physicians from performing abortions not necessary to save the life of a woman, could prohibit abortions not necessary to save the life of a woman from being performed in state facilities, and could require physicians to determine fetal viability at or after 20 weeks gestation.

None of these three statutory restrictions are inconsistent with *Roe*, although the first two, like the previous Medicaid funding decisions, will make it more difficult for poor women to actually obtain abortions. If this technical holding was all the case did, it would have occasioned almost no comment. The reason it is so important is that five of the Justices, writing three separate opinions, made it clear that they no longer believe the "trimester" scheme of *Roe* is tenable, and four of them were ready to permit states to heavily regulate, and perhaps even prohibit outright, most abortions at any point in pregnancy.

Roe v. Wade was based on two conceptual foundations: first, that there is a fundamental constitutional right of privacy that is broad enough to encompass a woman's decision to have an abortion and, second, that the state's interests in abridging the exercise of this right are related to the stage of pregnancy. The plurality opinion in *Webster* (which only three Justices agreed on) ignored the right of privacy altogether. Although the scope of the constitutional right of privacy was the issue on which most *amici* who filed briefs argued this case, the Court did not seek to contract this right in areas other than abortion. Instead, the plurality concentrated exclusively on *Roe*'s trimester scheme. The plurality said, for example, that "the key elements of the *Roe* framework — trimesters and viability — are not found in the text of the Constitution." Rather than having to balance individual rights and state interests, the plurality concluded that states have a compelling interest "in protecting human life throughout pregnancy." If this is true, of course, then the fact that women have a fundamental constitutional right to make an abortion decision does not help them in a state that wants to outlaw abortion to protect fetal life, because compelling state interests trump individual rights.

Four Justices indicated that they would uphold any state restriction on abortion that "permissibly furthers the state's interest in protecting potential human life." Four other Justices would continue to uphold a *Roe* balancing scheme. The Justice with the ability to make a 5 to 4 majority by joining either side of this debate was Justice O'Connor. She had previously indicated her displeasure with the trimester scheme and suggested that the Court should instead determine the constitutionality of state abortion laws on the basis of whether they "unduly burden" the woman's right to have an abortion.[15] But because she believed that the three provisions in the Missouri law were consistent with *Roe*, she refused to use *Webster* as an opportunity to reverse or restrict *Roe*.

This is why constitutional law on abortion before *Webster* remained the same after *Webster*. On the other hand, anyone who could count knew that one more change in the U.S. Supreme Court's membership, or a shift in Justice O'Connor's thinking, could result in *Roe*'s reversal and wide powers to restrict abortions being given to the individual state governments. This is the central reason why the appointments of Justices David Souter and Clarence Thomas to replace Justices Brennan and Marshall were viewed with such dismay by the supporters of *Roe*.

WHAT IS AT STAKE IN ABORTION RIGHTS

The scope of the constitutional right of privacy is analytically the most challenging and ultimately the most central issue at stake in the abortion debate. The plurality in *Webster* simply ignored it, even though, as Justice Blackmun properly noted in dissent:

> These are questions of unsurpassed significance in this Court's interpretation of the Constitution, and mark the battleground upon which this case was fought, by the parties, by the Solicitor General . . . and by an unprecedented number of *amici*. On these grounds, abandoned by the plurality, the Court should decide this case.

"Privacy" has come to be simply a one-word legal description of individual liberty (or self-determination) to make decisions that involve marriage, sterilization, contraception, and abortion. As Ronald Dworkin has aptly described the core of self-determination in the privacy right, decisions that affect marriage and childbirth are "so important, so intimate and personal, so crucial to the development of personality and sense of moral responsibility" that individuals must be allowed to make them "consulting their own conscience, rather than allowing society to thrust its collective decision on them." Abortion, the Court has consistently reaffirmed, is substantially identical to these decisions. In Dworkin's words:

> In many ways it is more private, because the decision involves a woman's control not just of her connections to others, but of the use of her own body, and the Constitution recognizes in a variety of ways the special intimacy of a person's connection to her own physical integrity.[16]

The real constitutional issue is defining the boundaries of this right. If abortion is removed from the compass of this cluster of privacy rights, is there an alternative principle that explains why the abortion decision is not constitutionally protected, but marriage, contraception, and sterilization decisions are? Some contraceptives, such as the IUD, operate to prevent the embryo from implanting. Protection of the embryo from conception would prohibit not only abortion, but methods of contraception that prevent the implantation of embryos as well. And if an embryo can be protected immediately after fertilization, why cannot the act of fertilization itself be protected by prohibiting the use of contraceptives? Why should the line be drawn at the point where the sperm enters the egg? What *constitutional* principle tells us why we can require women to protect and nurture all embryos, but cannot prohibit women (or men) from taking steps to prevent embryos from being formed in the first place? Because the *Webster* plurality had no answer to this question, and was not eager to provoke a constitutional crisis over contraception, it simply ignored the core issue of the boundaries of the right of privacy.

COMPROMISE ON *ROE*

In 1992, reviewing the Pennsylvania Control Act, the Court surprised almost all observers by refusing to reverse *Roe*. Three Reagan-Bush appointees joined together to reinterpret and uphold *Roe*, making it clear that the twelve-year attempt to overturn *Roe* by packing the Court with ultraconservative, anti-*Roe* Justices had failed. In the twenty years since *Roe* was decided, only two Justices willing to vote to actually reverse *Roe* had been appointed (Scalia and Thomas). In this regard, the decision in *Planned Parenthood of Southeastern Pennsylvania v. Casey*,[17] which has been condemned by activists on both extremes of the abortion rights debate,[18] is extremely important.

Like *Roe v. Wade*, to which it is faithful in spirit if not in letter, *Casey* recognizes the constitutional right of pregnant women to make the ultimate decision about continuing or terminating a pregnancy prior to viability free from substantial government interference. There *are* real differences between *Roe* and *Casey*, but Justice Blackmun is correct in observing, "now, just when so many expected the darkness to fall [on *Roe*], the flame has grown bright."

The Pennsylvania Statute

At issue in *Casey* were a series of provisions of the Pennsylvania Abortion Control Act of 1982 (as amended in 1988 and 1989). These provisions require that all women seeking an abortion give informed consent after being told, at least 24 hours before the abortion, by the referring physician or the physician who will perform the abortion, of the nature, risks and alternatives of the procedure; the probable gestational age of the "unborn child" at the time the abortion will be performed; and the medical risks of carrying "her child" to term. Either the physician or an assistant must also inform the woman (again, 24 hours before the abortion) that the state has prepared printed materials which describe the "unborn child" and agencies which offer alternatives to abortion; that medical assistance may be available for prenatal care, childbirth, and neonatal care; and that the father of the "unborn child" is liable to assist in the support of her child. The printed material must be made available to the woman, and she must certify in writing that she has been given the above information orally and given a chance to view the printed materials if she so chooses.

There are also provisions in the Pennsylvania law for parental consent, spousal notice, and reporting requirements. As a general rule, an unmarried, financially dependent pregnant woman under the age of 18 must have the consent of either one parent, a guardian, or certification of maturity or a best interest finding by a judge. A married woman must give notice to her husband about her intention to have an abortion (unless the spouse is not the father, cannot be located, has criminally assaulted her, or she fears bodily injury as a result of notice). As with informed consent, any physician who fails to obtain a written confirmation from the woman that she has so notified her husband, or meets an exception, shall be guilty of "unprofessional conduct" and subject to license revocation. In addition, the physician shall be civilly liable to the spouse "who is the father of the aborted child" for any damages caused and for punitive damages in the amount of $5,000, and for reasonable attorney fees. Required reports on each abortion must include such information as the name of the physician performing the abortion, the facility where it was performed, and the name of the referring physician, agency or service, the county and state where the woman resides, the woman's age, the number of prior pregnancies and abortions, the gestational age of the "unborn child," the type of procedure used, and the weight "of the aborted child." Finally, all these requirements are waived in a "medical emergency."

The Joint Opinion in Casey

In a very unusual move, three Justices, Sandra Day O'Connor, Anthony Kennedy and David Souter, wrote a joint opinion reframing *Roe*, and under *Roe*'s new contours, upheld the constitutionality of all the provisions of the Pennsylvania law except spousal notification. Since Justices Harry Blackmun and John Paul Stevens agreed that the aspects of *Roe* that these three justices retained should be retained (they would have retained it all), there were five votes for retaining what the joint opinion called the "essential holding" of *Roe*. As recast by the joint opinion's authors, *Roe* now stands for the proposition that pregnant women have a "personal liberty" right to choose to terminate their pregnancies prior to viability that the state cannot "unduly burden."

The nature of the constitutional right to choose an abortion is seen as not only being derived from the "right of privacy" regarding family and personal decisionmaking, but also from cases restricting the government's power to mandate medical treatment or to bar its rejection, such as *Cruzan* (see Chapter 7). Such post-*Roe* medical treatment cases protecting bodily integrity "accord with *Roe*'s view that a state's interest in the protection of life falls short of justifying any plenary override of individual liberty claims," and prohibit the state from forcing either continued pregnancy or abortion on a pregnant woman.

The joint opinion concludes this substantive due process approach by holding that a woman's constitutional "right to choose to terminate her pregnancy" continues to fetal viability. Viability is chosen because it was the most important line drawn in *Roe*, because "there is no line other than viability which is more workable," and because at viability "the independent existence of the second life can in reason and all fairness be the object of state protection [although *not* a person under the constitution] that now overrides the rights of the woman." The joint opinion continues:

> The woman's right to terminate her pregnancy before viability is the most central principle in *Roe v. Wade*. It is a rule of law and a component of liberty we cannot renounce.

The joint opinion, however, rejects the Court's post-*Roe* cases that struck down most attempts by states to ensure "that a woman's choice contemplates the consequences for the fetus . . . " as misconceiving "the nature of the pregnant woman's interest; and . . . undervalu[ing] the state's interest in potential life. . . ." In this regard, the joint opinion insists that not every law that makes a right more difficult to exercise "is, *ipso facto*, an infringement on that right," even if such laws make the actual exercise of the right more difficult by increasing its expense or even decreasing the availability of the procedure. "Only where state regulation imposes an *undue burden* on the woman's ability to make this decision does the power of the State reach into the heart of the liberty protected by the Due Process Clause." (emphasis added) The phrase "undue burden" is "a shorthand for the conclusion that a state regulation has the *purpose or effect* of placing a substantial obstacle in the path of a woman seeking an abortion of an nonviable fetus." (emphasis added)

Applying the Undue Burden Test

As to informed consent, the joint opinion held that it is not unconstitutional to require physicians to present *"truthful, nonmisleading information,"* (emphasis added) not only about the basic information needed to gain consent to the abortion, but also as to the probable gestational age of the fetus, to attempt "to ensure that a woman apprehends the full consequences of her decision. . . ." Making available additional materials relating to the fetus is also acceptable, much the way the joint opinion believes it would be acceptable "for the State to require that in order for there to be informed consent to a kidney transplant operation the recipient must be supplied with information about risks to the donor as well as risks to himself or herself." None of these requirements present a "substantial obstacle to obtaining an abortion, and, it follows, there is no undue burden."

The 24-hour waiting period was found by the lower court to be burdensome for poor, rural women who must travel long distances to a clinic. The joint opinion, however, concluded that a "particular burden is not of necessity a substantial obstacle" and the waiting period, as part of the informed consent requirement which "facilitates the wise exercise" of the right to choose, is not an undue burden on the exercise of that right. Likewise, the requirements of having one parent consent or judicial review for a woman under 18 years of age, and of requiring the reporting of certain information to the Department of Health, were found not to be undue burdens on the woman's right to choose.

On the other hand, the joint opinion found that the requirement of spousal notification could not meet the undue burden test. Because its exceptions were so narrow (not including, for example, psychological abuse, and assault not reported to the police), it would "likely prevent a significant number of women from obtaining an abortion." This is because "the significant number of women who fear for their safety and the safety of their children are likely to be deterred from procuring an abortion as surely as if the Commonwealth had outlawed abortion in all cases." As to the husband's undoubted interest in the pregnancy (when he is the father), the joint opinion concluded: "A State may not give to a man the kind of dominion over his wife that parents exercise over their children . . . Women do not lose their constitutionally protected liberty when they marry."

The Concurring/Dissenting Opinions

Justices John Paul Stevens and Harry Blackmun both wrote opinions concurring in the affirmation of *Roe*, but dissenting from the approval of the provisions of the Pennsylvania law. The remaining four justices all would have overturned *Roe* and upheld all of the provisions of the Pennsylvania law. They expressed themselves in two opinions, one by Chief Justice William Rehnquist and the other by Justice Antonin Scalia, each of which was concurred in by the four dissenting Justices (the two authors and Justices Byron White and Clarence Thomas).

Of these two opinions, the most illuminating portions are their remarks on *Roe* and on the undue burden test. In the Rehnquist opinion, the four dissenters say bluntly:

> We believe that *Roe* was wrongly decided, and that it can and should be overruled consistently with our traditional approach to *stare decisis* in constitutional cases.

In their view, the state should be able to prohibit abortion, or to regulate it in any "rational" way, throughout pregnancy. The undue burden test is dealt with in detail in Justice Scalia's opinion. He argues (persuasively, I think) that the test is ultimately "standardless" and "has no principled or coherent legal basis," noting that "defining an 'undue burden' as an 'undue hindrance' (or a 'substantial obstacle') hardly 'clarifies' the test." Justice Scalia then tries to define the test operationally. He concludes that as applied in the joint opinion the "undue burden" standard means that "a State may not regulate abortion in such a way as to reduce significantly its incidence."

THE CURRENT STATE OF THE LAW

Justice Scalia's reading of the undue burden test seems correct: under *Casey* states cannot regulate abortion in ways that will prevent a significant number of women from obtaining them. It is in this sense that the Court has affirmed *Roe v. Wade* in *Casey*. In addition, the always problematic emphasis in *Roe* on the right of the physician to practice medicine has been replaced by emphasis on the pregnant woman and her right to make the abortion decision. In *Roe*, for example, the Court had said:

> The decision [*Roe*] vindicates the *right of the physician* to administer medical treatment according to his professional judgment [prior to viability] . . . the abortion decision in all its aspects is inherently and primarily, *a medical decision*, and basic responsibility for it must rest with the physician. (emphasis added)

It is primarily for this reason, I believe, that the Court had previously consistently struck down detailed informed consent requirements, waiting periods, and reporting requirements: they interfered with the physician's judgment and discretion.

Casey properly focuses on the pregnant woman. It is *her* decision that the constitution protects, not her physician's. This makes requiring an informed consent conversation with the physician perfectly reasonable:

> Whatever constitutional status the doctor-patient relationship may have as a general matter, in the present context it is derivative of the woman's position. The doctor-patient relation does not underlie or override the two more general rights under which the abortion right is justified: the right to make family decisions and the right to physical autonomy.

This shift in emphasis, from doctor to patient, should be applauded by physicians. It *is* the woman, not the physician who is pregnant, the woman who is making the decision, and the woman who is responsible for the decision. The problem with the joint opinion is not its emphasis on women, but its view of women. The Pennsylvania "informed consent" requirements are based on the supposition that women who decide to have abortions do not think very much about their decision, and if they had some additional information about the procedure and the development of the fetus, as well as 24 hours to think about it, many would continue their pregnancies to term. This view is extraordinarily patronizing to pregnant women, has no empirical support, and the consent requirements apply to no other medical procedure. Further, since it must be assumed that the authors of the joint opinion understand the "undue burden" test as well as the four dissenters, the approved requirements are expected to have little effect on the actual number of abortions in Pennsylvania. If they do affect a significant number of women, the Court will hear a further challenge to the restrictions on the basis of their practical impact on obtaining abortions, rather than, as here, solely on theory.

The Court's approval of the Pennsylvania "informed consent" requirements highlights two major flaws in the approach of the joint opinion. First, the joint opinion seems to rest on the proposition that it is acceptable for the state to require physicians to "inform" women that childbirth is much preferable to abortion, as long as this does not inhibit many women from actually choosing abortion. This suggests that this value judgment and inculcation of guilt feelings based on it is a legitimate state function in the abortion arena—an inconsistent, bureaucratic, and pointless position. Second, the Pennsylvania rules *will* affect some women—notably the rural poor and the very young. This is, however, consistent with prior abortion-related opinions of the Court: government action that in its application is restrictive only to the poor and disadvantaged will, as discussed in Chapter 1, be assumed to be constitutionally acceptable absent very specific evidence of its impact on this group. The only way out of this discriminatory impact on the poor is to ensure that birth control services as well as abortion are fully covered in any national system of health care.

Casey has many implications for physicians. The most important one is that states cannot outlaw abortion prior to viability, although they can increase the "hassle factor" for patients and their physicians significantly. Record keeping and consent requirements like those approved in *Casey* will be enacted in some other states for abortion, and could be required for *any* medical procedure. This is because no other medical procedure is as constitutionally-protected as abortion, and thus any restriction a state can place on a physician who performs an abortion, it can place on a physician who performs any other medical procedure. Physicians who believe these and similar record-keeping requirements are bureaucratic, burdensome, and nonbeneficial, must oppose them both in state legislatures and in Congress.

The holding that it is constitutionally-acceptable to require physicians to personally present certain information to patients for informed consent could be made applicable to all medical procedures. This is not likely to be useful to patients in all medical contexts. Additionally, the holding that physicians can be required to tell patients specific "truthful, nonmisleading information" is troublesome in that it assumes that the state has some objective way to define these terms. In the abortion context, for example, do phrases like "abortion is immoral" and "the fetus is a human being" qualify? And under a national health program, would phrases like "this treatment is not worthwhile for patients your age [or condition]" or "this treatment does not contribute to quality of life" meet this test? Again, physician input in legislative and regulatory forums will be more critical from now on.

Since *Roe* still lives, efforts to overturn it will continue. Should one of the members in the five-person majority retire, the next Supreme Court Justice will be able to join the four *Roe* dissenters to overturn the decision. Because of this, Congress seems likely to pass a version of the Freedom of Choice Act, which is designed to codify the constitutional law of *Roe v. Wade* in statutory form.[19] Using its authority to legislate for the country under the interstate commerce clause (because a patchwork of state regulation would cause some women to cross state lines to obtain abortion services), its power to enforce the Fourteenth Amendment, and its primacy under the Supremacy Clause, the federal government could preempt the Court's influence in abortion and write uniform standards for the country. There is no constitutional prohibition to such legislation since all nine Justices agree that the fetus or unborn child is *not* a person under the U.S. Constitution. And it would, of course, be a product of democracy at work.

With or without such legislation, some states will continue to try to further regulate abortion in ways that discourage it—either by adopting the approved Pennsylvania restrictions, or by expanding on them to test the limits of the vague and unsatisfactory "undue burden" test. They may also test the language of the Freedom of Choice Act, which, when Congress passes it, President Clinton has said he will sign. In short, the joint opinion's attempt to call "the contending sides of a national controversy to end their national division by accepting a common mandate rooted in the Constitution" will, sadly, fail.

Ultimately abortion must remain a moral decision for the individual woman unless sexual inequality is to be governmentally enforced. *Roe* is to a large extent a technologically based decision, relying as it does on "viability" for choosing it as a constitutionally relevant boundary. Thus it will be perfectly fitting if technology, in the form of a drug like RU 486, ultimately makes early abortion readily available to all women in a way that is de facto unregulatable by government. The danger is that this will make abortion seem like birth control, and thus less morally troubling. The advantage is that it will eliminate governmental involvement in this personal, moral decision.

5

The Short, Happy Life of
Commercial Surrogacy

How did surrogate motherhood evolve from a "harebrained, fly-by-night" idea of the late 1970s, to one that had middle-class support in the mid-1980s, to at best a fringe activity in the early 1990s?[1] Many explanations have been suggested. Although the rate of infertility had not increased, infertility in the 1980s was no longer a secret, and major public support groups, like RESOLVE, had developed to advocate for infertile couples. New and powerful techniques, like IVF (in vitro fertilization) had been developed and had been widely publicized and approved. And babies were fashionable in the mid-1980s. As one movie critic put it: "Men and women do not fall in love with each other in the movies anymore. They fall in love with babies. Babies are the new lovers—unpredictable, uncontrollable, impossible and irresistible."[2]

These explanations all have some merit. But the core of surrogate motherhood lies in the birth and death of the modern fairy tale that babies can properly be viewed as a consumer product for those with money to purchase them, and that by permitting this transaction we will all live happily ever after. Hyped by slick, white, middle-class professionals, and advertised as a product in the free market environment of the 1980s, we were asked not to look behind the resulting children to see their lower middle-class and low economic class mothers. But the core reality of surrogate motherhood has always been that it is both classist and sexist: a method to obtain children genetically related to white males by exploiting poor women. Although it was promoted as simply supplying babies for those who "desperately" want them, in fact it always subverted any principled notion of economic fairness and justice, and it undermines our society's commitment to equality and the inherently priceless value of human life.

We all have myths to comfort us when reality is untenable. Surrogate motherhood is just one such myth. But the myth of surrogate motherhood is not sustainable in the 1990s, and without its fairy tale veneer surrogate motherhood will revert to a marginal activity at best. The thesis of this chapter is that the death of commercial surrogacy should not be mourned. Our attention should turn instead to planning for the future to avoid the commercialization of human embryos, the degradation of pregnancy, and the further exacerbation of class distinctions and economic violence that the use of embryos genetically unrelated to the "surrogate mothers" who bear them could bring.

THE BIRTH OF "SURROGATE MOTHERHOOD"

Attorney Noel Keane, the self-proclaimed "father of surrogate motherhood," first got the idea when Jane and her husband Tom visited him in September 1976.[3] Tom had "this harebrained idea of finding another woman to carry a child for them" (Jane was infertile) but didn't know how to go about it. He had ruled out adoption:

> Maybe it's egotistical but I want my own child. Adoption leaves me cold. I guess for some women, as long as they have a child, it's fine. But for me, it's like if I see my child do something, I need to know that he's *really mine*. (emphasis added)

Tom had met Jane during the Vietnam War. He had seen a lot of men get killed and told Keane:

> Say, if a woman had a couple of children and her husband was killed in the war, and say, she needed a few extra dollars for the family, well, then maybe she could help someone out who couldn't have children. *The Lord intended women to have children and I thought maybe one would want to do what came naturally* and maybe help somebody else out while helping herself and her family. Like I say, *it's just a fly-by-night idea* I had. (emphasis added)

Tom needed an attorney because he wanted anonymity; otherwise, he said, "I could just go out and look for a woman." While Keane was thinking it over, an article appeared in the *San Francisco Chronicle* about a man who had successfully advertised to find a woman to bear a child for him through artificial insemination. He had paid $7,000 to the woman and another $3,000 in legal and medical expenses. The child was born September 6, 1976. Shortly thereafter a medical newspaper reported the story, headlining it: "'Surrogate Mother' is recruited by Ad for Artificial Insemination." Noel Keane made his decision: "I had never done as much as an adoption, but if they can do it in California, I thought, what the hell, we can do it here."

Tom and Jane eventually made a deal with Carol to be inseminated. There was no fee involved, because Keane had been properly advised by a probate court judge that fees were illegal in Michigan. Carol, who was divorced, recalls making the decision with her three sons: "I told them what good parents Tom and Jane would be, and, from the start, we agreed we would call *it* Tom and Jane's baby, *never mother's baby*." When Carol became pregnant, Jane recalls: "*I wanted to put Carol under a glass bowl. You know, don't do this, don't do that. Are you eating right? Are you drinking enough? Are you taking your vitamins?*" (emphasis added) The contract that Tom and Jane had signed with Noel Keane stated explicitly, "if a surrogate is found and is, in fact, inseminated, there is no assurance she will give up the child."

Carol did give up the child. But Keane's first case illustrates most of the problems and pitfalls of so-called surrogate motherhood that remain unresolved more than fifteen years later: the use of fairy tale language, the commodification of children, and the degradation of pregnant women.

THE REALITY BEHIND THE FAIRY TALES

Fairy tale language is not unique to surrogate motherhood. In the mid-1980s we witnessed glitzy TV evangelists preach that they must have our money because God has demanded it, national security advisers surreptitiously trade arms for Iran-held hostages in the name of democratic values, and insatiable stock manipulators use inside information for personal gain in the name of free enterprise. Touted as family building for infertile couples, surrogate motherhood stems from the same greed that continues to threaten the best impulses and values in our society. The truth about surrogacy's "family building" is that it can only create one parent–child relationship by destroying another parent–child relationship. As Elizabeth Kane, the country's first openly paid "surrogate mother" has put it: "Surrogate motherhood is nothing more than the transference of pain from one woman to another."[4] Even its strongest supporters freely admit that if they could not pay women a large fee for giving up their children, they would be out of business.

The brokers, like Noel Keane, usually charge much more for their own services ($20,000 or more) than they are willing to pay women to undertake a pregnancy and give up their child. The broker's fee is guaranteed, whereas the woman's fee is dependent on delivering a healthy child. Nor is it "just like adoption." Adoption seeks to find rearing parents for children without them; surrogacy seeks a child for would-be rearing parents. Adoption places the interests of the child first; surrogacy places the interests of the adults first. Adoption is child welfare; surrogacy is adult welfare. The exclusive use of this method by rich and upper-middle class white couples proclaims its economic class and racial characteristics. For example, although black couples are *twice* as likely as white couples to be infertile, this method is not promoted for black couples, nor has anyone openly advocated covering the procedure by Medicaid for poor infertile couples.

The central deception, of course, is the term itself. The term "surrogate motherhood" seems purposely designed to dehumanize the mother and alienate her from her child. Noel Keane said, in commenting favorably on the lower court *Baby M* case: "She [the surrogate mother] has to realize she is carrying *their child*."[5] (emphasis added) The New Jersey Supreme Court, on the other hand, noted simply and forcefully, in the *Baby M* case, "the natural mother [is] inappropriately termed the 'surrogate mother.'"[6] Whenever we decide not to give something its rightful, descriptive name (in this case, mother or birthmother), it seems fair to assume that we are at least uncomfortable with the reality we are describing and want to believe some myth instead. In this case, the phrase surrogate mother actually comes from Harlow's monkey studies, in which newborn monkeys were separated from their mothers and placed in cages with either a wire or a cloth covered inanimate "surrogate mother" to test their responses.[7] Indeed, this identification of the surrogate mother as inanimate object is often complete, the so-called surrogate mother being referred to simply as the "surrogate" and sometimes as a "surrogate womb" or a "surrogate uterus."

Finally, although an attempt is almost always made to connect surrogate motherhood with new science and technology and with new reproductive techniques, in fact, the only thing new about this method is the introduction of attorneys into human reproduction. Moreover, the lawyer's role is inherently deceptive. Drafting a contract all parties sign, the lawyer usually assures them that it is "not enforceable," but nonetheless accepts a large fee for his draftsmanship. It seems overtime to ask why it's not legal malpractice and fraud for attorneys to charge clients large fees to draft contracts they publicly describe as unenforceable. Of course, it is not the role of contract drafter that the lawyer actually plays—that's just another fairy tale for the adults. The lawyer's real role is that of procurer, obtaining a woman willing to bear a child for the couple and to give it up to them at birth. As Barbara Katz Rothman has noted, although debate on surrogate motherhood and prostitution continues among feminists, "There is virtual unanimity [among feminists] on the inappropriateness of other people selling our bodies."[8] She goes on to term brokers "the pimps" of the surrogacy business. Like all pimps, their main motivation is greed, and their primary concern about women is how much money they can make by using them.

The reality of surrogate motherhood is that a lawyer-broker agrees, for a fee, to locate a woman who will, for a fee, agree to be inseminated with the sperm of a man, have their baby, and give the child up to the father (or relinquish her parental rights to the child) at birth. This is artificial insemination coupled with baby selling. But what's wrong with baby selling?

BABY SELLING

Baby selling comes complete with its own fairy tale, Grimms' *Rumpelstiltskin*. Having agreed to give her firstborn to Rumpelstiltskin if he would spin a room of straw into gold for her (a feat that helped make her queen), the queen changed her mind on the birth of her son and sought to get out of the contract. Rumpelstiltskin gave her a way out: three days to discover his name. Fortunately for her she did, and Rumpelstiltskin was so distressed to lose the child that "he tore himself in two." Grimms' sympathy was obviously with the mother, even though she was rich, had entered into the contract voluntarily, and had profited greatly by it. So is the sympathy of most readers. But the baby brokers (and even some women) have argued that "a deal is a deal" and that women, almost always poor women, who have agreed in advance to sell their babies at birth should be forced to go through with the deal so that the ability of women to enter contracts is not compromised.

Must we force women who change their minds to sell children they want to raise to satisfy some unrealistic and nonlegal notion of specific performance? This is economic violence at its starkest and is properly labeled economic brutality. The simple answer might be that since we have outlawed the sale of human kidneys (and other organs) because of the degrading prospect of having the rich live off the body parts of the poor, it follows *a fortiori* that the sale of children should also be outlawed. If and when uterine transplants become feasible, it is doubtful we would (or should) permit fertile women to sell their uteruses to women (or men) who need them to become pregnant and give birth. But many would treat children with less respect than kidneys or uteruses, and at least are willing to permit fathers to buy the mother's interest in rearing the child from her and give that interest to their own wife. Should this be permitted? Sale was not involved in Carol's case, but it was the key to the much more celebrated case of Mary Beth Whitehead (*Baby M*).

This highly publicized case involved a custody dispute between a father and a mother. The father, William Stern, had contracted with the mother, Mary Beth Whitehead, to bear him a child using artificial insemination. The contract, among other things, provided that she would receive a fee of $10,000 upon terminating her parental rights and giving up the child to him. The New Jersey Supreme Court had no problem in concluding (as did the Michigan judge Noel Keane had consulted) that payment to place a child for adoption (even with the spouse of its father) violated the state's adoption laws. The court declared that "the evils of baby bartering are loathsome for a myriad of reasons." There is coercion, lack of counseling, and exploitation of all parties (including desperate infertile couples), as well as the fact that "the child is sold without regard for whether the purchasers will be suitable parents" and the lack of any protection of the natural mother. Making money takes precedent even over predictable human suffering. For example, the broker in the *Baby M* case failed to make further inquiry when a psychological evaluation of Mrs. Whitehead revealed that she might change her mind. In the court's words, "It is apparent that the profit motive got the better of the Infertility Center . . . To inquire further might have jeopardized the Infertility Center's fee."

The selling of babies that has been so slickly glazed over by others properly disgusted the court. The court noted that the originator of this scheme to circumvent the law by private contract is "a middle man, propelled by profit" who "promotes the sale. . . . The profit motive predominates, permeates, and ultimately governs the transaction." What's wrong with profit and using money as the sole measure of the value of children? The court did not hesitate to say: "There are, in a civilized society, some things that money cannot buy. . . . There are . . . values that society deems more important than granting to wealth whatever it can buy, be it labor, or life." Not the least of these values is the protection of children from the vicious exploitation that treating them as commodities would bring, exploitation of the poor by the rich, and the demeaning of pregnant women by treating them as breeders indentured to their "employers."

There has been much confusion about constitutional rights in the surrogacy arrangement. The only real rights at stake are those involving the rights to custody of a child resulting from an unwed pregnancy, and in this contest the rights of the child properly take precedence. There is no constitutional right to purchase a child, even your own. And whatever procreation rights might be raised to a constitutional level in the area of custody, the rights of the mother must be at least as strong as those of the father. Indeed, they should be stronger since fertile men need a nine-month commitment on the part of a woman to procreate, whereas fertile women only need sperm to procreate.

The constitutional right of privacy is founded on liberty interests in intimacy and freedom of association, along with notions of self-identity and self-expression. Privacy is *not* a technocrat's toy that requires the government to keep its hands off any method of procreation inventors can devise. Treating men and women equally in the realm of noncoital reproduction may require egg donation to be treated like sperm donation, but no principled argument can equate (as the trial judge in *Baby M* did) nine months of gestation and ultimate childbirth with sperm donation. As the U.S. Supreme Court has ruled, states cannot even permit husbands to prohibit their wives from having abortions since, among other things, "it is the woman who physically bears the child and she is the most directly affected by the pregnancy."[9] An Oklahoma court has also noted that husbands have no right to prevent their wives from becoming sterilized. In the court's words:

> We have found no authority and the plaintiff has cited none which holds that the husband has a right to a childbearing wife as an incident to their marriage. We are neither prepared to create a right in the husband to have a fertile wife nor to allow recovery for damage to such a right. We find the right of the person who is capable of competent consent to control his own body paramount.[10]

If husbands have no constitutional right to fertile wives, it follows that they have no constitutional right to contract with unrelated women for purposes of reproducing themselves. The *Baby M* court saved for another day the question of whether a woman can irrevocably waive her constitutional right to the companionship of her children by a preconception contract (assuming such a contract is "legalized" by future legislation). But there would seem to be no basis that would allow the courts to enforce such an agreement. Even the lower court *Baby M* judge, for example, recognized that a woman could not irrevocably waive her right to terminate her pregnancy under the U.S. Constitution because judicial enforcement of such an agreement would be an intolerable burden on the woman.[11] The argument against permitting an irrevocable prebirth waiver of maternal rearing rights seems at least as strong. Both decisions are so intimately related to the individual's personhood and human dignity that it would be an intolerable violation of personal integrity to force compliance with either. This is because pregnancy and childbirth may predictably and radically change self-image and self-fulfillment aspirations that are central features of identity and personhood.

The *Baby M* court could have gone further. It did not, for example, even discuss the images of slavery inherent in enforcing contracts in commercial surrogate motherhood. Selling children conjures up the indignity and degradation of selling any human being; more than that, specifically enforcing contracts that lead to the involuntary breakup of a family unit is at the heart of what many Americans found most repulsive about slavery prior to the Civil War. As James McPherson, one of the war's great historians, has noted: "This breakup of families was the largest chink in the armor of slavery's defenders." McPherson tells us that one of the most powerful "moral attacks" on slavery was Theodore Weld's *American Slavery as It Is*. First published in 1839, it was made up mainly of newspaper excerpts and advertisements. An example:

NEGROES FOR SALE. — A negro woman 24 years of age, and two children, one eight and the other three years. Said negroes will be sold separately or together as desired.[12]

He also notes that the influential *Uncle Tom's Cabin* was itself based on the forced breakup of the family: "Eliza fleeing across the ice-choked Ohio River to save her son from the slave-trader and Tom weeping for children left behind in Kentucky when he was sold South are among the most unforgettable scenes in American letters."[13] Surrogacy is not slavery. But our inability to seriously discuss the relevancy of selling children and forcibly removing them from their mothers to one of the core aspects of 19th-century American slavery indicates our preference for dealing with fairy tale versions of surrogacy.

Since the sale of children can lead to their commodification or reification, and since this will devalue all children and put all children at risk, it is quite reasonable to outlaw the sale of children, even to their fathers. But if greed is the real root of evil, isn't surrogacy motivated by love rather than by money (as in the case of Carol) acceptable?

THE DEGRADATION OF PREGNANCY

Margaret Radin has noted that whether surrogacy is paid or unpaid it may still involve "ironic self-deception." In her words:

> Acting in ways that current gender ideology characterizes as empowering might actually be disempowering. Surrogates may feel they are fulfilling their womanhood by producing babies for someone else, although they may actually be reinforcing oppressive gender roles.[14]

She goes on to note that would-be fathers can also be seen as oppressors of their wives, who, believing it is their duty to mother their husband's genetic child, "could be caught in the same kind of false consciousness and relative powerlessness as surrogates who feel called upon to produce children for others."

These arguments seem intuitively correct: Another key to surrogate motherhood is the traditional (and oppressive) female role it reinforces. The male's right to have a child is seen as paramount, and any interest the mother might have in their child is subordinated to it. But there is no more right for a male to have a child than there is a right to have a fertile wife, or a right to prevent one's wife from being sterilized or from having an abortion. Men simply don't have this power over women, and we do not advance sexual equality by promoting a scheme that subordinates females so completely to male interests.

The surrogate mother is asked not only to perform this "service" for the male, but also to engage in purposeful self-deception. Like Carol, she is asked to pretend that the child she is carrying is not her own, but only the father's. The country's most famous surrogate mother, Elizabeth Kane, told her fairy tale simply during her pregnancy: "It's not my baby, it's the father's. I'm just growing it for him."[15] Another has proclaimed on national television: "Motherhood is not biological."[16] Nor is the father's wife unaffected. As one infertile wife proclaimed in support of surrogacy: "The most rewarding thing a woman can do is raise her husband's child."[17] The supposition that the women in surrogacy are involved in a "liberating" experience is akin to the supposition that selling one's kidney gives one the freedom to control one's body.

But surrogacy involves more than just fairy tale–like self-deception. It involves real degradation of the pregnant woman by proclaiming that the most important concern is not for her welfare, but for that of the fetus she is carrying. And this is what makes this "harebrained" idea both so offensive and so potentially important symbolically for women. The lower court judge in the *Baby M* case, for example, termed surrogacy a "viable vehicle" to help deliver a baby to the Sterns; and the Sterns' expert witness termed Mrs. Whitehead simply a "surrogate uterus." The contract Noel Keane drafted, and which she signed, gave rights over her activities and body during the pregnancy to the father (William Stern), who could require not only that she undergo amniocentesis but also that she abort a handicapped child at his demand, or his contract obligation ended.

This untenable proposition—that a pregnant woman's life is not her own, but that others should be able to determine her activities based on what they think is in the best interests of the fetus she is carrying—underlies surrogacy. The contract attempts to get the mother to fantasize that she is simply a container carrying a precious cargo that she dare not injure. Since surrogacy did not take place in a vacuum, other physicians and courts in the 1980s adopted the view that pregnancy is just for the fetus and ordered women to submit to cesarean sections for the sake of their fetuses[18] and, in the shameful case of Angela Carder (discussed in Chapter 3) even forced a dying woman to undergo emergency surgery to deliver a fetus that was of questionable viability. These cases were wrongly decided. But they are consistent with the notion that pregnant women are not fully human and can properly be viewed as containers.

The New Jersey Supreme Court was on solid ground in holding that surrogate mother contracts can never be specifically enforceable and that women must have the right to change their minds and assert their maternal rights to rear their children (at least up to the time after birth specified in the state's adoption statute). When the woman does assert her maternal rights, the New Jersey Supreme Court also seems correct in decreeing that she should retain custody during the legal battle over permanent custody, a decision that ultimately must be based on the best interests of the child. Arguing that we should try to prevent such custody battles by contract is tangential: the way to prevent them entirely is simply not to engage in this arrangement. Objecting to making decisions after birth in the child's best interests, and ignoring the interests of the child before birth, simply exposes the fact that the surrogacy arrangement *never* considers the child's welfare, only the welfare of the contracting parents. Nor is the argument that the child is always better off existing than not existing sufficient to justify surrogacy from the child's perspective[19]: unconceived children have no "right to exist," and we do not harm them by not conceiving them or by prohibiting such practices as polygamy. We do, however, harm real children by commodifying them, forceably separating them from their natural mothers, and arranging situations that predictably lead to unstable and uncertain family relationships.

WHAT SHOULD BE DONE?

I understand those who would prohibit not just commercial surrogacy, but voluntary surrogacy as well. But just as we permit organ donations among living family members, we may also wish to permit relatives (especially sisters), to have children for each other. My own preference is for legislation aimed at what has been mistermed "full surrogacy,"—the hiring of a woman to carry a fetus to whom she is not genetically related. This will involve "high tech" IVF and embryo transfer (and probably freezing), and could become more popular since the resulting child will be the genetic child of both the husband and wife (assuming they supply the gametes). Use of this technology could much more radically alter our notions of pregnancy and motherhood, as discussed in the next chapter.

If one must choose between the genetic and gestational mother, then to prevent the gross exploitation of poor women, to prevent pregnant women from being viewed simply as vessels, to recognize the greater contribution of gestation to the child, and to ensure that the child is protected by having at least one parent with responsibility for it available at birth, the gestational mother should be irrebuttably considered the rearing mother for all legal purposes. She should be permitted to give the child up to the genetic mother and father after birth, but only by acting in conformity with the state's adoption laws. Permitting the gestational presumption to be modified by contract could make *all* pregnancies and *all* births suspect. No one would know who the newborn's "mother" was until contracts were examined and genetic testing was performed. This "suspended motherhood" model is (or should be) societally insupportable since it endangers all mothers and children. A statute that irrebuttably presumes the gestational mother to be the child's legal mother for all purposes would be protective of gestational mothers and children and should be enacted in all states.[20]

The second statute I endorse is one that would outlaw the sale of human embryos. A few states have already enacted legislation to do this. Embryo freezing is already commonplace. The attempted commercialization and sale of frozen embryos will not be far behind. Like children, embryos will be bought and sold in the belief that they will produce a healthy child, and probably one with a certain physical type, IQ, stature, and so on. All of these characteristics will command a specific market price—thereby monetizing the characteristics of all live children. Because of this, and the fact that selling human embryos brings with it almost all of the problems and evils of selling children, their sale should be prohibited by statute.[21]

Commercial surrogate motherhood deserves the death without dignity that Rumpelstiltskin suffered. Legislation to try to resuscitate it and put it on temporary life-support systems would not be in the best interests of children, families, or society. But it has given us the opportunity to anticipate and plan for the next generation of issues brought to us by real science. We should act now to support economic and sexual equality and to protect future children and families from commercial exploitation.[22] We should work for a future in which pregnant women retain their personhood—a future of economic and social justice, rather than a future based on economic violence and social inequality. The fairy tales surrogate mothers (and brokers) tell must not be taken seriously.

6

A French Homunculus in a Tennessee Court

Law has become part of popular culture, and this is probably good.[1] *The People's Court* brings Judge Joseph P. Wapner into our homes five days a week to decide disputes between real people. *L.A. Law*, properly described as one part L.A. and one part law, has been said to have had "a beneficial influence on popular conceptions of law and legal ethics."[2] To sustain audiences, *L.A. Law* has had to ignore the more than 95 percent tedium of a typical law practice and concentrate instead on the spectacularly controversial cases that make the national press, such as "medical ethics" issues involving the termination of life support, a psychiatrist's duty to warn others of his patient's dangerousness, and forcing a terminally ill pregnant woman to have a cesarean section. One can argue persuasively that all of these cases were dealt with ineptly from a legal perspective, but they were presented in an entertaining manner, and entertainment is what television is all about.[3]

Judge Wapner does not "do" bioethics issues in his courtroom. In real life, however, bioethics issues do come to court. Unfortunately, few lower court judges have had exposure even to television's version of these issues, and the record of lower court judges in resolving them has been mixed at best. In some of the best-known cases, including the cases of Karen Ann Quinlan, Elizabeth Bouvia, William Bartling, and Baby M, lower court judges issued opinions that were very wide of the mark and that led to unanimous and vigorous reversals by appellate courts. The trial court judges in all of these cases could be severely criticized for their reasoning, and, as a result of their opinions, it could even be suggested that trial courts are institutionally incompetent to deal with bioethics issues. Professional standards, blue ribbon commissions, and legislative bodies may be more appropriate. I'm not ready to give up on trial court judges yet, but the

71

performance of Circuit Judge W. Dale Young of Tennessee's Fifth Judicial District in the case of *Davis v. Davis*[4] provides a powerful example of what can go wrong when a trial court judge takes it upon himself to "solve" a major bioethical dispute on the basis of what he hears in his courtroom.

DAVIS v. DAVIS

Junior L. Davis and Mary Sue Davis decided to divorce after nine years of marriage. After five tubal pregnancies, Mrs. Davis had her fallopian tubes severed to prevent further risk to her. She and her husband thereafter decided to attempt pregnancy through in vitro fertilization (IVF). The couple went through six attempts at IVF before deciding to try adoption. After their efforts to adopt also failed, they returned to IVF. In their seventh attempt, two embryos were transferred, and seven additional embryos that had been created were frozen for future attempts. The seventh attempt was also unsuccessful. The couple agreed to all aspects of their divorce settlement with the exception of the disposition of the seven frozen embryos. Mrs. Davis wanted to use them to attempt to have a child after their divorce; Mr. Davis objected to this use. They therefore sought a judicial determination of what should be done with the seven frozen embryos.

The case was heard by Judge W. Dale Young, in Maryville, Tennessee, and almost immediately attracted the attention of the national press. Judge Young opined that it was the first time anyone but the litigants cared about any decision he'd ever made. In fact, it seems fair to say that the case attracted more national notoriety than any case in Tennessee history since the trial of Joseph Thomas Scopes for teaching evolution in defiance of Tennessee creationist law.[5] It also seems fair to say that the level of science professed by the judge was even more rudimentary than that espoused by the antievolutionary preachers of the 1920s.

Judge Young can be seen as reviving the untenable theory of the homunculus, the fully formed miniature person once held to reside in every sperm, which is making a comeback. Although the following description was written by Laurence Sterne in *Tristram Shandy* (1760), it bears a disquieting resemblance to expert scientific testimony recently in Young's Tennessee courtroom:

> The Homunculus, Sir, in however low and ludicrous a light he many appear, in this age of levity, to the eye of folly or prejudice; —to the eye of reason in scientific research, he stands confessed —a Being guarded and circumscribed with rights. —The minutest philosophers . . . shew us incontestably, that the Homunculus is created by the same hand, —engendered in the same course of nature, —endowed with the same locomotive powers and faculties with us: —that he consists as we do, of skin, hair, fat, flesh, veins, arteries, ligaments, nerves, cartilages, bones, marrow, brains, glands, genitals, humerus, and articulations; —is a being of as much activity, and, in all senses of the word, as much

and as truly our fellow creature as my Lord Chancellor of England. He may be
benefitted, — he may obtain redress; — in a word he has all the claims and rights
of humanity, which Tully, Puffendorf, or the best ethic writers allow to arise
out of the state and relation. (Bk. 1, ch. 2)

To decide this case, Judge Young could simply have determined either
which of the litigants had a greater interest in the embryos or which had
the most reasonable expectation that their wishes regarding the disposition
of the embryos would be followed. Accordingly, the judge could have
awarded the embryos to Mrs. Davis, either on the basis that she had contributed more to them than Mr. Davis (because she had to undergo a surgical procedure to have the ova removed) or on the basis that her reasonable
expectation in agreeing to have the seven embryos created and frozen was
that they would be used by her in future attempts to have a child, should
the immediate attempt fail. He could, alternatively, have decided that in
absence of agreement, the embryos should be destroyed.

For reasons he never explains, and that may be more related to the media
value of the case than its fair resolution, the judge stated the case not as
who should get the embryos, but, rather, whether the embryos were people
or products. This, of course, is *not* an outcome-determining categorization
(since, either way, the question of who gets them remains). Moreover,
stating the question this way is very misleading: embryos could just as easily
be considered *neither* products nor people, but put in some other category
altogether. There are many things, such as dogs, dolphins, and redwood
trees that are neither products nor people. We nonetheless legally protect
these entities by limiting what their owners or custodians can do with them.
Every national commission worldwide that has examined the status of the
human embryo to date has placed it in this third category: neither people nor products, but nonetheless entities of unique symbolic value that
deserve society's respect and protection. By setting up a false dichotomy,
Judge Young doomed himself from the outset to write an unsound opinion.
This structural mistake led to a more serious error.

The judge believed that it was up to him to decide for the rest of the
world whether or not embryos were people. In an interview granted after
his opinion was issued, Judge Young said that the U.S. Supreme Court had
"ducked" this issue in *Roe v. Wade*, but that he had to decide it. This is a
rare combination of hubris and ignorance. Nor was the method the judge
chose to decide whether embryos were people one that brings much credit
to the judiciary: he decided to rely exclusively on the testimony of one
witness, a physician from France.

The Testimony of Jerome Lejeune

As summarized by the judge, Jerome Lejeune, the discoverer of the genetic
basis of Down syndrome, testified, among other things, to the following
"facts":

Each human being has a unique beginning, which occurs at the moment of conception.

What is reproduced and transmitted as a result of fertilization is information by way of the DNA molecules; the information then animates matter.

[In cryopreservation] time is frozen, not embryos.

When the first cell exists, all the "tricks of the trade" (or "tricks of Mother Nature" as he later called it) to build itself into an individual already exists.

At the three cell stage "the tiny human being . . . exists . . . and it is now an experimentally-demonstrated fact that at the three cell stage every individual is uniquely different from any other individual."

When the ovum is fertilized by the sperm, the result is "the most specialized cell under the sun," specialized from the point of view that no other cell will ever again have the same instructions in the life of the individual being created.

"[A]s soon as he has been conceived a man is a man."

According to the Hippocratic Oath it does not matter what the size of the patient, a patient is a patient.

No scientist has ever offered the opinion that an embryo is property.[6]

The judge did not quote other testimony of Lejeune's that, "Putting tiny human beings in a very cold space, deprived of liberty, deprived even of time, they are as it were in a concentration camp. . . . It is not a hospitable place as the secret temple of a woman's womb."[7] Nor did he recall the cross-examination by Mr. Davis' lawyer, Charles Clifford, who pulled a chicken egg from his pocket and asked: "Can you tell me, doctor, what this is?" Lejeune replied: "It looks to me like it's an egg." To which Clifford responded: "I thought you would have told me that it was an early chicken."[8]

Judge Young's Conclusion

On the basis of Lejeune's testimony, the judge concluded that "the life codes for each special, unique individual are resident at conception and animate [*sic*] the new person very soon after fertilization occurs." Judge Young continued:

The argument that the human embryo may never realize its biologic potential, it appears to the Court, is statistically and speculatively true, but is a hollow argument. A newborn baby may never realize its biologic potential, but no one disputes the fact that the newborn baby is a human being. And if it is a part of the logic that an embryo . . . is not a being because it cannot sustain itself, then we must also reason that a newborn baby . . . also lacks a necessary criteria to qualify as a human being, for surely it is good logic that a newborn human being left naked in a field without the sustenance, aid and assistance of another human being will surely die; it is utterly helpless; it, too, lacks the capacity to sustain itself.

He then went on to conclude that the seven frozen embryos "are human beings . . . not property" and that "human life begins at the moment of conception." Based on these conclusions, the court was left only to determine "the best interests of the children." The conclusion followed naturally: "The Court finds and concludes that it is to the manifest best interest of the children, in vitro, that they be made available for implantation to assure their opportunity for live birth; implantation is their sole and only hope for survival." Temporary custody of the "children" is awarded to Mrs. Davis for purposes of implantation, while "all matters concerning, support, visitation, final custody and related issues" are reserved by the court until "such time as one or more of the seven cryogenetically preserved human embryos are the product of live birth."

What Does it Mean?

The overwhelming attribute of this opinion is that it makes almost no attempt to deal with the law. It cites only a handful of cases and makes no attempt to analyze any of them. The most remarkable thing about the opinion is that its holding that embryos are children is simply a conclusion based exclusively on the unsubstantiated opinion of one French witness. And, although the judge spends all his time deciding that the embryos are people, not property, he ends up treating them like property. Instead of deciding custody, visitation, and support issues (which he would have to do if the embryos *were* children), he instead awards them to Mrs. Davis in exactly the way he would award a dresser or a painting. Of course, if these embryos really were children, the public would not have cared which parent got custody of them, and the case would not have been newsworthy.

The decision itself trivializes and devalues children by treating them no better than embryos. Physicians were tried, convicted, and sentenced to death at Nuremberg for freezing experiments performed on human beings during World War II. If these embryos really were children, people, or human beings it would not be lawful to conduct potentially deadly experiments on them, such as freezing, and the physician who did so would have engaged in criminal conduct. The Nazi concentration camp experience was suggested as the proper analogy by Lejeune. Nonetheless, the judge nowhere in his opinion suggests that there is anything wrong with freezing embryos, and thus he cannot really believe that embryos are children (unless, of course, we are to believe that he thinks freezing children with a view to thawing them out at a later date when the parents might be better able to care for them is an acceptable activity).

It seems that the judge was dazzled with Lejeune's testimony even though the "science" in it is less sophisticated than that of *Mr. Rogers' Neighborhood*. The embryos are frozen, not time, as is apparent from the assertion that they can only remain frozen for two years (a dubious assertion itself, but one that admits that time continues to run for the embryos). Saying that an individual exists when one cell exists makes the same mistake as saying an oak tree exists when an acorn exists. Focusing on the "three cell" stage is wonderfully curious since there is nothing to distinguish three cells from two or four cells, and this "stage" exists only because the two cells do not split simultaneously. The term "specialized" seems to have been used by Lejeune in a way entirely different from the way other witnesses used it, and this seems to have confused the judge. Lejeune says "specialized" means unique; the other witnesses used specialized to mean specific.

Finally, if the judge really believed that he had to decide this case based on the "best interests of the children" he would have had to at least determine if Mrs. Davis was a fit mother to gestate them. Given her past history of inability to carry a fetus to term, there is little probability of her successfully gestating any of the seven embryos. Requiring her to hire a surrogate mother to gestate them would almost certainly enhance their chances to be born.

The Homunculus

The judge bows to the wonders of modern DNA techniques, but his opinion harkens back to the old theory of the homunculus, or "little man." This theory held that a fully formed miniature person resided in every sperm, and when it united with the egg it began to grow larger, always maintaining its fully formed human shape. In commenting on this case columnist Ellen Goodman was reminded of the movie "Honey I Shrunk the Kids."[9] The image is correct. Judge Young and his favorite witness, Lejeune, each see embryos as space capsules containing miniature astronauts. This is why Lejeune could testify that a patient is a patient "no matter what the size of the patient" and that embryos are "tiny human beings."

Many "right-to-life" activists applauded Judge Young's opinion that embryos are children. But those who equate embryos and children show cold disrespect and lack of concern for children. To use a simple example: if a fire broke out in the laboratory where these seven embryos are stored, and a 2-month-old child were in one corner of the laboratory and the seven embryos in another, and you could only save either the embryos or the child, I doubt you would have any hesitancy in saving the infant. Saving the infant, however, acknowledges that the child is *not* to be equated with the embryo.

Likewise, if embryos are children, there have been many more children in the world than we have thus far acknowledged—approximately 35 percent of all human embryos either do not implant or abort spontaneously early in pregnancy. If we valued children, we would have to do something about this. To save these children, we would have to consider requiring women to strain their menstrual blood every month that they either had intercourse or were artificially inseminated to try to "rescue" the "children" that would otherwise be lost. Those that could not be saved could nonetheless be named and mourned and added to the list of "deceased" brothers and sisters.

If readers are either amused or horrified at this scenario, it can only be because we know both rationally and intuitively that embryos are *not* children, even though some embryos will become children. The judge's long exegesis on infants not being able to survive alone is, of course, logical nonsense. Embryos are not children simply because they share with children an inability to survive without help, any more than elephant embryos are children because they cannot survive without help. Neither elephant embryos nor human embryos are children because they do not possess the characteristics of children in either form or function. The fact that embryos possess the *information* that *may* be translated into a child at some future date does not make the embryo a child, any more than a fertilized chicken egg is a chicken.

Celebrity Judges

The trial court judges in *Quinlan, Bouvia, Bartling*, and *Baby M* mostly stayed out of the press. Judge Young, on the other hand, seems to have done almost everything he could to insure that the media's spotlight was on him. His opinion, for example, reads more like a press release than judicial opinion. Not only is there almost no law in it, but "Appendix A" is simply a general essay on how courts work that can only be read as background information for the press. The judge also had himself filmed for television when he presented his written opinion to the clerk, and then proceeded to give interviews to TV, radio, and the print media on the opinion after it was filed, a virtually unprecedented performance by a judge, and injudicious behavior at best.

Judge Young seems to have been auditioning for Judge Wapner's job. Perhaps he wanted to play himself in the modern version of *Inherit the Wind* (tentatively titled "The Tennessee Embryo Massacre"), or perhaps he really thought that the primary function of law is to entertain and that it is his job to demonstrate that "TN Law" can be as entertaining as *L.A. Law*. If the latter, he is correct: his opinion is as entertaining as *The Beverly Hillbillies*.

It was predictable, but still comforting, that Judge Young's opinion was soundly reversed on appeal. The appellate court sensibly observed that even though embryos at law have been "accorded more respect than mere human cells because of their burgeoning potential for life, . . . even after viability they are not given legal status equivalent to that of a person already born."[10] The court ruled that the couple "shared an interest in the seven fertilized ova" and concluded that they should be given "joint control . . . with equal voice over their disposition." In other words, the genetic contributors, not the court or anyone else, will decide what to do with the embryos. If they fail to agree, the embryos will remain frozen. This nondecision, which has been affirmed by the Tennessee Supreme Court, strikes me as a reasonable one, although it challenges us to give content to the phrase "worthy of respect," as in "human embryos are worthy of respect." Embryos are neither children nor furniture, but have a unique, exotic status that demands unique rules. The gene-based "solution" is probably as good as we can do for now. But should the genetic contributors get to make all the decisions even after the embryo becomes a baby by virtue of being nurtured in a "surrogate" mother's womb? Lower courts are unlikely to resolve this issue, as is well illustrated by the case of Anna Johnson.

THE ANNA JOHNSON CASE

Part of the answer to "who's the mother?" is the status we accord the embryo gestator, the woman we used to simply call "mother." The identity of the mother was the central issue in a California case in which Crispina and Mark Calvert hired a young, single, black nurse to gestate an embryo composed of their egg and sperm and to give the resulting child to them for a fee of $10,000. Mrs. Calvert was unable to bear a child because of a hysterectomy. Near the end of her pregnancy, Anna Johnson sought to retain custody of the child. Genetic testing confirmed that the child, Christopher, born September 19, 1990, had no genetic relationship to Ms. Johnson. Following a hearing, Judge Richard N. Parslow, Jr., rendered an oral opinion from the bench, concluding that Crispina alone should be considered Christopher's mother:

> Anna Johnson is the gestational carrier of the child, a host in a sense. . . . She and the child are genetic hereditary strangers. . . . Anna's relationship to the child is analogous to that of a foster parent providing care, protection and nurture during the period of time that the natural mother, Crispina Calvert, was unable to care for the child.[11]

The judge bolstered this opinion by mentioning twin studies that showed that genetics was more important than environment, by finding that the contract was valid, and by concluding that giving the child exclusively to the Calverts was in the best interests of the child. As to the contract, the judge said that the "relinquishment" provision was "enforceable by either specific performance, arguably even by habeas corpus, if necessary."

On the issue of the child's interests, the judge said:

> I think a three-parent, two natural mom claim in a situation is ripe for crazy making, as they say nowadays, involving a high probability of that happening in this case given the parties we have involved. . . . This will create confusion in a child having a three-parent arrangement.

The judge went on to make "some suggestions for the legislature," including a state law that required the following: intensive psychological evaluation of the parties by an independent agency; the genetic mother must be medically unable to carry a child to term; a clear understanding that the "surrogate" will have no parental rights; and the "surrogate" must have previously given birth to at least one child.

Baby Selling

Having initially said that this case "is not a baby selling case, it's not a *Baby M* type case where we had natural parents on two sides of a situation. It's none of those things," the judge nonetheless returned to baby selling near the end of his opinion:

> I see no problem with someone collecting, the general going rate appears to be $10,000, getting paid for your pain and suffering, shall we say. I haven't carried a child myself, but from what I've seen, it's a tough program. And I think altruism aside, there is nothing wrong with getting paid for nine months of what I understand to be a lot of misery and a lot of bad days. . . . They are not selling a baby, they are selling, again, the pain and suffering, the discomfort, that which goes with carrying a child to term.

The judge concluded with a quotation from Democritus: "Everywhere man blames nature and fate, yet his fate is mostly but the echo of his character and passions, his mistakes and weaknesses."

Like the trial court decision in *Davis*, this opinion seems simply wrong. The judge's denial of any relevance of the *Baby M* case is particularly unpersuasive. As discussed in the previous chapter, that case declared that contracts of this type could not be specifically enforced and were void because they amounted to baby selling. The New Jersey Supreme Court correctly determined that money is being spent for a child, *not* for nine months of gestational services. If all that was being purchased was "pain and suffering," Anna Johnson earned her money without giving up the child. Moreover, the pain and suffering of being forcibly separated from one's child lasts a lifetime.

It has been suggested that society knowingly employs a double standard here: we see it as much worse to sell a child than to buy one. This may be because we view any woman who is willing to sell her child (even if she later changes her mind) as suspect and a poor risk to raise the child. It may also be because of the common class difference between purchasers and sellers: the middle class approves of their members buying babies from poor women.

The case is, of course, different from *Baby M* in one critical way: Anna Johnson is not genetically related to the child she bore. The legal and social policy question is whether this is a distinction that should matter. The trial judge seems to have been overwhelmed by pop genetics in reaching his opinion that the genetic mother should prevail. In the judge's words: "Who we are and what we are . . . is a combination of genetic factors. We know more and more about traits now, how you walk, talk and everything else, all sorts of things being equal, when your immune system is going to break down, what diseases you may be susceptible to." Referring to an article in *Science*[12] that had been published during the last week of the trial, he observed: "They have upped the intelligence ratio of genetics to 70 percent now." He then went on to compare genetics not to environment, but to "gestational environment," although by this he seems to mean "uterine bonding" rather than the impact of the mother's health, smoking, drug taking, and nutrition on the child. Genetics is clearly relevant, but just as clearly it does not supply an unequivocal answer to the question of legal and social policy.

The Appeals Court Decision

It would be comforting (and consistent with the general thesis of this chapter) to report that the appeals court did a better job with the genetics question than the trial court. Unfortunately, quite the opposite occurred. The opinion was unanimously affirmed, with the appeals court concentrating exclusively on determining which of the two women was "the child's 'natural' mother, the woman who nurtures the child in her womb and gives birth—or the otherwise infertile woman whose egg [embryo] is implanted into the woman who gave birth?"[13] The court decided that a blood test should determine maternity, just as it could determine paternity under California's 1975 Uniform Parentage Act:

> We must "resolve" the question of Anna's claim to maternity as we would resolve the question of a man's claim to (or liability for) paternity when blood tests positively exclude him as a candidate. . . . In light of Anna's stipulation that Crispina is genetically related to the child and because of the blood tests excluding Anna from being the natural mother, there is no reason not to uphold the trial court's determination that Crispina is the natural mother. She is the only other candidate!

The court also concluded that California law violates no constitutional liberty interests in any relation with the child that Anna Johnson might have gained through pregnancy and childbirth. The appeals court relied exclusively on the U.S. Supreme Court case of *Michael H. v. Gerald D.* for the proposition that only liberty interests that have been "traditionally protected" have constitutional stature.[14] In *Michael H.* Justice Antonin Scalia, who wrote the Court's plurality opinion, decided that California could constitutionally refuse to grant a paternity hearing to a man who had had a daughter with a married woman because U.S. laws had not traditionally protected the relation between an unwed "adulterous natural father" and his daughter. Similarly, the appeals court determined that Ms. Johnson could not claim a constitutionally protected liberty interest because "our society has never 'traditionally protected' the right of a gestational surrogate."

As to a possible violation of equal protection, the appeals court ruled that using genes instead of gestation to determine parenthood for both mothers and fathers was sex-neutral and rational because:

> As the evidence at the trial showed, the whole process of human development "is set in motion by the genes." There is not a single organic system of the human body not influenced by an individual's underlying genetic makeup. Genes determine the way physiological components of the human body, such as the heart, liver, or blood vessels operate. Also, according to the expert testimony received at trial, it is now thought that genes influence tastes, preferences, personality styles, manners of speech and mannerisms.

Implications of the Opinions

These opinions contribute little to the resolution of whether the genetic or the gestational mother should be considered the legal mother of a child. Calling the genetic mother the "natural" mother simply begs the question; it does not answer it. The court's equation of paternity testing with maternity testing is, of course, correct if one is trying to determine who the genetic parent is, but in this case that was never an issue. In human reproduction men contribute only genes; women contribute both genes and gestation. The question is what rules society should adopt now that these maternal contributions can be separated.

Anna Johnson never claimed to be the child's genetic mother. The only question she asked was whether her pregnancy and childbirth gave her a mother–child relationship with Christopher. Thus, the court's exegesis on statutes defining parenthood that were passed before the advent of in vitro fertilization is as irrelevant as the statutes concerning motherhood that were passed before in vitro fertilization and the statutes concerning artificial insemination, passed before embryo transfer, that the court discounted. The relevant question was the relation of Ms. Johnson to Christopher; labeling Mrs. Calvert Christopher's "natural mother" does not answer it.

The appeals court acknowledged early in its opinion that words were often used to color questions regarding the new reproductive techniques. Calling a woman a surrogate, for example, tends to objectify and dehumanize her. The lower court judge referred to Ms. Johnson as a "carrier" and as a "host" who provided a "gestational environment," all terms that suggest an impersonal, interchangeable service role, like providing a taxi or a hotel room. The appeals court, even recognizing the potential pitfalls of language, could not help adopting the adjective "natural." Having labeled Ms. Calvert the natural mother, the court in effect relegated Ms. Johnson to an "unnatural," almost alien status. In this regard the case is similar to that of *Michael H.*, in which the U.S. Supreme Court, upholding the same statute relied on by the appeals court, referred to a natural father as an "adulterous natural father." That decision has been properly criticized for adopting the indeterminate test of "traditional protection" to identify currently protected constitutional liberties.[15] Appeal to tradition does not answer the question of which traditions merit protection. It probably escaped no one's notice, for example, that there is no legal tradition of protecting the contributors of ova in the United States, whereas there is a long tradition of protecting gestational mothers.

The judges ultimately decided that the genetic mother is the natural mother because "the whole process of human development 'is set in motion by the genes.'" But, of course, the same statement can be made on behalf of the gestational mother. Without her body and her pregnancy, human development would not have continued. Similarly, "there is not a single organic system" in Christopher's body that was not influenced by Ms. Johnson's body during the pregnancy. Thus, many of the same arguments that the court used to favor genes over gestation could be used to uphold an opposite decision. The problem, of course, is that the genetic and gestational mothers have more in common than judges care to acknowledge. As discussed in the previous chapter, there is a tidiness in designating one the natural mother and the other an unrelated stranger. But such a designation will never be satisfactory, since whichever woman is chosen, the other is depersonalized and marginalized. The opinion of the appeals court marginalizes and devalues pregnancy and childbirth, but an opposite opinion would devalue and marginalize genetics.

We currently live in an age when genes are seen, as all of the California judges in this case saw them, as the key to human existence. But what is the status of women who are capable of carrying a child to term but who cannot produce ova? They now rely on donated ova (rather than gestational surrogacy) to enable them to give birth to children.[16] If the judges are correct, the "natural" mothers of these children are the donors of the ova, not the women who gave birth to them. This conclusion would make current ovum donation programs unworkable.[17] A related question involves fatherhood. Under California's Uniform Parentage Act, if we consider the donor of the ovum the natural mother, then her husband, and not the husband of the woman who gives birth (who is also the genetic father), is the natural father of the child. Likewise under the act, if Ms. Johnson had been married, Christopher would have been "conclusively presumed" to be a child of her marriage. These results are, of course, the very type of "crazy making" the judges thought they were avoiding by ignoring the claims of the gestational mother. They have done even worse than ignore her, however. They have taken part in exploiting her. As in virtually all "surrogate motherhood" arrangements, Ms. Johnson was poor and needed the $10,000 fee literally to pay her rent. Poor women will probably continue to be used by middle class couples to perform this "service" for them.

What Role Should Genes Have in Defining Motherhood?

It is unfair to criticize the courts too harshly for not arriving at the ultimate solution to this unique and complex question, in which three adults are intimately involved in producing a child to whose development all have contributed biologically and emotionally (if not genetically). Although the appeals court's approach seems both misdirected and unfair, the best solution is not obvious. I argued in the previous chapter that the traditional definition of motherhood should be maintained — that is, that the woman who gives birth to a child should be irrebuttably presumed to be the mother of that child. Although she could relinquish her parental rights to the child after birth, she would have the option to raise the child if she so chose. This would make commercial surrogacy less attractive, but the United States is now the only country to endorse it in any case. This rule would protect all women who go through pregnancy and childbirth, including the recipients of donated ova. Birth certificates would continue to name only the gestational mother.

On the other hand, the reality of this case and others like it is that the child has two mothers, a gestational mother and a genetic mother.[18] Society should acknowledge this biological fact and take it into account in allocating the rights and responsibilities of parenthood. We might decide to treat donors of ova the same way we treat sperm donors, but we cannot treat gestational mothers this way.

My own preference is to legally acknowledge the existence of all three parents (two mothers and one father) in the case of ova donation followed by embryo transfer. If these three individuals could not work out a mutually agreeable living arrangement for themselves and their child, a custody hearing would have to be held. During this hearing, the gestational mother should have temporary custody of the child. Permanent custody should be determined on the basis of the best interests of the child. Because custody does not determine parenthood, however, the noncustodial mother should continue to have her status as gestational or genetic mother legally recognized, and should be granted specific visitation rights as well. As we work out the proper approach, all physicians and clinics must maintain careful records of the identities of donors of both sperm and ova. Public policy must acknowledge the complexity of gamete donation and ultimately take into consideration the best interests of the child.

The California appeals court rejected the position of the Committee on Ethics of the American College of Obstetricians and Gynecologists that gestation determines motherhood, regardless of genetics.[19] The court said that the committee had failed to provide an adequate explanation for its conclusion, adding that "the operation of the Parentage Act does not depend on what a group of doctors, however distinguished and learned in their field, think the law ought to be." On this latter point, the court is correct. But this should not dissuade medical and other professional groups from formulating policy recommendations — provided they are supported with a well-articulated rationale that focuses on the best interests of parents and children and are not self-serving. It will be especially important for physicians to be actively involved as this issue moves from the courts to the state legislatures, which currently have the constitutional authority to enact any laws that are "rational."

We may actually want to see our fate determined by our genes so that we can avoid responsibility for problems of our own invention. But this will not do. Judge Parslow's quotation of Democritus is ironic in view of his genetically determined decision. Shakespeare improved on Democritus in *Julius Caesar*, but the words of Cassius to Brutus began a period Roman "crazy-making" as well:

> Men at some times are masters of their fates.
> The fault, dear Brutus, is not in our stars,
> But in ourselves . . . (I.ii)

7

The Insane Root Takes Reason Prisoner: The Supreme Court and the Right to Die

The United States Supreme Court has dealt with issues at the beginning of life almost every term since 1973. But it was not until 1990 that the Court first faced a so-called "right to die" decision.[1] The Court, however, chose to deal with the case of Nancy Cruzan[2] almost as if it were just another abortion decision—and, like its decision in *Webster* (discussed in Chapter 4) the Court continued to recreate America's legal landscape by transferring traditional rights from its citizens to state legislatures and other government officials. *Webster* may have made the decision in *Cruzan* inevitable. But its inevitability does not make its consequences any more desirable than the devastation caused by a predicated and inevitable tornado or tidal wave. This chapter summarizes the *Cruzan* decision and suggests how to contain its potentially destructive force.

NANCY CRUZAN AT THE TRIAL COURT (ROUND I)[3]

On a clear, cool January night in 1983, Nancy Cruzan, then 25 years old, was driving alone when her car went off a Missouri country road and she was hurled into a ditch. She was found lying face down, not breathing, and apparently dead. Paramedics arrived, commenced CPR, and spontaneous respiration was restored after about ten minutes. She never regained consciousness.

Nancy Cruzan's parents were appointed her guardians in January 1984. There was no real dispute about her medical condition. She was in a persistent vegetative state, oblivious to her environment except for reflexive responses to sound and perhaps painful stimuli. Her cerebral cortical atrophy was irreversible, permanent, progressive, and ongoing. She could not move her body and would never recover her ability to swallow. With gastrostomy feeding she was expected to live for thirty years or more. Her medical bills were the responsibility of the state of Missouri.

Ms. Cruzan's parents eventually asked that the gastrostomy feedings be withdrawn, and in 1988 they sought a court order when the doctors and hospital refused to carry out their request. The trial court's opinion is not a model of clarity. But Judge Charles E. Teel granted their petition, finding, among other things, that:

> Her expressed thoughts at age twenty-five in somewhat serious conversation with a housemate friend that if sick or injured she would not wish to continue her life unless she could live at least halfway normally suggests that given her present condition she would not wish to continue on with her nutrition and hydration.

Judge Teel authorized "the coguardians to exercise [Nancy's] constitutionally guaranteed liberty to request the withholding of nutrition and hydration" and instructed the coguardians to exercise their legal authority consistent with Nancy's "best interests." The state and the guardian ad litem appealed.

THE SUPREME COURT OF MISSOURI[4]

Justice Edward D. Robertson capsulized the court's opinion at the end of the first paragraph: "A single issue is presented: May a guardian order that all nutrition and hydration be withheld from an incompetent ward who is in a persistent vegetative state, who is neither dead . . . nor terminally ill? Because we find that the trial court erroneously declared the law, we reverse."

It is difficult to discern the basis for the court's decision. The court almost immediately noted, for example, that this is a "case of first impression" in Missouri and cited more than fifty cases from sixteen other states that had dealt with similar cases. The court concluded that "nearly unanimously, those courts have found a way to allow persons wishing to die, or those who seek the death of a ward, to meet the end sought." But this erroneously states the question posed by these cases: almost none of the patients involved wished to die, and their guardians did not "seek" their deaths. Rather, the core issue was the right to refuse treatment that was unwanted or intolerably burdensome for the patient. Life was almost always preferred if it could be lived without intrusive and undesirable medical intervention.

The Missouri Supreme Court thus decided *Cruzan*, and rendered the uniformity of prior opinions from other states irrelevant, by inventing a new and artificial question. This made the opinion almost impossible to write. Justice Robertson acted like someone asked to write the fiftieth chapter of a novel who begins by declaring that the first forty-nine chapters are irrelevant to his endeavor. Instead of doing a reasoned analysis of these cases, and explaining why the principles on which they stand are wrong, the court simply asserted that it had found all of them "wanting." Given the dearth of legal authority to support its characterization of prior cases, it bolstered its conclusion by citing only *Macbeth*: "[We] refuse to eat 'on the insane root which [sic] takes the reason prisoner.'"

This quotation can be more aptly used to demonstrate exactly the opposite point the court wanted to make. Banquo speaks the words to Macbeth after the witches, who have accurately foretold their futures, vanish. The entire statement is: "Were such things here as we do speak about? Or have we eaten on the insane root that takes the reason prisoner?" The answer, of course, is that the witches were real; Banquo and Macbeth had not "eaten on the insane root." The Missouri court seems to say, however, that the fifty cases from other states "were not there." This leads to the conclusion that the four-person majority in this 4 to 3 opinion has itself "eaten on the insane root."

Because the court labeled *Cruzan* a "right-to-die" case rather than a "right to refuse treatment" case, it frequently dealt with irrelevant and misleading issues. For example, it focused on death and terminal illness without an apparent appreciation of the implications of either. It used the phrase "Nancy is not dead" almost like a mantra in the opinion. Although the court seems to view this as a major discovery, no one was arguing that the law could or should require guardians to provide artificial feeding to corpses.

The court also repeatedly stated that the *Quinlan* case was irrelevant because Karen Quinlan was "terminally ill" even though the New Jersey Supreme Court *never* used that phrase to describe her and this description is factually incorrect. Karen Quinlan was in almost every way identical to Nancy Cruzan: a young woman in a persistent vegetative state who could live indefinitely with mechanical assistance, but who would never regain consciousness. In fact, the only real difference between Ms. Quinlan and Ms. Cruzan is that while Karen had been maintained on both a mechanical ventilator and artificial feeding, Nancy required only the latter.[5] But as the New Jersey Supreme Court held in two subsequent opinions,[6] this is a legally meaningless distinction.

Although the court was skeptical about using the right of privacy as a basis for medical treatment decisions, and about treating artificial feeding as medical care, it ultimately did not reject either view. Instead it focused almost exclusively on the state's legitimate interest in preserving life, at least when continued care "does not cause pain" and is not particularly "burdensome to the patient" the patient "is not dead" nor "terminally ill" and cannot render a decision because of present incompetence. The court never determined, however, if or how these conclusions would apply to antibiotics, CPR, or other medical interventions Ms. Cruzan might need to survive.

A recurring theme was the state's interest in life, regardless of its quality. If there was a holding to the Missouri Supreme Court decision, it was that the state can *never* take quality of life into consideration in acquiescing to a decision to withdraw treatment from an incompetent individual, as long as the individual's life can be medically sustained without pain. This can be gleaned from statements like: "Were quality of life at issue, persons with all manner of handicaps *might find the state seeking to terminate their lives.* Instead, *the state's interest is in life; that interest is unqualified.*" (emphasis added)

This is the central theme of the case, and seems to be the major reason why "right-to-life" groups applauded it so vigorously. Both they and the court are correct to want to protect handicapped individuals from being denied proper medical care by the state. But the state of Missouri was not trying to deprive Nancy Cruzan of anything. As other courts have noted, we protect the rights and human dignity of handicapped people, not by denying them options but by trying to afford them the same rights we afford competent people. By treating all handicapped persons like treatable children who just need some simple medical intervention to live a normal life, they make the same mistake the New York Court of Appeals made in *Storar.*[7] In Ms. Cruzan's case, the state protects only her interest in avoiding pain, but ignores her interests in autonomy and personal dignity. Therefore the state degrades and dehumanizes her.

Why have almost all other courts permitted patients or their surrogates to refuse treatment under similar circumstances? The reason is that those courts focused on the liberty interests of handicapped citizens, whereas the *Cruzan* court focused instead on laying the groundwork for a possible reversal of *Roe v. Wade*. The Missouri Supreme Court, for example, expended great effort criticizing the entire concept of the right of privacy. To argue for the state's unqualified interest in life, the court relied heavily not only on the state's new Rights of the Terminally Ill Act but also on its new abortion act. As amended in 1986, its statement of purpose reads:

> It is the intention of the . . . state of Missouri to grant the right to life to all humans, born and unborn, and to regulate abortion to the full extent permitted by the Constitution of the United States, decisions of the United States Supreme Court, and federal statutes.

The act defines "unborn child" as "the offspring of human beings from the moment of conception until birth" and viability as "when the life of the unborn child may be continued indefinitely outside the womb by natural or *artificial life-support systems*." (emphasis added)

Cruzan was thus transformed into an abortion opinion. The court seemed to say that it would be difficult to explain why the state could permit parents to withdraw artificial life support from their adult daughter, but not from an extracorporeal embryo. Instead of appreciating the distinctions between these cases, the court concluded simply that if life can be supported "indefinitely . . . by natural or artificial life-support systems" then it *must* be because of Missouri's unlimited interest in "the right to life of all humans." Thus, the court, allegedly protecting Nancy Cruzan, transformed her not just to the status of a child, but to the status of an embryo.

THE U.S. SUPREME COURT OPINION[8]

Chief Justice William Rehnquist wrote the opinion of the United States Supreme Court, which was split 5 to 4. Adopting the Missouri Supreme Court's mistake, he mischaracterized the case as one about the right to die and the right to cause death: "This is the first case in which we have been squarely presented with the issue of whether the United States Constitution grants what is in common parlance referred to as a 'right to die.'" Without deciding the issue, he said, "for the purposes of this case" the Court would "assume that the United States Constitution would grant a competent person a constitutionally protected right to refuse lifesaving hydration and nutrition." Such a right was seen as implicit in previous Court decisions based on the liberty interest delineated in the Fourteenth Amendment, not on the right of privacy. It should be noted, however, that both rights derive from the same source, and their content in this context is unlikely to be different. The core of the case was determining whether the state could restrict the exercise of the right to refuse treatment by surrogate decision-makers acting on behalf of previously competent patients. In the Court's words, the question was "whether the U.S. Constitution forbids a state from requiring clear and convincing evidence of a person's expressed decision while competent to have hydration and nutrition withdrawn in such a way as to cause death." The Court concluded that the Constitution did not prohibit this procedural requirement. Four basic reasons were given.

The first reason was that this heightened evidentiary standard promotes the state's legitimate interest "in the protection and preservation of human life." The second was that "the choice between life and death is a deeply personal decision." The third was that abuses can occur in the case of incompetent patients who do not have "loved ones available to serve as surrogate decisionmakers." And the fourth was that the state may properly "simply assert an unqualified interest in the preservation of human life."

There is no mathematical formula for the "clear and convincing" standard of proof, which is somewhere between the usual civil standard of "preponderance of the evidence" and the criminal standard of "beyond a reasonable doubt." Courts have described it in this context as "proof sufficient to persuade the trier of fact that the patient held a firm and settled commitment to the termination of life support under circumstances like those presented"[9] and evidence is "so clear, weighty and convincing as to enable [the fact finder] to come to a clear conviction, without hesitancy, of the truth of the precise facts in issue."[10] The use of this strict standard of proof was justified by the Court on the basis that it is better to make an error on the side of continuing treatment:

An erroneous decision not to terminate results in a maintenance of the status quo; the possibility of subsequent developments such as advancements in medical science, the discovery of new evidence regarding the patient's intent, changes in the law, or simply the unexpected death of the patient despite the administration of life-sustaining treatment, at least create the potential that a wrong decision will eventually be corrected or its impact mitigated. An erroneous decision to withdraw life-sustaining treatment, however, is not susceptible of correction.

In conclusion, the Court held that Missouri could require clear and convincing evidence of Nancy Cruzan's wishes before permitting surrogates to authorize the termination of treatment. Even though Nancy's mother and father are "loving and caring parents," Missouri may "choose to defer" only to Nancy's wishes, and ignore both her parents' own wishes and their views about what their daughter would want.

Justice Brennan's Dissent

Justice William Brennan wrote a dissent for three of the four dissenting members of the Court. Following traditional constitutional jurisprudence, Justice Brennan argued that if a fundamental right of a citizen is at stake, state action restricting it "cannot be upheld unless it is supported by sufficiently important state interests and is closely tailored to effectuate only those interests." He chided the Court for not being more forceful in defining the nature of the liberty interest competent adults have in refusing treatment. Instead of simply assuming the liberty interest to be free of unwanted medical treatment, he clearly characterized it as a "fundamental right," one that "is deeply rooted in this Nation's traditions." To restrict such a right, the state must allege more than a general interest in life, because "the State has no legitimate general interest in someone's life, completely abstracted from the interest of the person living that life, that could outweigh the person's choice to avoid medical treatment."

Moreover, Justice Brennan asserted that even if the preservation of life is a legitimate state interest in this context, the Missouri restriction is irrational since it would probably lead to more deaths than would current medical practice. This is because medical measures to sustain life, once begun, cannot now be terminated without clear and convincing evidence of th patient's wishes as long as continued treatment prolongs life. Trials of therapy are thus effectively discouraged by the Missouri rule, a result that is irrational.

Justice Brennan argued that the only legitimate interest the state can assert in Nancy Cruzan's case is an interest in accurately determining her wishes. In his view, the Missouri rules were designed not to determine her wishes, but to frustrate them. By permitting only her own statements as probative of her wishes and by using a "clear and convincing" standard to permit them to be determinative, the state effectively deprived her of all other evidence, including the best judgment of those who knew and loved her, as to what decision she would make (substituted judgment) or what decision would be in her best interests. Instead of furthering the citizen's right to decide, the Missouri rules impose "an obstacle to the exercise of a fundamental right."

Justice Brennan also found untenable the notion of erring on the side of life by preserving the status quo. As he noted, the status quo proposition itself begs the question: had artificial respiration and feeding not been undertaken in the first place, the status quo would have been death from the accident. Moreover, the majority improperly implied that continued existence and treatment in a persistent vegetative state is either beneficial or neutral, whereas, in fact:

> An erroneous decision not to terminate life-support robs a patient of the very qualities protected by the right to avoid unwanted medical treatment. . . . [A] degraded existence is perpetuated; his family's suffering is protracted; the memory he leaves behind becomes more and more distorted.

Finally, Justice Brennan argued that the Missouri rules are simply out of touch with reality: people do not write elaborate documents about all the possible ways they might die and the various interventions doctors might have available to prolong their lives. Friends and family members are most likely to know what the patient would want. By ignoring such evidence of a person's wishes, the Missouri procedure "transforms [incompetent] human beings into passive subjects of medical technology."

Justice Brennan Got It Right

I think Justice Brennan got it right. But it hasn't escaped my notice that he was in the minority and that the opinion required Nancy Cruzan to continue to be "treated." It has been argued that the Court found no fundamental constitutional right to refuse treatment. This argument can be made, but it is no more persuasive than the argument that Justice Brennan was writing the majority opinion. This is because on the issue of a fundamental constitutional right to refuse life-sustaining treatment, five Justices (the four dissenters and Justice Sandra Day O'Connor) explicitly acknowledged this right. There is no holding here, but it is wrong to continue to assert that the Court found that there is no fundamental constitutional right to refuse any and all medical treatment.

The argument that the Court did not decide that fluids and nutrition, artificially delivered, are medical treatment like all other medical treatment is also technically correct (its holding did not require this). But six of the nine Justices explicitly found that there was no distinction to be made, and none of the other three found a constitutionally relevant distinction. Moreover, as previously noted, even the Missouri Supreme Court ultimately did not hold that there was a constitutionally relevant distinction. Thus it is highly unlikely that the Justices will reopen the fluids and nutrition issue in the future. There will undoubtedly be more litigation, but the result now seems as inevitable as *Cruzan* seemed to many conservative commentators: attempts by states to restrict the ability of competent adults to reject artificially delivered fluids and nutrition, while other similar forms of medical treatment may be refused, will likely be struck down as a violation of equal protection guaranteed by the U.S. Constitution.[11]

THE TRIAL COURT (ROUND II)

Commenting on the Missouri Supreme Court decision, conservative attorney Thomas Marzen wrote: "So Nancy Cruzan will live — Because Missouri Supreme Court Judge Edward Robertson refused to accept reflexively a line of previous decisions authorizing the lethal withdrawal of foods and fluids from people with severe mental disabilities."[12] That prediction, thankfully, turned out to be wrong. Nancy Cruzan died on December 26, 1990, approximately two weeks after Judge Charles E. Teel ruled again (as he had in 1988) that her parents could order the feeding tubes removed from their daughter's body. There were three major differences in the 1990 hearing. First, three of Nancy's friends testified that Nancy had told them she would never want to live "like a vegetable" on medical machines. Second, her attending physician, James C. Davis, testified that continued treatment was no longer in Nancy's best interests. Third, the state of Missouri withdrew from the case, leaving no one with legal standing to oppose the family's petition or appeal the judge's finding that "clear and convincing evidence" demonstrated that Nancy would not have wanted tube feeding continued.

THE PROBLEM WITH THE ABSOLUTIST
"RIGHT TO LIFE" POSITION

The problem with the "right to life" position is that it is exclusively a slippery-slope argument that ignores the current rights of real people in favor of the speculative harms that may be visited on future people. In the short period of history since *Cruzan*, we can already observe its destructive results rather than speculate about them. We can observe first that the state of Missouri never had Nancy Cruzan's interests at heart, only its own anti-abortion agenda. When it became clear to Missouri Attorney General William Webster, for example, that most people could distinguish an adult in a permanent coma from an embryo or a fetus, he dropped his opposition to the Cruzan family. He announced on national television on the day of the oral arguments before the U.S. Supreme Court that he agreed that Nancy's parents should be able to make the decision about her medical treatment themselves. So when the parents went back to court, the state of Missouri had abandoned its hypocritical "unqualified" interest in Nancy's life.

The same state that had in effect used Nancy Cruzan as a human shield to protect its absolutist and vitalist "right to life" ideology (its "unqualified interest in human life"), has since gone one step further. The state in effect took another patient, Christine Busalacchi, hostage and refused to permit her father to have her transferred to another physician (in another state) for medical evaluation. Worse, the state released a videotape of its hostage to the media,[13] a ploy substantially identical to the one used by Iraq with the first prisoner-of-war pilots it captured. This shameless invasion of privacy by the state of Missouri was embraced by the "right to life" movement, which republished Ms. Busalacchi's photo on the cover of their February 11, 1991, issue of the "National Right to Life News."

Both the state of Missouri and the U.S. Supreme Court's antifamily position virtually mirror the Reagan administration's position in setting forth "Baby Doe" rules and squads: families and doctors are out to kill the handicapped, and only strong state intervention will prevent them from carrying out their agenda. As Thomas Marzen has put it:

> The purpose behind "right to die" litigation and legislation is plain, certain, and obvious. It is to assure that those persons deemed to *lack* some requisite "quality" of life (especially consciousness or "cognitive sapience," but even sometimes the capacity to move, to feel, to see, or to hear) or people who *possess* some "quality" (pain, anguish, "mental suffering," or a diminished life span) should forthwith depart from the company of the living.[14] (emphasis in original)

This is a gross distortion of the "right to die" movement, just as it was a gross distortion of the Baby Doe problem. It *was* horrible for physicians not to treat Baby Doe (a child with Down syndrome), but the Reagan administration's reaction was counterproductive overkill. Instead of concentrating on real problems of prematurity, maternal and infant health care, and nutrition, the administration acted in a police-like fashion, describing physicians as child abusers and parents as accessories before the fact. This politically expedient characterization was a lie: what was really going on in America was overtreatment, not undertreament. Moreover, this lie permitted policymakers to avoid real problems of access to medical care and concentrate publicly on a fictitious problem that would cost no money to address. Thus after more than 100 formal Baby Doe reports and investigations, the federal government was unable to document even one violation of its Baby Doe rules. The Supreme Court ultimately voided the Baby Doe rules themselves. The Child Abuse Amendments of 1984 leave the law exactly where it was before the Baby Doe fiasco began: child abuse and neglect is an issue for the states, and the failure to provide children with "reasonable, appropriate, beneficial, or indicated" medical care can be child neglect.[15]

The Missouri scheme, which *Cruzan* holds is constitutional, goes even further than the Baby Doe regulations. It is an uncompromising Baby Doe-type rule that forbids the discontinuance of medical care which prolongs life from any child or never-competent individual in the state. Moreover, if the state has an interest in sustaining Nancy Cruzan's life regardless of its quality, antibiotics, CPR, kidney dialysis, and even organ transplantation *could* have been ordered over her parents' objections, had any of these interventions been needed to sustain her life. These bizarre results illustrate how radical a departure this antifamily opinion is from the traditional American practice that defers such decisions to the family, and it indicates that the United States Supreme Court believes that no matter what the state of Missouri does to her, Nancy Cruzan herself has no right to respect or dignity and cannot be harmed by any medical intervention that could prolong her life.

As the identical five U.S. Supreme Court Justices decided in *Webster* concerning abortion, so they have decided here: the interests of the state outweigh those of its individual citizens. The sweeping powers the Court cedes to states to control the private lives of their citizens can be illustrated by contrasting the state rationales put forward, and approved by the Court, for keeping Nancy Cruzan alive on the one hand, and for requiring pregnant teenagers to notify their parents about an abortion decision on the other. In both cases the Court ruled that the state could exercise power over individuals based on the state's view of the importance of the family. In *Cruzan*, the Court determined that Missouri could "legitimately and rationally" assume that all families of incompetent patients are a lethal danger to them. In *Ohio v. Akron*,[16] upholding the constitutionality of a statute that required notification of parents prior to a minor obtaining an abortion, *the same Court on the same day* decided that Ohio could "legitimately and rationally" assume that all families are loving and supportive in order to uphold the "dignity of the family." The only value the Court seems interested in fostering is unbridled state power to control the lives of individual citizens.

WHERE DO WE GO FROM HERE?

The vast majority of Americans are appalled by what the state of Missouri put the Cruzan family through.[17] In many states, state supreme courts will continue to find a constitutional right to refuse medical treatment that is not automatically lost when an individual becomes incompetent. (Divergent approaches of the highest courts in New York and New Jersey, taken just prior to *Cruzan*, are discussed in the next chapter.) In other states, legislation will be introduced to broaden the rights of individuals. And, although *Cruzan* did not change the law as it existed prior to the opinion in any state, its grant of authority to states to restrict the role of surrogate decisionmakers will encourage some attempts to restrict such decisionmaking. The problems with living wills are well illustrated by the *Cruzan* case, even though Nancy Cruzan did not have one. Even had she signed a living will, it seems likely that neither the Supreme Court of Missouri nor the U.S. Supreme Court would have honored it unless it had specified that she did not want tube feeding in the event she was in a permanent coma. This type of predictive specificity is both unrealistic and unlikely. The inherent difficulty of prediction led Justice Sandra Day O'Connor to discuss, in her concurring opinion, an issue the Court specifically declined to address: designating a surrogate decisionmaker. Since she agreed that few people will provide explicit instructions, she suggested that everyone appoint a proxy decisionmaker, noting that *Cruzan* "does not preclude a future determination that the Constitution requires the states to implement the decision of a duly appointed surrogate."

Every state now has durable power of attorney laws, and all of these can be used to name a proxy to make health care decisions.[18] If we take autonomy and self-determination seriously, we must take Justice O'Connor seriously as well: such delegations should be constitutionally protected, and the state should not be able to substitute its "official" decisionmaker for the one chosen by the patient. Many states will pass specific health care proxy laws in response to *Cruzan*, as discussed in detail in Chapter 8; New York and Massachusetts have already done so. Other states, like Florida,[19] will act through their courts, guaranteeing the right of individuals to use the health care proxy method to help assure that they will not be victims of the state's technology-imposed vitalism. The growth of the durable power of attorney for health care, and the shrinking use of living wills, is an "inevitable" outgrowth of the *Cruzan* opinion.[20]

Another inevitable and constructive outgrowth is the passage of statutes designed to authorize specific family members to make decisions for their loved ones. Such decisions will not always be precisely those that the patient would have made, but the overwhelming majority of Americans will agree that it is more likely that family members will make decisions consistent with their wishes and best interests than that state officials will make decisions in the interests of the state that are congruent with their personal interests. Not only should such statutes be passed, but the standard for challenging family decisions under such statutes should also be the reverse of the "clear and convincing evidence" standard. The burden should be on the state to prove by clear and convincing evidence that the decision of the authorized family member is not consistent with the wishes of the individual, or (if these are unknown) is not in the individual's best interests, in order to interfere with it.

The Role of Physicians

The U.S. Supreme Court did not consider the professional or personal role of Nancy Cruzan's physicians at all, simply referring to them as "hospital employees" who refused to honor her parents' request without a court order. Because the Court ignored physicians, it never discussed the doctor–patient relationship or whether it matters if the physician had a long-standing relationship with the patient and understood what treatment the patient wanted. This is consistent with the Court's new view that there is nothing Constitutionally special or protected in the doctor–patient relation-ship. Even though the Court ignored physicians, lawyers will not, and physicians across the country have been deluged with conflicting opinions regarding what they should do and what they must do in the wake of *Cruzan*. The reality is that *Cruzan* did not change the law in any state or in any way alter what physicians could or could not do before the opinion.

It remains good medical practice for physicians to discuss future care with patients and to document their wishes. It is also good practice to encourage patients to execute a durable power of attorney for health care, and to encourage them to discuss their wishes with their designated agent and their doctor. These discussions and documents will help, but they will obviously not solve all the real treatment problems for all patients, and, of course, will have no application to children and the never-competent. Medi-cal care will continue to require the compassion, and often the courage, to act in a manner consistent with the patient's wishes, and if these are not known, consistent with the best interests of the patient and good medical practice. Outside Missouri and New York (thankfully) there is no legal obligation to provide incompetent patients with medical care that is either unwanted or not medically indicated.

Conclusion

Michel Foucault insisted that the real political struggles of the 20th century have not been over legal rights but over control of the way individuals live their lives. The modern state, in his view, uses its technological power to homogenize and normalize life, not just through law, but through edu-cation, military training, medicine, public health and housing, and other regulatory mechanisms. Constitutions, far from protecting against such normalization, "were forms that made an essentially normalizing power acceptable."[21] In Foucault's words, since the last century it has been

> life more than the law that became the issue of political struggles, even if the latter [was] formulated through affirmations concerning rights. The "right" to life, to one's body, to health, to happiness, to the satisfaction of needs, and beyond all the oppressions or "alienations," the "right" to rediscover what one is and all that one can be, this "right"—which the classical juridical system was utterly incapable of comprehending—was the political response to all these new procedures of power which did not derive, either, from the traditional right of sovereignty.

Foucault wrote of disciplining the body on the individual level and of regulating populations on the societal level (the "biopolitics of the popula-tion") shortly before *Quinlan*. Although he did not have the *Quinlan* case in mind, he would likely have predicted its outcome. I think he would have been surprised, however, by *Cruzan*—surprised to see the state so publicly and aggressively demand to make all decisions about the medical treatment of an incompetent person with a loving family. He would have been equally surprised to see the state openly seeking to control individual decisions about continuing a pregnancy (as the United States did during the Reagan and Bush presidencies). But he would agree with the *Webster* and *Cruzan* Court that the Constitution offers citizens no real protection from state control.

Our challenge is to resist the state's inherent normalization program by striving to give meaningful content to our stated goals for forming our country: "life, liberty and the pursuit of happiness." We cannot, of course, have liberty or pursue happiness without life. But life without liberty or happiness, in the sense of self-realization and benevolence, translates into mindless vitalism: life reduced to the biology of cell division. The case of Nancy Cruzan provides us with a public warning as to how much control we have already ceded the state over our lives, and how far the state has already gone in redefining the "life" it seeks to "normalize" and control. It is past time to reclaim control for ourselves and our families. In the words of Adam Smith: "All constitutions of government [should be] valued only in proportion as they tend to promote the happiness of those who live under them."[22]

8

In Thunder, Lightning, or in Rain: In the Laboratory of the States

In her concurring opinion in *Cruzan*, discussed in the previous chapter, Justice Sandra Day O'Connor opined that it was appropriate to return the right to refuse treatment issue to the laboratories of the states where further experimentation could go on. This chapter examines decisions of the highest courts in two states that have as much experience in this area as any in the United States: New York and New Jersey.[1] Neither suggests that state supreme courts are likely to be the source of reasonable solutions in this area. It also looks to state legislatures with only a bit more optimism. State judicial and legislative strategies both portray some of the fragmentation of, and destructiveness to, human rights inherent in the U.S. Supreme Court's movement to undercut the U.S. Constitution by expanding the power of states to regulate the lives of their citizens. As such they illustrate the increasing need for a code of medical ethics that is not founded solely on U.S. law.

NEW YORK

Nostradamus allegedly said, "Prediction is difficult, especially about the future." For more than a dozen years a steady stream of appellate courts had forcefully affirmed the right of competent individuals to refuse treatment, and the right of incompetent individuals to have their previously expressed treatment directions followed. I would have predicted New York would join in. Nonetheless, in 1988 the New York Court of Appeals became the first state supreme court to break with the trend, refusing to honor the wishes of an incompetent 77-year-old widow (as expressed when she was competent) to refuse to have a nasogastric tube inserted to deliver nourishment to her body. What can we learn from this aberrational opinion?

The Case of *Mary O'Connor*[2]

Mary O'Connor was, according to the only two physicians to testify about her condition, "severely demented" and "profoundly incapacitated." She had suffered a series of progressively debilitating strokes that rendered her bedridden, paralyzed, and unable to care for herself. She responded to some simple questions and commands, but her neurological damage was irreparable, and there was no hope for any significant improvement in her mental or physical condition.

Her two daughters, both nurses, had cared for their mother since her health began to deteriorate in 1985. She had been hospitalized or in a nursing home since her latest stroke in December 1987. They reported that since this stroke their mother had never spoken or responded to them in any way, even by facial expression or movement, although they visited her daily. The hospital to which she was transferred in June 1988 asked permission of the daughters to place a nasogastric tube for artificial feeding. Her attending physician "guessed" that this might prolong her life for several months to "perhaps a year or two." The daughters refused on the basis that their mother would not want to be treated under these circumstances. The hospital then sought court authorization to insert the nasogastric tube.

The trial court denied the petition on the grounds that there was clear and convincing evidence that O'Connor would not want the tube inserted, and the Appellate Division affirmed. A stay was granted, which permitted O'Connor to be fed intravenously while an appeal to the state's highest court was taken. The Court of Appeals reversed the decision and, in an opinion authored by Chief Justice Sol Wachtler, ordered the nasogastric tube inserted because "On this record there is not clear and convincing proof that the patient had made a firm and settled commitment, while competent, to decline this type of medical assistance under circumstances such as these."

What Mary O'Connor Wanted

Mary O'Connor had been employed in hospital administration until 1983, when she retired. Her husband had died of brain cancer, and the last two of her nine brothers died of cancer. She visited all of them regularly and cared for them at home. She had had several conversations with a hospital co-worker over the years concerning prolongation of life by artificial means. These conversations were prompted by deaths and illnesses in their families. She consistently expressed her view that artificial means should not be used to sustain life. In one conversation she stated she would, if ill, never want to be a burden or "lose her dignity," that "nature should take its course" without using "artificial means," and that it was "monstrous to keep someone alive . . . by using machinery and things like that when they were not going to get better." She also told her daughters, after her husband died, and again when she was hospitalized for heart failure in 1984, that she "would never want any sort of intervention, any sort of life support system." Her daughters had no doubt that their mother would not want her life prolonged by artificial means in her present condition.

My guess is that almost every other appellate court in the United States would find this evidence sufficient to deny the hospital's request to insert the nasogastric tube. Thus this court's opinion is astonishing. How can it be explained?

The "Brother Fox Rule"

One superficial explanation is New York's leading case, which involved Brother Fox. He was an 83-year-old member of the Society of Mary, who suffered a heart attack during otherwise uneventful surgery, sustained substantial brain damage, and wound up in a permanent coma able to breath only with the assistance of a respirator. There was no reasonable possibility he would regain consciousness. His confessor, Father Eichner, testified that he had discussed both the *Quinlan* case and Pope Pius XII's *allocution* with him, and that Brother Fox wanted no "extraordinary means" to sustain him if he were ever in a condition similar to that of Karen Quinlan. Since he did in fact wind up exactly like Karen Quinlan (on a respirator and in a permanent coma), and since his oral declarations were considered "solemn pronouncements and not casual remarks" by the Court of Appeals, the court ruled that they constituted clear and convincing evidence of intent that had to be honored.[3] Can it be that the Brother Fox case only applies to members of religious orders who accurately predict the manner of their deaths and discuss it with a credible religious superior? This almost comical interpretation is one way to read the *O'Connor* opinion. In the words of the majority opinion:

> Although Mrs. O'Connor's statements about her desire to decline life-saving treatments were repeated over a number of years, there is nothing, other than speculation, to persuade the factfinder that her expressions were more than immediate reactions to the unsettling experience of seeing or hearing of another's unnecessarily prolonged death. Her comments . . . are in fact, no different than those that many of us might make after witnessing an agonizing death.

Such comments, the court concluded, "are often made casually" by others. Her daughters, moreover, candidly admitted that, although they were certain their mother would not want the nasogastric tube, she had never specifically discussed either artificial feeding or dying from lack of nutrition with them:

> Her statements with respect to declining artificial means of life support were generally prompted by her experience with persons suffering terminal illnesses, particularly cancer. However, Mrs. O'Connor does not have a terminal illness,

except in the sense that she is aged and infirm. . . . She is simply an elderly person who as a result of several strokes suffers certain disabilities, including an inability to feed herself or eat in a normal manner.

Although an extraordinarily narrow-minded interpretation of the Brother Fox case is supported by the language of the opinion, it is not the key to it. Rather, the Court seems extremely concerned, as the *Conroy*[4] court in New Jersey was before it, with protecting nursing home patients. It sees these patients as especially vulnerable and subject to abuse by those who would deny them treatment, especially fluids and nourishment, for their own selfish purposes.

This perfectly appropriate and laudable goal, however, causes the court to rewrite the facts of the case (an extremely unusual move by an appeals court), to construct an argument that seems to suggest that death is optional, to conclude that individuals who have lost their ability to think can change their minds, and to rule that doctors may treat patients without their consent, even over their previously expressed objections and those of their family.

Life versus Liberty?

The essence of this case is the majority's view of it as a case of life (on artificial support) versus liberty. And this framing of the issue is ironic because, although the court believes that almost everyone in the United States would agree with Mary O'Connor that it is "monstrous" to use life-support machinery to prolong death when recovery is not possible and that almost all of us who witness an agonizing death would not want our own deaths prolonged by artificial means, the court nevertheless concludes that it would be wrong to protect our autonomy in this respect. Two reasons for this counterintuitive conclusion are given: (1) such imprecise statements should not be accepted "because if an error occurs it should be made on the side of life" and (2) even if such precatory statements are clear, "there always exists the possibility that, despite his or her clear expression in the past, the patient has since changed his or her mind."

Neither of these reasons stands scrutiny. First, if the court is correct that "few nursing home patients" have not made similar expressions to that of Mary O'Connor, the solution is not to ignore them all, but to accept them all. It is because technology is indiscriminately used that most elderly citizens have had to witness friends and relatives have their lives painfully and pointlessly prolonged, and have therefore expressed their own desire not to have their own lives so prolonged. The answer is not to try to make it procedurally harder for all of us to refuse unwanted treatment, but to make it easier. To say we want to "err on the side of life" is a meaningless slogan when the price of that err is the individual's involuntary suffering and indignity. My guess is that most Americans would rather have the court system err (if at all) on the side of liberty and personal autonomy. When all the close relatives agree on what the patient would want, and there is no conflict of interest, those wishes should be honored. Only when real disputes about wishes exist should court resolution be needed.

Likewise, the notion that patients who are permanently incompetent and incapable of thought can nonetheless change their minds is a fiction worthy of only the most fantasy-affected lawyers. People who have lost the ability to think have no minds to change. For these individuals, as for the dead and the permanently comatose, the idea that they might change their minds if they could is meaningless. The fact is that they can't. If this notion of mindless mind change were taken seriously, for example, probate courts could not simply follow wills, but would have to try to determine if their authors would have changed their minds if they had known how the heirs would behave. The same, of course, would apply to living wills no matter how specific they are drafted. The court's scheme is also blatantly biased: clear and convincing evidence is required to refuse treatment, but any "possibility" that the person without a mind may have changed it is sufficient to justify treatment.

These two fictions are rationalizations that permit physicians and judges to impose their own wills on incompetent patients and their families, requiring them to mimic choices the physicians and judges would make. The rule announced by this case is that unless the now incompetent person precisely predicted how she would die and what medical interventions might be employed to prolong her dying process, and clearly and "solemnly" rejected these interventions, the patient and her family lose all authority regarding treatment decisions, and the attending physician can treat her without obtaining consent, informed or otherwise. This result destroys personal autonomy for previously competent patients, denying them their rights. This is the opinion's most grotesque feature: it simply refuses to acknowledge that all incompetent individuals have constitutional rights. Mary O'Connor's body is treated like that of a mollusk which, it seems to be assumed, can neither be harmed nor degraded by unconsented-to invasive medical interventions. Further, by rejecting the substituted judgment approach (based on other than specific predictions), and the best interests approach, this opinion threatens their welfare by subjecting them to involuntary medical interventions that may be cruel, painful, pointless, and degrading.

The Dissent

Judge Richard Simons' dissenting argument was simple and persuasive. If Mary O'Connor cannot refuse nasogastric tube feeding by her statements, it is unlikely that anyone (other than a religious person like Brother Fox) will ever be able to refuse treatment in New York after they become incompetent, "with the result that the right of self-determination is reduced to a hollow promise." Simons instead argued for a broadening of the *Eichner* and *Storar* rule that would permit decisions based on substituted judgment and on best interests. This would put New York in conformity with almost every other court that has ruled on similar cases.[5]

Judge Simons correctly noted that the majority had effectively rewritten the facts to make it appear that Mary O'Connor's condition was much better than it really was, and that it could even be improved. Simons noted that although her pneumonia and urinary infection had been treated, there was no significant change in her underlying condition:

> While she may not be terminally ill in the sense that death is imminent, she is dying because she has suffered severe injuries to her brain and body which, if nature takes it course, will result in death. Full medical intervention will not cure or improve her, it will only maintain her in a rudimentary state of existence.

The majority also, and more significantly, reversed a factual determination by both lower courts that Mary O'Connor demonstrated her desire to reject nasogastric feeding under these circumstances by clear and convincing evidence and "trivialized" her statements by suggesting "possible" reasons to discount them.

Finally, Judge Simons argued that the majority's strict rule is "unworkable because it requires humans to exercise foresight they do not possess." The majority did this by requiring people to do better than reject "all" artificial or mechanical means of support: they must anticipate and specifically state those they wish not to use, and categorize them in ways that are "qualitatively" the same as the intervention sought by the hospital or physicians. In addition, the disease or injury with which one is afflicted must also be predicted with some qualitative certainty: incapacitation by stroke, for example, will not qualify for statements made in the presence of relatives dying of cancer or suffering from heart attacks:

> Mary O'Connor expressed her wishes in the only terms familiar to her, and she expressed them as clearly as a lay person should be asked to express them. To require more is unrealistic, and for all practical purposes, it precludes the right of patients to forego life sustaining treatment.

Judge Simons concluded, correctly I think, that the majority had simply rejected Mary O'Connor's expressed wishes and, instead,

> made its own substituted judgment by improperly finding facts and drawing inferences contrary to the facts found by the courts below. Judges, the persons least qualified by training, experience or affinity to reject the patient's instructions, have overridden Ms. O'Connor's wishes, negated her long held values on life and death, and imposed on her and her family their ideas of what her best interests require.

NEW JERSEY

Kathleen Farrell was 37 years old, competent, and suffering from amyotrophic lateral sclerosis (ALS) when her case came to court. After all effective treatments were exhausted, and she had been discharged home, she asked that the mechanical ventilator that sustained her breathing be disconnected. Her physician refused, and her husband was forced to seek a court authorization to order treatment ceased. The lower court granted the request but stayed its order until it could be reviewed by a higher court. Farrell died, still connected to the ventilator, before the appeal could be heard.

Hilda Peter was a 65-year-old nursing home patient in a persistent vegetative state whose life was being sustained by a nasogastric feeding tube when her case first came to court in 1985. She had executed a durable power of attorney granting her close friend authority to make all medical decisions for her. A court also appointed this friend Peter's legal guardian, but required him to obtain the acquiescence of the Ombudsman for the Institutionalized Elderly before making any decision to terminate treatment. The Ombudsman agreed that Peter would not have wanted to be maintained in a persistent vegetative state, but refused permission to withdraw treatment because he believed Hilda Peter did not meet the profile of a "Claire Conroy type case" since, although she was an elderly nursing home patient, she was not expected to die within a year. The guardian appealed this decision.

Early in 1980 Nancy Jobes was in an auto accident. She sustained severe loss of blood flow to her brain during otherwise routine surgery and had been in a persistent vegetative state in a nursing home ever since, her life sustained by a surgically implanted feeding tube. She was 30 years old when, in 1986, her husband requested that the tube feedings be ceased. The nursing home refused, and he brought suit. A lower court agreed that use of the tube could be ended.

What links these three tragic cases is that they were all heard and decided together by the New Jersey Supreme Court. All three opinions were written by Justice Marie Garibaldi, and all but *Jobes* (which was 6 to 1) were unanimous.[6] The court decided that treatment could be terminated in all of these cases; in *Farrell* and *Peter* because this is what the patient clearly wanted, and in *Jobes* because this was the family's best judgment of what the patient wanted. As it had done before in *Quinlan* (discussed in Chapter 7) and *Conroy*, the court forcefully articulated the rights of patients to refuse any intervention:

> *All patients*, competent or incompetent, with some limited cognitive ability or in a persistent vegetative state, terminally ill or not terminally ill, *are entitled to choose whether or not they want life-sustaining medical treatment*. . . . Medical choices are private. . . . They are not to be decided by societal standards of reasonableness or normalcy. Rather *it is the patient's preferences—formed by his or her unique personal experiences—that should control*. The privacy that we accord medical decisions does not vary with the patient's condition or prognosis. (emphasis added)

Moreover, "A competent person's interest in his self-determination generally outweighs any countervailing interest the state might have."

These are powerful substantive rulings, and they give patients, physicians, families, and guardians a clear message: patients have a right to refuse any treatment, regardless of prognosis, age, place of residence, or any other arbitrary characteristic. Efforts should be focused not on categorizing individuals or granting their physicians immunity, but on determining and following patient wishes. In this regard, the court makes some very helpful procedural suggestions.

Helpful Suggestions

Two questions that have plagued patients, physicians, and courts are, how can competent patients make their wishes known regarding treatment when they are no longer competent to participate in decisionmaking, and, what legal authority does the family have to make treatment and nontreatment decisions? As to the first, the court explicitly states that "the best evidence is a 'living will,' a written statement that specifically explains the patient's preferences about life-sustaining treatment." This has been said before. However the court went further, holding that New Jersey's statutes, although not specifically designed to permit the individual designated by a durable power of attorney to make medical decisions, "should be interpreted that way." Thus an individual in New Jersey (without any additional legislation) can legally delegate medical decisionmaking to another person. This delegation is most effective when it is accompanied by explicit instructions concerning the types of treatment the person wants and the types refused. The court virtually pleads with the citizens of New Jersey to use living wills and durable powers of attorney to attempt to avoid placing the decisionmaking burden on others, including the courts:

> Ideally, each person should set forth his or her intentions with respect to life-supporting treatment. This insures that the patient's own resolution of this extraordinarily personal issue will be honored. Failure to express one's intentions imposes an awesome and painful responsibility on the surrogate decisionmaker.

In the absence of a living will or other "clear and convincing evidence" of the patient's wishes, the family's role becomes central. The court believes "family members are best qualified to make substituted judgments for incompetent patients. This is not only because of their peculiar grasp of the patient's approach to life, but also because human experience informs us that family members are generally most concerned with the welfare of the patient." The court prefers "close" family members, like a "spouse, parents, adult children, or siblings." However, physicians can rely on the judgment of another relative ("a cousin, aunt, uncle, niece, nephew") if the "attending health care professionals determine [that this person] functions in the role of the patient's nuclear family." Thus, although the court found no clear and convincing evidence of Nancy Jobes' wishes, it concluded that her family was "the best qualified" to make the substituted judgment decision.

If the physician suspects that the family member is not acting in the patient's best interests, a guardian petition should be filed. A close friend can only be substituted for the family member if that close friend was designated by the patient himself or herself as the surrogate decisionmaker. Eliminating any guardianship requirement when there is involved family acting in the patient's interests eliminates the court's role in choosing the decisionmaker. This is the court's goal. Having set forth the legal rules for making a decision, and having identified the proper decisionmaker, a good argument can be made that the court's job is concluded. Why isn't this the end of these opinions?

Categorizing Patients

Although recognizing that it is not helpful to patients to arbitrarily limit their rights to refuse treatment based on factors like prognosis, age, and place of residence, the court nonetheless seems to have done so, albeit with patient protection in mind. The entire legal analysis in *Quinlan* is founded on the rights any competent patient would have. Nonetheless, the court now seems to categorize that case as one involving a young person in a persistent vegetative state who is in a hospital. A "Claire Conroy–type case," on the other hand, involves an individual over the age of 60, in a nursing home, and likely to die within one year. Thus there was a "trick" to deciding what to do in the Hilda Peter case. The Ombudsman refused to authorize the withdrawal of treatment because Peter did not meet the "Claire Conroy criteria," in that she was not likely to die within a year. The court, however, held that Peter was actually a *Quinlan*-type case, since Peter was in a persistent vegetative state and her medical condition was more relevant than her time of likely survival. Since she was also over the age of 60 and in a nursing home, she also fell under the jurisdiction of the Ombudsman for the Institutionalized Elderly.

The question the court had to struggle with is how much difference, if any, medical condition, age, and place of residence should make in medical decisionmaking. In *Conroy* the court had held that being over 60 years of age and institutionalized in a nursing home was sufficient justification for involving the ombudsman in a decision to terminate treatment.

The court now says as well that the persistent vegetative state diagnosis is important for everyone, regardless of age, because patients in persistent vegetative states are beyond having any interests in that they "do not experience any . . . benefits or burdens." But focusing on medical condition seems just as arbitrary as making age or place of residence determinative. Indeed, by placing individuals in persistent vegetative states in a separate category, these people become less human than people suffering from other conditions; the operative word is "vegetative," vegetable in the vernacular.

The family of such patients seems to be permitted to treat them almost as if they were plants: to be fed and watered (or not) at the behest of the family. Families and physicians should be *required* to honor the previously expressed wishes of patients in persistent vegetative states to terminate treatment.

Developing elaborate categories based on age, place of residence, and medical condition, and permutations of these factors, is both intellectually unsatisfying and conceptually flawed. Why then does the court use these factors?

What Three Doctors Can Do

By categorizing patients, the court is following its *Quinlan* precedent of focusing on physician behavior. In *Quinlan* the court asserted that physicians refused to remove Karen Quinlan's mechanical ventilator, not because they thought removal was wrong, but out of fear of being sued. The court defined its problem as devising "a way to free physicians, in the pursuit of their healing vocation, from possible contamination by self-interest or self-protection concerns which would inhibit their independent medical judgments for the well-being of their dying patients."[7] The *Quinlan* court's solution to frightened and timid physicians, who would rather inflict unwanted medical interventions on their patients than take the virtually nonexistent risk of being sued, was to adopt an immunity model that did not require judicial involvement. Specifically, the court ruled that if the physician's diagnosis of a persistent vegetative state was confirmed by an "ethics committee" (now properly labeled a "prognosis committee" and consisting entirely of medical consultants), then discontinuation of treatment could occur and all involved would be immune from lawsuits. The *Quinlan* court suggested that "the most appealing factor" in this review mechanism was "the diffusion of professional responsibility for decision."

More than a decade has passed since *Quinlan*, and the problem is no longer getting timid physicians to do what they think is right. In these cases the New Jersey Supreme Court sees the problem as preventing dangerous physicians from doing what the court views as wrong. The solution proposed by the court for controlling rogue physicians is fundamentally the same, except that its purpose is now to provide a public check on otherwise secret acts. Since neither nursing homes nor private homes have "prognosis committees," the same thing (the court seems to think) can be accomplished by requiring the involvement of two outside physicians.

In the two persistent vegetative state cases (*Jobes* and *Peter*), this calls for the surrogate decisionmaker to "secure statements from at least two independent physicians knowledgeable in neurology that the patient is in a persistent vegetative state and that there is no reasonable possibility that the patient will ever recover to a cognitive, sapient state." The attending physician, if there is one, must also so certify. The purpose of these medical consultations is to "substitute for the concurrence of the prognosis committee for patients who are not in a hospital setting and thereby prevent inappropriate withdrawal of treatment."

For the competent patient at home, the "three physician rule" works like this: "To protect the patient who is at home, we require that two nonattending physicians examine the patient to confirm that he or she is competent and is fully informed about his or her prognosis, the medical alternatives available, the risks involved, and the likely outcome if medical treatment is discontinued." In a footnote, the court extends this procedure for determining competence to hospital and nursing home patients as well. As in *Quinlan*, physicians who follow these procedures "in good faith" (which includes the "obligation to act in accordance with generally accepted medical practices") are immune from any civil or criminal liability.

This "three physician rule" seems totally arbitrary and misguided, since doctors can make *every* other medical decision with their patients or appropriate surrogates without required consultation. On the other hand, three is a magical and mystical number that can evoke comfort and signal power. Shakespeare, for one, used the number to devastating effect in *Macbeth*, and one can almost see the three doctors at the patient's bedside echoing the words of the first witch: "When shall we three meet again? In thunder, lightning, or in rain?" The judges don't seem to care, as long as their meeting doesn't take place in the courtroom.

Where We Are

The law in New Jersey regarding physicians in termination of treatment cases is now almost precisely what it was prior to *Quinlan*: follow accepted medical practice, with your patient's consent, and you will incur no criminal or civil liability. The only novel part is that there are now procedures that can be used to obtain prior immunity. On the surface it might appear that there is a procedural difference in that medical consultations are now *required* (while before they were optional) in cases involving refusals of life-sustaining medical treatment. But this overstates the cases, since although the court uses words like "we require" the additional two medical consultants, it seems more legally correct to read the cases as saying "we recommend" their use. This is because there is no specific crime of not getting two medical consultants; instead, what the court has said essentially parallels what it said in *Quinlan*: if you want prospective legal immunity for honoring treatment refusals that might result in death, don't come to court; instead, follow the "three doctor rule." If you don't follow it, and in the unlikely event that you are sued or prosecuted, you will be judged by traditional methods. Specifically, did you follow accepted medical practices with your patient's informed consent? Of course, even to claim immunity, one must prove in court that one acted in "good faith"—that is, followed good and acceptable medical practice with informed consent. Thus the immunity provisions themselves are illusory.

Moreover, interpreting these cases as *requiring* two independent medical consultants prior to honoring the patient's informed decision would be unconstitutional. In *Doe v. Bolton*,[8] the companion case to *Roe v. Wade*, the U.S. Supreme Court examined a Georgia statute that required a licensed physician to obtain the written concurrence "of two other physicians duly licensed" that the abortion is "necessary." The U.S. Supreme Court found this three doctor rule unconstitutional as an unwarranted interference with the doctor–patient relationship. The Court concluded that the clinical judgment of the attending physician alone was sufficient and that the decision of whether to call in other medical consultants was itself a medical decision that the attending physician should make:

> If a physician is licensed by the State, he is recognized by the State as capable of exercising acceptable clinical judgment. If he fails in this, professional censure or deprivation of his license are available remedies. Required acquiescence by co-practitioners has no rational connection with a patient's needs and unduly infringes on the physician's right to practice. The attending physician will know when a consultation is advisable.

This language is, of course, directly applicable to these treatment refusal cases, which are based on the exercise of one's constitutional right of privacy. The U.S. Supreme Court is certainly correct to stress physician responsibility and accountability rather than "diffusion of responsibility." The best protection a patient is likely to have is a physician responsible for his actions. And just as it is unconstitutional to allow police to search the bedroom for telltale signs of contraceptive use, it should be unconstitutional for the state, even in the form of two "independent physicians" to invade an individual's home to examine his competence without either his consent or probable cause that a crime is being committed. The New Jersey Supreme Court seems to have come up with procedural "rules" that are likely to make it more difficult for patients to exercise their substantive rights.

The most constructive thing courts could do is to more directly and clearly state that physicians' legal authority to treat or not treat derives from the constitutional and common law rights of their patients, and that acts and omissions in the doctor–patient relationship that honor these rights are always legally sanctioned. Because even experienced and well-intentioned courts like those in New York and New Jersey have had such a difficult time articulating the rights of patients, it is perhaps inevitable that both Congress and the legislatures of the individual states have begun to move to support the autonomy rights of their citizens in the doctor–patient relationship.

Pushed to act by the public's reaction to *Cruzan*, Congress and the President decreed, with the Patient Self-Determination Act, that all hospitals, nursing homes, and HMOs that serve Medicare or Medicaid patients must provide all their new adult patients with written information describing the patient's rights under state law to make decisions about medical care, including their right to execute a living will or durable power of attorney.[9] New forms have been added to the practice of medicine. Their purpose is to help implement a right that has been universally recognized: the right to refuse any and all medical interventions, even life-sustaining interventions. The challenge is to use these forms to foster substantive doctor–patient communication and respect for patient autonomy.

THE LIVING WILL[10]

The term living will was coined by Luis Kutner in 1969 to describe a document in which a competent adult sets forth directions regarding medical treatment in the event of future incapacity.[11] The document is a will in the sense that it sets forth the individual's directions. It is "living" because it takes effect prior to death. Public interest in this document has always been high, and a national organization, Concern for Dying, has devoted most of its resources for the past twenty years to educating the public and professionals about the living will. A sister organization, Society for the Right to Die (which merged with Concern for Dying in 1991 to form Choice in Dying), had devoted itself to encouraging states to pass legislation to give formal legal recognition to the living will.

Karen Quinlan's story prompted enactment of the nation's first living will statute, California's 1976 Natural Death Act. The California statute is very narrow. A legally enforceable declaration can only be executed fourteen days or more *after* an individual is diagnosed as having a terminal illness, which is defined as one which would cause the patient's death "imminently," whether or not life-sustaining procedures are continued. Thus, even though this statute was inspired by her story, it would not have helped Quinlan because she was not terminally ill.

By 1993, more than forty states had enacted living will statutes. All of them provide immunity to physicians and other health care professionals who follow them. Most of them also suffer from four major shortcomings:

1. They are restricted to the "terminally ill."
2. They limit the types of treatment that can be refused (usually to "artificial" or "extraordinary") and sometimes exclude fluids and nutrition.
3. They do not make provisions for the person to designate another person to make decisions on their behalf, nor do they set forth the criteria on which such decisions should be made.
4. They do not require health care providers to honor the patient's wishes.[12]

These problems led to a call for "second generation" living will legislation.[13] But other shortcomings were also noted: living wills require an individual to accurately predict their final illness or injury, as well as what medical interventions might be available to postpone their death, and living wills require physicians to make decisions based on an interpretation of a document rather than on a discussion of the treatment options with a person acting on behalf of the patient. The proposed solution to these problems was not to modify the living will, but to replace it with another form: the durable power of attorney, also known, in this context, as the health care proxy. The person named in the document is variously known as the attorney, the agent, the surrogate, or the proxy, four terms that are synonyms in this context.

Every state has a durable power of attorney law that permits individuals to designate another person to make decisions for them after they lose decisionmaking capacity.[14] Although these statutes were enacted primarily to permit the agent to make financial decisions, no court has ever invalidated a durable power of attorney specifically designated for health care decisions. Moreover, as discussed in Chapter 7, Justice Sandra Day O'Connor has advised individuals to use this device. She also observed that *Cruzan* "does not preclude a future determination that the Constitution requires the States to implement the decisions of a duly appointed surrogate." The *Cruzan* case itself (which involved facts essentially identical to *Quinlan*) energized the health care proxy, just as the *Quinlan* case had previously energized the living will.

Physicians are legally and ethically bound to respect the directions of a patient set forth in a living will. But living wills are limited because no one can accurately foretell the future, and interpretation may be difficult.[15] Attempts to make the living will less ambiguous by developing comprehensive checklists with alternative scenarios may be too confusing and abstract to be useful to either patients or health care providers, although opinions on this differ.[16]

THE HEALTH CARE PROXY

Although *not* legally required in any state (because of existing durable power of attorney laws), the current trend in the United States is for each state to enact a proxy law that specifically deals with health care. Such health care proxy laws generally specify the information that must be included in the proxy form, outline the standards by which treatment decisions must be made, and grant good faith immunity for all involved in carrying out the treatment decision. A health care proxy law also has the advantage of trying to return some rights-based uniformity to American health law, and all such laws should recognize health care proxy documents properly executed in other jurisdictions. Two of the best-written proxy laws became effective at the beginning of the decade: in New York in January 1991 and in Massachusetts in December 1990. The New York law is based on a recommendation of the New York State Task Force on Life and the Law, and that group's booklet describing its rationale is still the best introduction to the health care proxy concept.[17] The Massachusetts health care proxy law[18] is largely modeled on the New York law.

The heart of both laws (and of all proxy laws) is the same: enabling a competent adult (the "principal") to choose another person (the "agent") to make treatment decisions for him after he becomes incompetent to make them himself. The agent has the same decisionmaking authority the patient would have if competent. Instead of a document to decipher, the physician is able to discuss treatment options with a person who has the legal authority to grant or withhold consent on behalf of the patient. The manner in which the agent must exercise this authority is also crucial. The agent must make decisions consistent with the wishes of the patient, if known, or, if they are not known, consistent with the patient's best interests.

Proxy laws also permit the principal to limit the authority of the agent in the document (for example, no authority to refuse CPR or tube feeding), but the more limitations the principal puts on the agent, the more the health care proxy resembles a living will. In addition, because every limitation is subject to interpretation, the likelihood of a dispute about the meaning of the document is increased. One compromise that makes sense to me is to give blanket decisionmaking authority to the agent, and to give the agent a private letter detailing one's values and wishes with as much precision as possible. The agent could use this letter when relevant to the actual decision and keep it private when it was not relevant or helpful.

Implementing the Health Care Proxy

The goal of the new forms is to simplify decisionmaking by making it more likely that the patient's wishes will be followed, not to complicate existing problems. If hospitals and hospital lawyers cooperate, this goal will be attained because the vast majority of physicians will welcome the ability to discuss treatment options with a person chosen by the patient who has the legal authority to provide or withhold consent. Hospitals can help their patients by making a simple form available, by educating their medical, nursing, and social service staff about the health care proxy, and by supporting decisions based on it. Hospitals, on the other hand, can be obstacles to good decisionmaking by concentrating on the paperwork rather than on the substance of decisionmaking. After Massachusetts enacted its health care proxy law, for example, some attorneys drafted a thirteen-page, single-spaced, proxy form that is all but unintelligible to nonlawyers. Others began exploring and cataloging all the reasons why physicians and hospitals might want to seek judicial review before honoring a health care proxy. Neither of these strategies is constructive. The use of complex forms and obstructive strategies makes it likely that treatment decisions will be made by the hospital lawyer and the agent's lawyers, not by the agent and the physician. This will make the document frustratingly counterproductive by adding another layer of bureaucracy and another outsider to the decisionmaking process, instead of focusing the decision on the patient and the patient's wishes, where it belongs.

The most useful form for both patients and providers is a simple one-page document that sets forth all necessary information in easily comprehensible language. Such a form, which is easily understood and meets all the legal requirements of the new Massachusetts proxy law (as well as those of the New York law) was developed by a broad-based task force made up of representatives from all of the major health care organizations in the state, including the Medical Society, Hospital Association, Nurses Association, Federation of Nursing Homes, and Department of Public Health, as well as the Executive Office of Elder Affairs and the Bar Association. This model form, which also includes attached instructions and optional spaces for the signature of the agent and alternative agent (naming an alternate agent is not required) was distributed across the state.[19] Cooperation in its development was virtually unprecedented, and it may provide a model for future cooperation and coordination. A similar strategy was used in California.

Adding to the Proxy

Perhaps concerned with tidiness, some commentators have advocated combining an organ donor form with the health care proxy. This is a serious mistake for at least two reasons. First, much effort has been expended over the past twenty years to untangle organ donation and treatment decisions, since the leading reason why individuals don't sign organ donor cards is because they believe doctors might "do something to me before I'm really dead."[20] Tying organ donation to treatment refusals that might lead to death only heightens this concern and is likely to lead individuals to use neither form. Second, the proxy form takes effect upon the patient's incompetence; the organ donor form takes effect only upon death. The health care agent will have nothing to say about organ donation, because the agent can only make treatment decisions, and the agent's authority dies with the principal. Organ donation is laudable, but it has nothing to do with the health care proxy, and organ donation should be done by the principal on a separate form designed for that purpose. The principal may designate the agent to also implement his or her wishes regarding organ donation—but these two issues should be kept separate to avoid counterproductive confusion. Organ donor forms may teach another lesson as well. U.S. physicians will not honor an organ donor form over the objections of the patient's family. Likewise, physicians have difficulty honoring a patient's living will over the family's objections. By giving the physician a person with legal authority to talk with, the health care proxy is likely to be a more effective mechanism to implement patient wishes.

It should be stressed that health care proxy laws do not substantively change existing law: they merely make it procedurally easier for a person to designate an agent to make whatever health care decisions the person could legally make if competent, and they give health care providers legal immunity for honoring such decisions. The patient can, for example, give the agent the authority to refuse any and all medical care, but the agent has no more legal authority than the principal to insist on assisted suicide or to demand a lethal injection. The proxy also solves the problem of a dispute among family members concerning treatment, since the agent has the legal and ethical right and responsibility to make the decision. When the long "lost" relative arrives and demands that "everything be done or I'll sue," the physician can refer that person to the agent, rather than try to get all the relatives to agree on what the patient would want.

Limits of the Proxy

Medical ethics remains more important than medical law here for many reasons. The health care proxy only applies to competent adults who actually execute the document. Since fewer than 10 percent of Americans have either living wills or organ donor cards, few may use this mechanism. They certainly will not unless physicians encourage their use. It has no application to children, the mentally retarded, and others unable to appreciate the nature and consequences of their decisions. Treatment decisions for these populations will continue to be governed by the vague "best interest" standard, which is the functional equivalent of "reasonable medical care," "appropriate medical care," and "indicated medical care." The document will also be of limited use in the emergency department, although there may be rare cases when the health care agent arrives with the principal and there is time for consultation and informed consent before a specific intervention is tried. Nor will the document solve problems of futility. Physicians retain the right and responsibility not to offer treatment they believe is contraindicated, useless, or futile. Finally, some people will not have a person they trust sufficiently to designate them as their health care agent. For them the living will remains the primary vehicle available to document their wishes in advance of incompetency.

Physicians and lawyers should make health care proxy forms available to the public and their clients free of charge as a public service and then encourage them to complete them. Forms must be written in language that both patients and health care providers can easily understand: the form does not require a lawyer to write and should not require a lawyer to interpret.

Like soldiers in past wars, American soldiers who went to the Persian Gulf wrote their wills. Unlike past wars, however, many also wrote living wills or executed durable powers of attorney. It was not just a formality. In the words of one observer: "In the process, the soldiers had to clarify ambiguous personal relationships, chart out their children's lives, and, in some cases, confront their own mortality for the first time."[21] The health care proxy gives us all the opportunity to confront our mortality and to determine who among our friends and relatives we want to make treatment decisions on our behalf when we are unable to make them ourselves. A clear focus on these substantive issues, rather than on forms or formalities, can help individuals feel more secure that their wishes will be respected regarding medical treatment. It can also help health care professionals feel more secure that the treatment decisions made for incompetent patients actually reflect their patient's wishes. These are worthy goals.

II

PRIVATE SECTOR BIOETHICS

9

Not Saints, but Healers:
Legal Duties of Physicians
in the AIDS Epidemic

Albert Camus closes his narrative of *The Plague* by observing of those who "fought against its terror and relentless onslaughts" that, although they were "unable to be saints," they refused "to bow down to pestilences, [and strove] their utmost to be healers." Neither law nor ethics expects sainthood or martyrdom of physicians. Nor can the law force people to be courageous or virtuous. But the law does set a minimum standard of conduct below which physicians cannot fall without risking lawsuits, loss of license, or loss of employment. This chapter explores the legal framework within which physicians must work as healers in the AIDS epidemic, and suggests ways in which the law can reinforce an ethic of professionalism in the face of this modern plague.[1]

VALUES IN HEALTH CARE

It has been persuasively suggested that the only shared ends that any longer matter in our society are "the desire to be affluent [and] avoiding the risk of cancer."[2] This suggestion was made to explain society's reaction to new technology that promises a better life. And it parallels Camus' description of the population of Oran almost a half century ago: "Our citizens work hard, but solely with the object of getting rich." In view of the failure of our science and technology to effectively address the AIDS epidemic, we can reformulate our "shared goals" as accumulating wealth and avoiding cancer *and* AIDS. In the medical profession, some physicians have openly espoused this view. It has been asserted, for example, that "the

119

contractual model" is the proper one for medicine, and that there is (and should be) no professional obligation for physicians to treat patients with AIDS.[3]

Outright refusals to treat AIDS patients or those infected with HIV remain rare and have generally been condemned.[4] But as the number of AIDS patients relentlessly increases, such refusals will become much more commonplace if they are countenanced by the public health, nursing, or medical communities. Many surgeons suggest that their patients should be screened for HIV on a routine basis, so that surgeons can take added precautions during surgery. Former Surgeon General C. Everett Koop, for example, proposed voluntarily screening surgical patients; and said those who refuse should be given a blank medical record regarding their HIV status and treated by the surgeon as if they are infected.[5] Syndicated columnist Ellen Goodman agreed, arguing that "If we are going to trust the health-care profession to treat the sick, part of that trust is to give them privileged information, the tools of their job."[6] She, and others, argue that the proper risk/benefit analysis to apply to procedures is no longer one that focuses exclusively on the patient's welfare, but, rather, "We need to assess more fully the benefit to the patient against the risk to health care workers."

This is a strange and novel type of risk/benefit analysis, focusing as it does on the risk to the physician of treatment, rather than the risk to the patient. And although proposals to screen surgeons for HIV infection are based on protecting patients from surgeons, the risk of transmission is so low that fear and prejudice rather than reasonable risk assessment seems to be the primary motivation for such proposals.[7] But it is one thing to label routine screening of surgeons and patients as useless and unprofessional; it is another thing to effectively influence conduct. The law is often seen as exacerbating the problems of health professionals, but it can be used constructively to reinforce a caring ethic that can help insure that HIV-infected individuals and those with AIDS will get the care and treatment they need and deserve. Indeed, by helping to prevent the most blatant types of discrimination, lawyers may be as helpful to patients in the AIDS epidemic as physicians.

The law's influence can be seen most relevantly by examining common law principles relating to emergency treatment and the obligations inherent in a provider–patient relationship, statutes dealing with discrimination, and contractual agreements related to treatment obligations. In addition, professional associations, state licensing boards, hospitals, and medical schools can articulate standards of professional conduct that have legal implications for practitioners. In discussing each area, a critical distinction between treating AIDS and treating a person who is infected with HIV should not be lost: the first involves knowledge and skill in treating a specific disease; the second involves knowing what precautions to take to avoid infection while treating a different condition.

COMMON LAW OBLIGATIONS TO TREAT

American common law supports the traditional proposition that, absent some special relationship, no citizen owes any other citizen anything. Even though a communitarian view based on obligations to those in need makes more modern sense, our law continues to reflect 19th century frontier values in this regard. As applied to health care and medicine, the general rule, sometimes denoted the "no duty rule," is that a health professional is not obligated to treat any particular patient in the absence of a consensual professional–patient relationship.[8] Put another way, in the absence of some prior agreement or specific legal requirement, physicians are free to accept or reject the requests of individual sick people who come to them for treatment.

Emergency Treatment

On the other hand, physicians, nurses, and allied health professionals working in emergency departments must treat *all* patients who arrive suffering from a medical emergency. Virtually every modern court has repudiated the ancient doctrine that an emergency room physician need accept for treatment only those patients the physician or hospital chooses. The relevant issue is not whether the person can pay, what color the person's skin is, or even if the person has reached the age of consent; the only legally relevant issue is whether the person is experiencing a medical emergency. If so, the individual has a legal right to be treated, and physicians, nurses, and others working in the emergency room have a legal obligation to provide this treatment.[9] There is no suggestion in the case law of an exception based on a specific virus (like HIV) the patient might also be harboring or a specific disease (like AIDS) from which the patient may be suffering.[10] This rule is essentially universal and noncontroversial. Of course, emergency department personnel have the right to take reasonable precautions to protect themselves from harm, and their employers should comply with recommendations from the Centers for Disease Control regarding appropriate protective procedures and clothing.[11] But protection does not include acts that would amount to refusing treatment or would compromise good patient care.

Initial care is almost always given. Nonetheless, patients are sometimes "dumped" or transferred to other hospitals for nonmedical reasons. For example, early in the AIDS epidemic, a Florida hospital chartered a plane to fly a terminally ill patient to San Francisco to die.[12] And in 1988 a San Francisco hospital was sued for allegedly "dumping" a patient after testing for HIV without patient consent. The hospital denied the charge, saying that it was a small hospital and thus not equipped to properly treat the patient because it did not have adequate infection control guidelines to protect its other patients.(!)[13]

Health professionals are not expected to be saints, but they are legally obligated to act as other qualified professionals would act in the same or similar circumstances. Thus, if a patient threatened an emergency room physician with a gun or a knife, he or she would be acting lawfully in refusing to treat the patient who was putting their life and health at substantial risk. Likewise, if the patient's medical condition exposed the physicians to great risk, and if it was the accepted practice of qualified physicians not to treat the person under the same or similar circumstances, the physician could be legally justified in refusing to treat the patient. Although AIDS is a fatal, infectious disease, it is not accepted medical practice to refuse to treat people with AIDS because of the risk they pose to providers.

The obligation to treat in an emergency does not usually apply outside of the emergency department setting. Only one state, Massachusetts, has adopted licensing regulations that require its physicians to render emergency care to any person experiencing a medical emergency, no matter where that emergency occurs.[14] Even under this rule, however, physicians who are not competent to treat in an emergency are required only to try to find another physician who can.

In the absence of some contractual or statutory right (discussed below), AIDS and HIV-infected patients, like all other persons, have no legal right to access to medical services in the United States, unless they are suffering a medical emergency and are able to get themselves to an emergency room. That this situation is still tolerated in the United States is a national disgrace; on the other hand, by refusing to grant universal access to health care and medical services to AIDS and HIV-infected patients, we are treating them no different from anyone else in need of medical care.[15]

Abandonment

A patient's right to treatment is greatly enhanced after the establishment of a relationship with a particular physician or hospital. This is because after a voluntary provider–patient relationship has been established, the provider has a duty not to abandon the patient. The general rule is that once a provider–patient relationship is established, it continues until one of the following occurs: it is terminated by mutual consent; it is terminated by the patient; the services are no longer needed; or the provider withdraws after reasonable notice to the patient.[16]

The creation of a provider–patient relationship, therefore, may be critical to the obligation of a provider to care for a particular patient. Such a relationship is always formed when a physician agrees to examine or treat a patient for a specific ailment. This will usually involve a face-to-face meeting. But at least one case has held that a doctor–patient relationship can be formed simply by making an appointment with the patient for an office visit, at least where the appointment relates to a specific condition mentioned by the patient over the telephone when seeking the appointment.[17] Relationships with hospitals are formed on the patient's admission.

The provider cannot abandon or refuse to treat a patient under his or her care simply because that person is infected with HIV or has AIDS, at least not without reasonable notice. On the other hand, if the physician is unqualified to treat the patient (and this is more likely to be true of a person with AIDS rather than a person who is simply infected with HIV), the physician usually has an obligation to refer the patient to a specialist or someone who is qualified to treat the patient's condition. Thus, under some circumstances a physician may be able (or even required) to transfer the care of an AIDS patient to another provider. Nonetheless, as long as the patient requires treatment for the condition that the physician is treating or attending, such as pregnancy, the physician cannot simply terminate the relationship without ensuring that the patient is able to obtain alternative care.

STATUTORY OBLIGATIONS TO TREAT

Private citizens can discriminate against their fellow citizens in the absence of prohibitory or antidiscrimination legislation. This is why both the state and federal governments have enacted statutes to protect against some of the most offensive forms of discrimination. The most noteworthy federal effort is the Civil Rights Act of 1964. Among other things, that act prohibits places of public accommodation involved in interstate commerce (such as transportation, food, and lodging establishments) from discriminating on the basis of race, religion or national origin. Later, Congress passed the Rehabilitation Act of 1973, which prohibits discrimination in federally assisted programs on the basis of handicap when the individual is "otherwise qualified." This law was interpreted by the U.S. Supreme Court to include a person with the contagious disease of tuberculosis as a "handicapped individual" and to provide that such a person cannot be discriminated against in employment covered by the act if the person is "otherwise qualified" for the position.[18] The Americans with Disabilities Act of 1990 (ADA) goes even further and "seeks to plug the holes left by prior law and exposed by the HIV epidemic."[19]

Even though the Supreme Court specifically declined to rule whether an individual who is infected with HIV is handicapped, the logic of the opinion requires the conclusion that HIV infection is a handicap. Even the U.S. Justice Department finally recognized this and reversed its previous position. The reason is that, as the Court noted in *Arline*, the purpose of the 1973 Act was to protect "handicapped individuals from deprivations based on prejudice, stereotypes, or unfounded fear, while giving appropriate weight to such legitimate concerns of the grantees [recipients of federal funds] as avoiding exposing others to significant health and safety risks." HIV-infected individuals certainly experience prejudice. The remaining issue is whether they pose a real threat of harm to others. Whether an exposure is "significant" in the context of a contagious or infectious disease will be up to the courts, but as the Court noted, "courts normally should defer to the reasonable medical judgments of public health officials." Thus, as long as public health officials continue to reasonably conclude that AIDS is not easily transmissible in specific settings and circumstances, those with AIDS and HIV infection should be protected from discrimination in federally assisted programs for which they are "otherwise qualified," both under prior law and the new ADA.

Most states have enacted laws, modeled after the federal civil rights legislation, that prohibit "public accommodations" from discriminating against individuals on the basis of handicap. These laws, of course, will provide the broadest protection for individuals if they are construed (as I believe they should be) to include HIV-infected individuals. Even under the most rigorously fair antidiscrimination law, for example, the most health professionals would ever have a legal obligation to do would be to refer patients that they are unqualified to care for to providers and facilities qualified to care for them. Antidiscrimination laws do *not* create a duty to treat any particular person, anymore than a hotel or restaurant is obligated to serve a particular person. What they do is make certain reasons (e.g., disability) unacceptable reasons to refuse to treat individuals. On the other hand, once care is commenced, it must be continued until the patient either no longer needs it or has been safely transferred to other competent care.

CONTRACTUAL OBLIGATIONS TO TREAT

Duties can also be created by contract, and private contracts between physicians and health care institutions or insurance plans (like health maintenance organizations) may be one of the most powerful ways to insure access to care. The employment contract generally requires employed health professionals to render medical care to any patient in the plan who applies for care in the regular course, or (in the case of nurses, medical students, interns, and residents) to any patient on their service or to whom they are assigned. As employees, they have the right to work together to change employment conditions under standard collective bargaining procedures and laws. Unless it is the private employer's nonemergency policy, they do not, however, have the right to arbitrarily discriminate against any particular class or category of patient.[20] As employees, they also have a right to insist that their employer take steps to provide them with a healthful work environment and to take steps to protect themselves from dangerous exposures.

Employees can claim protection under the Occupational Safety and Health Act (OSHA) guidelines, and they can refuse to work if these guidelines are not complied with.[21] In addition, federal OSHA legislation protects workers who complain of an OSHA violation, and it prohibits retaliation by the employer. The right not to work, however, may be constrained by collective bargaining agreements, which, for example, contain a no-strike clause that does not exempt refusals to work for health or safety matters or which contain a grievance mechanism that provides an exclusive method to present complaints. The only exception in this case would be the general rule under the law, which provides that both individual and concerted actions taken in "good faith because of abnormally dangerous conditions" will not be construed as violating a no-strike or collective bargaining agreement. Ultimately, however, unless there is some "ascertainable, objective evidence" of an abnormally dangerous condition, the employee must follow the policy or he or she can be lawfully fired.[22] Current evidence of the danger of HIV infection to health care providers does not meet this risk standard.

A more complex question is whether a hospital or other facility can have a policy of refusing to treat a patient solely because the patient is infected with HIV. This discrimination issue would be equivalent to refusing to treat a patient because the patient is black or gay, if there was no risk of transmission of the infection. The question, of course, is: How high must the risk to the health providers be before their employer should be lawfully permitted to discriminate against HIV-infected individuals by denying them nonemergency treatment? There is no easy answer, but a point of reference seems relevant. The risk of hepatitis B infection is real, and the disease is sometimes fatal, but this risk has never been seen as sufficiently high to justify discrimination against either patients or providers who are infected. Thus it would seem that at least as long as the reasonable scientific estimates are that the dangers of becoming infected with HIV and dying are significantly less than those of becoming infected with hepatitis B and dying, there is no objective data that would justify a policy of discriminating against an HIV-infected individual.

Nonetheless, some surgeons have argued that it is easy for internists, ethicists, lawyers, and others who do not have direct blood-to-blood contact with patients to argue against HIV screening, and that some circumstances should justify routine screening. Just what these circumstances are has yet to be determined. It seems irrational to screen all surgical patients routinely. Depending on one's assumptions, screening a low-risk population to protect surgeons would require falsely labeling as seropositive at least twenty-two and as many as 1,300,000 uninfected patients, to prevent one surgeon from becoming infected.[23] The authors of this study suggest that we cannot even begin to develop a rational surgical screening test procedure until we know the answers to some questions, including, "How many false-positive results are tolerable to protect one health care worker?"[24] Moreover, because of the problem of false negatives, screening may actually provide a false sense of security. More to the point, perhaps, is to suggest screening of high risk populations for surgery that pose special problems of personal protection for surgeons. This screening, however, can only be tolerated if the results of the screening do not affect *whether* the nonelective surgery is performed, but only affects *how* it is performed, and if confidentiality of the results can be maintained. Routine screening of patients makes no more sense than routine screening of surgeons—although the public is now demanding the latter, and some surgeons, like those in the New Jersey Medical Society, see this as a small price to pay to screen patients. Current risk data do not justify screening physicians, however, and politically inspired efforts to encourage such screening should be rejected. Infection control should concentrate on improving things (such as disposable needles) and infection control procedures, rather than on restricting the rights of people.[25]

PROFESSIONAL STANDARD SETTING

Medical Societies

Organized medicine has traditionally defended the right of individual practitioners to treat or not treat whomever they wish, except in an emergency. Ethical standards set by professional associations do not carry any formal sanctions other than loss of membership in the association. But courts can use these standards as evidence of a duty of care, since a physician's legal duty is primarily defined by medical custom. Thus specific ethical standards of medical and nursing associations can be used as evidence in a malpractice suit brought by a patient denied care by a physician or nurse, if the patient was harmed by the refusal. Perhaps more importantly, an ethical standard can help set the tone of the profession, and most practitioners will likely adhere to it if it is perceived as reasonable.

In 1986, a joint report from the Health and Policy Committee of the American College of Physicians and the Infectious Diseases Society of America urged "all physicians, surgeons, nurses, other medical professionals and hospitals to provide competent and humane care to all patients, including patients critically ill with AIDS and AIDS-related conditions." In their words, "Denying appropriate care to sick and dying patients for any reason is unethical."[26] In early 1987, the General Medical Council in Britain, responding to reports of physicians refusing AIDS patients, said: "it is unethical for a registered medical practitioner to refuse treatment . . . on the ground that the patient suffers, or may suffer, from a condition which could expose the doctor to personal risk."[27]

The American Medical Association (AMA) took longer, but in late 1987 its Council on Ethical and Judicial Affairs issued a report to the AMA House of Delegates saying that a physician "may not ethically refuse to treat a patient whose condition is within the physician's current realm of competence" solely because the patient has AIDS or is infected with HIV:

> A person who is afflicted with AIDS needs competent, compassionate treatment. Neither those who have the disease nor those who have been infected with the virus should be subjected to discrimination based on fear or prejudice, least of all by members of the health care community. Physicians should respond to the best of their ability in cases of emergency where first aid treatment is essential, and physicians should not abandon patients whose care they have undertaken.[28]

The report, which was accepted, stops short of saying that physicians must care for AIDS patients, but it does make refusal to do so unethical if such care is within the physician's competence and refusal is based solely on the patient's disease status. Explaining the report, Russell Patterson, the vice-chairman, quoted from Principle VI of the AMA's 1980 Principles of Medical Ethics, which says: "A physician shall, in the provision of appropriate patient care, except in emergencies, be free to choose whom to serve, with whom to associate and the environment in which to provide medical services." In Patterson's words:

> We never took that to mean that a physician could illegally or unethically discriminate against any group of patients, such as blacks, members of a religious group, or patients with AIDS. A physician doesn't have to care for AIDS if the disease process is out of his spectrum of knowledge but, for example, a surgeon should not refuse to operate because a patient has AIDS.[29]

Since the AMA has always stood for the rights of its members to treat whomever they wanted to (except in an emergency), this statement seemed astonishing. It would be, except that the AMA's top officials have made it clear that they have no plans to enforce it[30] and that, if doctors don't want to take care of AIDS patients, the AMA will consider them "incompetent" to treat and thus excuse them. In the words of AMA executive vice-president James Sammons: physicians with a "psychological hang-up" that interferes with their ability to treat AIDS patients are covered by the clause that excuses them as "not competent" to treat.[31] If this is an accurate portrayal of the AMA's position, it is the same as saying a doctor must treat an AIDS patient if the doctor wants to treat an AIDS patient.

Few state medical associations have addressed this issue, and at least in states with large HIV-infected populations, like New York, Massachusetts, Illinois, California, and Florida, they should. The Texas Medical Association adopted a standard that actively invites discrimination by giving the physician the option to treat the patient or to refer the patient, regardless of the physician's ability to treat the disease. Explaining the decision, James Mann, chairman of TMA's Board of Counselors, said:

> We didn't agree that a physician who diagnoses AIDS is mandated to treat the patient. I don't think it can be called discrimination when it's a matter of a guy laying his health and career on the line. A young man may spend 15 years of his life getting medical training and risk his life treating disease. You must think of the potential dangers and risks. . . . All it takes is a slip of a needle or a splash of secretions.[32]

The president of the Texas Medical Association explained that he thought physicians should continue to do business as usual even in the face of the AIDS crisis and that the "traditional freedom" physicians have to choose whom to serve should be maintained. In his words: "You and I don't want to be treated by someone who doesn't want to treat us."[33]

Strong and unequivocal ethical statements from organized medicine can help patients obtain access to needed services. Statements that encourage fear and prejudice, however, like that issued by the Texas Medical Association and the "clarifying" remarks of Sammons on the AMA standards can have precisely the opposite effect. Physicians should set their own ethical standards. But if they fail, or if the standards are too low, the law must operate to protect the public.

State Licensing Boards

Health professionals are licensed by state agencies in each of the fifty states. Licensing grants a monopoly and makes the practice of their profession without a license a crime. These agencies have statutory authority to issue regulations that govern the practice of medicine and nursing and to define "unprofessional conduct." Unlike private professional organizations, like the AMA and American Nurses' Association, the regulations promulgated by these licensing boards have the force of law, and violation of them could lead to license suspension or revocation.[34] Because of these potential sanctions, standards promulgated by licensing boards are much more powerful agents to affect behavior.

The most complete and comprehensive policy position of any state licensing board has been announced in Massachusetts by the Board of Registration in Medicine. In 1988, the Board adopted regulations (which it had helped to fashion with an Inter-Agency Task Force on AIDS in the Office of Consumer Affairs and Business Regulation), entitled "AIDS Guidelines."[35] The guidelines set forth physicians' obligations in relatively non-controversial general terms:

> Licensed professionals have a duty to care, treat or provide services to persons with AIDS or HIV-infection. Exceptions to this obligation may occur in clearly defined, unusual instances but as a general rule, all licensed professionals should be aware of their affirmative duty to treat, care for or deliver services to persons with AIDS or HIV-infection.

As is apparent from the common law, statutes, and various medical society policies, the major excuse not to treat a patient with AIDS is ignorance of how to treat such a patient. The Massachusetts board responds to this concern by declaring that it is the physician's obligation as a physician to learn how to care for AIDS patients:

> Caring for routine problems associated with AIDS is a skill all professionals need to master. . . . Therefore, when a person with AIDS develops problems that would normally be in the area of expertise of and be routinely handled by a skilled professional *referral to another professional would generally not be in conformity with the intent of these guidelines.* (emphasis added)

The Massachusetts board takes the AIDS epidemic seriously, and insists that physicians licensed to practice in Massachusetts take it seriously as well. Licensing agencies in other states have not been either so far-sighted or forceful. The Board of Medical Examiners in New Jersey, for example, issued its "AIDS Policy" in late 1987: "A licensee of this Board may not categorically refuse to treat a patient who has AIDS or AIDS related complex, or an HIV positive blood test, when he or she possesses the skill and experience to treat the condition presented." In those cases where the physician is unable to render care, "the licensee retains the responsibility to make alternative arrangements for the proper care of a patient." Taking an opposite stance, the Arizona Board of Medical Examiners has stated that their licensees have the right to refuse continued treatment to AIDS patients.

The licensing boards of states that have a significant number of AIDS patients have an obligation to clarify the legal obligation their licensees have to render care in a nondiscriminatory manner. They should do so before any movement to deny treatment or adopt either the "Texas solution" or the "Arizona avoidance strategy" develops. The Massachusetts model may seem just another example of overregulation, but it boldly attempts to deal with a problem that all physicians should rightly share, and Massachusetts deserves to be commended for its leadership in this area.

State Antidiscrimination Statutes and Private Employment Contracts

It would be useful for AIDS and HIV-infected individuals if each state antidiscrimination statute clearly included them in the category of handicapped individuals who could not be discriminated against in regard to employment, housing, and access to "public accommodations," including hospitals, clinics and physician and dental offices, as the ADA does.

Nonetheless, this will not solve all our problems because AIDS confronts us with a phenomenon much more complex than simple discrimination on the basis of an infectious, lethal disease. As others have correctly noted, even if fear of contracting AIDS is given as the reason for discrimination, the real motivation may be much more complex. Likely additional reasons may include (1) an aversion to gays or to intravenous drug users; (2) the fact that most sufferers are young and there is no effective treatment (so they are terminally ill); and (3) the fact that AIDS patients require intensive, expensive, and exhausting care.[36] As physician Douglas Shenson put it so well: "Inside the hospital I have learned to cope; the point, I know now, is not to be scared, but to be careful. The greatest occupational hazard in caring for my patients is not catching the disease, but rather in falling victim to the emotional brutalization that comes with the work."[37]

One of the most effective insurers of nondiscriminatory patient care can be the contract provisions set forth in employment contracts and hospital staff by-laws. These documents can bind physicians who are employees and physicians who have staff privileges to specific nondiscriminatory behavior regarding AIDS patients. The sanctions for noncompliance can also be spelled out. For employees, the ultimate sanction is dismissal. For attending physicians, it is usually loss of staff privileges. With interns and residents, it would be dismissal from the training program; and with medical students, it would be expulsion from school.

A powerful example of such a policy was adopted by the Associated Medical Schools of New York, which represents the state's thirteen medical schools. The association decreed that physicians had a "most fundamental responsibility" to treat AIDS patients and that any faculty member, hospital resident, or medical student who refused to treat an AIDS patient would be dismissed. Although there have been no reported cases of such refusal in the medical school system, the president of the association said he "felt it important to take a tough leadership position at a time of national crisis."[38] Other medical schools and hospitals in other states should follow this lead. In all of these cases, of course, physicians and medical students accused of discriminatory behavior should be given a fair hearing, including representation by legal counsel, prior to any punitive action against them.

CONCLUSION

Health providers in private practice have no legal duty to treat except in specific situations. Broad statements of ethical responsibility by organized public health, nursing, and medical associations and groups, state licensing boards, hospitals, and health schools, however, can transform the "no duty rule" into a "professional duty to treat or locate and refer to appropriate treatment rule." When such rules are promulgated, they should be followed by intense educational programs based in hospitals so that all heath care workers can be kept fully informed regarding the meaning of AIDS and HIV-infection, can realistically assess the risk of transmission, and understand the steps that can reasonably be taken to minimize that risk. Hospitals and prepaid health plans also need responsive employee grievance mechanisms, competent safety personnel, available safety clothes and equipment, safe methods of dealing with blood and bodily fluids, and adequate disability coverage. Antidiscrimination standards should also be adopted. But there is no quick legal fix to guarantee access to medical care to AIDS and HIV-infected patients, because the basic problems of health care access in the United States are economic and political, not legal.[39]

Health care professionals have special legal obligations because they have been granted special privileges by society. Their continued practice is voluntary, and their conduct is properly judged by standards higher than those we hold others to, even higher than those to which we hold firemen and policemen. Society could not tolerate firemen and policemen who refused to ever risk their lives in doing their jobs. Nor need it tolerate health care professionals who refuse to take risks to do theirs. Nonetheless, we must recognize that greed and fear of death are not just motivators of some health care professionals; they are the key shared "values" of contemporary society. In motivating health care professionals to care for AIDS and HIV-infected patients, we must take reasonable steps to address these issues if we want to be effective. Universal health insurance and disability coverage seems critical. Monetary and licensure suspension penalties for discrimination seem useful. And realistic methods to deal with prevention of HIV infection seem essential. Only a multifaceted approach is likely to prove effective in assuring access to medical care in the long run.

AIDS may be our first modern plague, but as the resurgence of tuberculosis assures us, it will not be our last. As Camus reminds us, plague "never dies or disappears for good." But in times of plague, he tells us, we learn an important lesson about ourselves—"that there are more things to admire in men than to despise."

10

Faith (Healing), Hope, and Charity at the FDA: The Politics of AIDS Drug Trials

AIDS forces us to confront our mortality, the limits of modern medicine, and the contours of our compassion.[1] How we respond is a measure of our society, as well as a reflection of our values and priorities. As a fundamentally death-denying society, our response has been hampered by denial and shaped by faith that a technological fix will make the AIDS epidemic go away. Technology is our new religion, our "modern" way to deal with death. As novelist Don Delillo has one of his characters in *White Noise* put it to another who is worried about death: you can deny it, you can put your faith in religion, or

> you could put your faith in technology. It got you here, it can get you out. This is the whole point of technology. It creates an appetite for immortality on the one hand. It threatens universal extinction on the other. . . . It's what we invented to conceal the terrible secret of our decaying bodies. But it's also life, isn't it? It prolongs life, it provides new organs for those that wear out. New devices, new techniques every day. Lasers, masers, ultrasound. Give yourself up to it. . . . They'll insert you in a gleaming tube, irradiate your body with the basic stuff of the universe. Light, energy, dreams. God's own goodness.

The less we understand about medical technology, the more we see it as magic. Nor are physicians immune from magical thinking. When medical science seems impotent to fight the claims of nature, "all kinds of senseless interventions are tried in an unconscious effort to cure the incurable magically through a 'wonder drug,' a novel surgical procedure, or a penetrating psychological interpretation."[2] In a parallel fashion, we speak of medical "miracles" in recounting techniques we cannot understand but nonetheless want to believe in. We have become modern believers in faith healing, faith based not in a Supreme Being, but in Supreme Science.

The AIDS epidemic has frightened us into "believing" that medicine will find a cure soon, and this faith in science has eroded the distinction between experimentation and therapy, has threatened to transform the U.S. Food and Drug Administration (FDA) from a consumer protection agency into a medical technology promotion agency, and has put AIDS patients, already suffering from an incurable disease, at further risk of psychological, physical, and financial exploitation by those who would sell them useless drugs. The not too subtle metamorphosis of the pre-Kessler FDA was abetted by an unusual political alliance between the antiregulation Reagan/Bush administrations and gay rights activists.

This chapter argues that the distinction between experimental and therapeutic interventions is crucial in terms of both science and individual rights; and that the FDA should continue to responsibly regulate experimental drugs and reassert its identity as a premier consumer protection agency. We should not permit the AIDS epidemic to be used as an excuse to dismantle the FDA or to put the integrity of our drugs and medical devices at risk. True compassion for AIDS patients does not involve dispensing false hope or unreasonable hype. It requires adequate funding and staffing of the National Institutes of Health (NIH) and their AIDS drug and vaccine testing programs, along with scientifically sound testing methodologies that can provide reasonable assurance that the drugs that are sold as therapies are safe and effective. To examine the politics of AIDS drug development, it is necessary to understand the purposes for the experimentation/therapy distinction in medicine, and the values that this distinction promotes and protects.

THE EXPERIMENTATION/THERAPY DISTINCTION

Perhaps the major source of controversy surrounding drug trials for experimental AIDS drugs is that investigators see these trials as *research*, whose purpose is to provide generalizable knowledge that may help others. On the other hand, most individuals suffering with AIDS see these trials as *therapy*, whose primary purpose is to benefit them. This confusion is not new, and a brief review of the history of human experimentation shows why it is important.

A reasonable summary of many of the major issues in human experimentation appears in Gustave Flaubert's realistic novel *Madame Bovary* (1857). Charles Bovary decides to try to make his name as a physician by curing the local stableman's club foot with experimental surgery. The experiment involved cutting the Achilles tendon and then screwing the foot and leg into "a kind of box, weighing about eight pounds, constructed by the carpenter and the locksmith, with a prodigal amount of iron, wood, sheet-iron, leather, nails and screws." The apothecary, an avid supporter of the experiment, helps convince Charles' wife, Emma: "'What risk is there? Look!'—and he counted the 'pros' on his fingers. 'Success, practically certain. An end of suffering and disfigurement for the patient. Immediate fame for the operator.'" The stableman is urged to consent by the entire town, but the "decisive factor was that it wouldn't cost him anything." The experiment does not go as planned, and another physician eventually must be called in to amputate the hideously painful and gangrenous leg.

Most experiments do not have such disastrous results for patients, but many share similar dangers, as well as the same motivations on the part of both physician and patient, the same inability to separate hopes from realistic appraisal of likely outcomes, and the same inability to distinguish voluntary consent from coercion. To protect subjects, rules have been developed regarding human experimentation.

The most comprehensive and authoritative legal statement on human experimentation is embodied in the Nuremberg Code. This ten-point code was articulated in a 1947 court opinion following the trial of Nazi physicians for "war crimes and crimes against humanity" committed during World War II, which included experiments designed to determine which poisons killed the fastest, how long people could live exposed to ice water and when exposed to high altitudes, and if surgically severed limbs could be reattached.[3] The Nuremberg tribunal rejected the defendant's contention that their experiments with both prisoners of war and civilians were consistent with the ethics of the medical profession as evidenced by previously published U.S., French, and British experiments on venereal disease, plague, and malaria, and U.S. prison experiments, among others. The tribunal concluded that only "certain types of medical experiments on human beings, when kept within reasonably well defined bounds, conform to the ethics of the medical profession generally."

These well-defined bounds are articulated in the ten principles of the Nuremberg Code. The basis of the code is a type of natural law reasoning. In the court's words: "All agree . . . that certain basic principles must be observed in order to satisfy moral, ethical, and legal concepts." Principle 1 of the Nuremberg Code thus requires that the consent of the experimental subject have at least four characteristics: it must be competent, voluntary, informed, and comprehending. This is to protect the subject's rights. The other principles have primarily to do with protecting the subject's welfare: They prescribe actions that must be taken prior to seeking subject enrollment in the experiment, and actions that must be taken to protect the subject during the experiment. These include a determination that the experiment is properly designed to yield fruitful results "unprocurable by other methods"; that "anticipated results" will justify performance of the experiment; that all "unnecessary physical and mental suffering and injury" is avoided; that there is no "*a priori* reason to believe that death or disabling injury will occur"; that the project has "humanitarian importance" that outweighs the degree of risk; that "adequate preparation" is taken to "protect the experimental subject against even the remote possibilities of injury, disability, or death"; that only "scientifically qualified" persons conduct the experiment; that the subject can terminate participation at any time; and that the experimenter is prepared to terminate the experiment if "continuation is likely to result in injury, disability, or death to the experimental subject." The code has been used as the basis for other international documents, such as the Declaration of Helsinki, it is a part of international common law, and I have previously argued that it can properly be viewed as both a criminal and civil basis for liability in the United States.[4]

Today the most likely subject of medical experimentation is not the prisoner or even the soldier, but the patient with a disease. As a leading medical commentator has put it:

> Volunteers for experiments will usually be influenced by hopes of obtaining better grades, earlier parole, more substantial egos, or just mundane cash. These pressures, however, are but fractional shadows of those enclosing the patient-subject. *Incapacitated and hospitalized because of illness, frightened by strange and impersonal routines, and fearful for his health and perhaps life, he is far from exercising a free power of choice* when the person to whom he anchors all his hopes asks, "say, you wouldn't mind, would you, if you joined some of the other patients on this floor and helped us to carry out some very important research we are doing?" When "informed consent" is obtained, it is not the student, the destitute bum, or the prisoner to whom, by virtue of his condition, the thumb screws of coercion are most relentlessly applied; it is *the most used and useful of all experimental subjects, the patient with disease.*[5] (emphasis added)

When the illness is fatal, pressures on both the physician-researcher and patient are much more acute, and the rules regarding research seem less relevant. Consent also seems a sham, since patients are "desperate" and are demanding to be research subjects, thinking that this is their best hope of getting "treatment" for their condition.[6] The assertion is made that patients have "nothing to lose" by engaging in all manner of experimentation, and that patients should have the "right" to be experimental subjects.[7] But it is when such political claims are made in the face of a fatal disease that consumer protection agencies like the FDA must stand firm and insist on scientific validity to those experiments that are performed. This is because, as important as informed consent is, the most important and prior question is whether the experiment should be done at all.[8] Only after this determination has been made, based on such things as prior animal and laboratory research, study design, risk/benefit analysis, and the alternatives, is it even legitimate to ask the subject to participate. And without such prior determinations, and the development of a sound research protocol, it is extremely unlikely that experimentation will yield any useful information, but, rather, will only serve to increase suffering and exploitation of desperate patients.

THE POLITICS OF AIDS DRUG TRIALS

AIDS politics has produced strange political allies. The antiregulation Reagan/Bush administrations and the gay community probably had only one interest in common: deregulating the drug approval process. The gay community's position is probably best summed up in a slogan used by ACT-UP (AIDS Coalition to Unleash Power): "A Drug Trial is Health Care Too." Of course, the truth is otherwise: a drug trial is research designed to test a hypothesis, not treatment meant to help individual patients. The reason for this strange alliance has little to do with shared love for those suffering with AIDS; rather, it is due to an administration composed largely of free-market advocates and the desire of drug companies for deregulation, both of whom see the AIDS epidemic as an opportunity to further their own interests. Unlike the experiment in *Madame Bovary*, experimental drugs are no longer universally delivered free, and there is tremendous pressure on the FDA to permit drug companies to sell "promising" experimental drugs to subjects. The sale of experimental drugs threatens to further erode the distinction between experimentation and therapy and makes it even more difficult for patients suffering from disease to distinguish recognized therapy from early experimentation, and false hope from reasonable expectation.

The administration's position was that drugs should be permitted to go on the market faster. President George Bush, while still Vice-President, urged the FDA to develop procedures to expedite the marketing of new drugs intended to treat AIDS and other life-threatening illnesses. In the fall of 1988, in his first debate with the Democratic presidential nominee, Michael Dukakis, Bush said that in response to his efforts FDA had "sped up bringing drugs to market that can help." He did, however, caution that, "you've got to be careful here because there's a safety factor."[9] Indeed there is, and the policy question is whether that safety factor should be ignored or radically lessened when the research subjects have a fatal illness for which there is no cure. Although the AIDS epidemic is new, this question is not. The FDA has faced it squarely before.

In the 1970s, thousands of cancer victims were traveling to Mexico and Canada to obtain laetrile, a substance derived from apricot pits. The drug was not available in the United States and was not even in experimental trials. In 1975 a group of terminally ill cancer patients and their spouses sued the federal government to enjoin it from interfering with the interstate shipment and sale of laetrile. The FDA vigorously opposed making laetrile available in the United States, even to terminally ill cancer patients, because "there were no adequate well-controlled studies of laetrile's safety or effectiveness."[10]

The United States Supreme Court upheld the FDA's position noting, among other things, that "In implementing the statutory scheme, the FDA has never made exception for drugs used by the terminally ill."[11] The Court also agreed with the FDA that effectiveness is not irrelevant simply because one is dying: "effectiveness does not necessarily denote capacity to cure. In the treatment of any illness, terminal or otherwise, a drug is effective if it fulfills, by objective indices, its sponsor's claims of prolonged life, improved physical condition, or reduced pain." Safety is also relevant to the terminally ill: "For the terminally ill, as for anyone else, a drug is unsafe if its potential for inflicting death or physical injury is not offset by the possibility of therapeutic benefit." The Court underlined that although the case involved laetrile, the logic adopted applied to all unproven drugs:

> To accept the proposition that the safety and efficacy standards of the Act have no relevance for terminal patients is to deny the Commissioner's authority over all drugs, however toxic or ineffectual, for such individuals. If history is any guide, this new market would not be long overlooked. Since the turn of the century, resourceful entrepreneurs have advertised a wide variety of purportedly simple and painless cures for cancer, including liniments of turpentine, mustard, oil, eggs, and ammonia; pear moss; arrangements of colored floodlamps; pastes made from glycerin and limberger cheese; mineral tablets; and "Foundation of Youth" mixtures of spices, oil and diet. . . . Congress could reasonably have determined to protect the terminally ill, no less than other patients, from the vast range of self-styled panaceas that inventive minds can devise.

Although the breast implant controversy may have caused some reassessment, since 1979 the FDA's public position on use of unproven drugs and devices in clinical settings has been shifting. In 1985, for example, the FDA decided to encourage the use of temporary artificial hearts, even though their use in clinical settings outside of a planned research project could generate no scientifically useful information on these devices (see Chapter 16). The justification was that the FDA should not stand in the way of a physician using an unapproved medical device in an "emergency." In 1987, in response to increasing political pressure to make experimental AIDS drugs more widely available, the FDA issued new regulations that permit the treatment, use, and sale of an investigational new drug (IND) that is not otherwise approved for treatment and sale, while the drug is still in clinical trials, if:

> The drug is intended to treat a serious or immediately life-threatening disease.

> There is no comparable or satisfactory alternative drug or other therapy available to treat that stage of the disease in the intended patient population.

The drug is under investigation in a controlled clinical trial under an IND in effect for the trial, or all clinical trials have been completed.

The sponsor of the controlled clinical trial, or all clinical trials, is actively pursuing marketing approval of the IND with due diligence.[12]

According to the then counselor to the Undersecretary of Health and Human Services, S. Jay Plager, the purpose of these new rules was to give "desperately ill patients the opportunity to decide for themselves whether they would rather take an experimental drug or die of the disease untreated."[13] Like ACT-UP, Mr. Plager and the FDA confused experimentation with treatment and seemed so intent on denying death that they believed it could be magically prevented with unproven drugs.

No one opposes cutting "red tape" or removing regulatory hurdles that do not improve safety and efficacy. Arguably, FDA's rules are not inconsistent with *Rutherford*. But in July 1988 the former FDA commissioner took a step that clearly is inconsistent, when he announced that the FDA would permit U.S. citizens to import unapproved drugs from abroad for their personal use. In attempting to justify this policy, Commissioner Frank Young said: "There is such a degree of desperation, and people are going to die, that I'm not going to be the Commissioner that robs them of hope."[14] The reaction of the scientific community to this new FDA position was well summed up in an article in *Science*: "The new directive stunned some AIDS researchers. One official in the federal government's AIDS program went so far as to suggest that the FDA commissioner had gone 'temporarily insane.'"[15] There are at least three reasons for this reaction.

First are all the arguments the FDA used in *Rutherford* to justify its central role as a consumer protection agency. All patients, particularly terminally ill patients, deserve protection from those who want to prey on their desperation for profit. People with AIDS have a lot to lose, including their health, their lives, their dignity, and their money. They can be and have been viciously exploited. Because many victims of AIDS are members of disenfranchised groups that have traditionally been rightfully suspicious of government's view of them, they may be at special risk for exploitation by those who proclaim that the government and orthodox medicine is in a conspiracy to deny them treatment. A few examples of harm to individuals from unapproved drugs illustrate the problem. The life and death of Bill Kraus frames Randy Shilts's chronicle of the politics of AIDS—*And the Band Played On* (1987). Kraus, like many other AIDS patients, including Rock Hudson (who left Paris in 1984 convinced he was cured of AIDS) traveled to Paris to be treated with HPA-23. When, in 1985, it became clear that the drug was not working, his doctor urged him to start taking another unproven medication (isoprinosine). Shilts writes: "The suggestion upset Bill because he had pinned his entire hope for survival on HPA-23. Even the possibility that it might not be a panacea enraged him, cutting to the core of his denial and bargaining with his AIDS diagnosis."[16] Almost a decade later, the efficacy of HPA-23 is still in doubt, and obviously the failure to prove or disprove its worth in France cannot be blamed on the FDA's regulations.

Suranim had been widely used to treat African sleeping sickness, and disabled HIV's ability to replicate in the test tube. When this information was made public, and the drug was touted as "promising," many patients wanted it. A subsequent trial in humans, however, found that suranim was extremely toxic in AIDS patients, worsening immune disorders and thus hastening death.[17] French researchers announced to the world that they had cured AIDS using cyclosporin. There was a clamor for the drug, and the announcement was later found to be premature hype: both patients were comatose and the drug did not improve their clinical course.[18] In late 1987 a Zairian scientist announced in a news conference that he had a possible cure for AIDS. In the aftermath of the announcement, the number of men in Zaire who believed AIDS could be cured doubled (to 57 percent), and educational efforts aimed at prevention were set back.[19] The lack of scientifically sound, carefully planned randomized clinical trials not only produces false hope but also can directly lengthen the time it will take to get a truly effective AIDS drug to those suffering from the disease.

The second reason why encouraging the use of unproven drugs is bad public policy is that denying death ultimately serves no purpose (other than providing temporary false hope). The FDA and other federal agencies (like the Centers for Disease Control) have recognized this in other aspects of the AIDS epidemic. For example, rather than continue to deny that teenagers engage in sexual activity, condom use and "safe sex" practices have been recommended to help prevent the spread of AIDS. Similarly, education about the science and epidemiology of AIDS has been used as the major weapon to fight fear and prejudice against those infected by others who would deny them education, housing, employment, and insurance. The scientific facts have been seen as the most powerful weapon against fear bred by ignorance. It is thus at least ironic that attention to scientific facts seems to have been jettisoned when it has come to research with AIDS drugs. It is not compassionate to hold out false hope to a terminally ill patient and thereby induce that patient to spend his last dollar on unproven "remedies." If anything, such a strategy seems aimed primarily at treating the guilt of a society that has done little to meet the real needs of AIDS victims by giving us the comforting illusion that we are doing something to help.

The third reason why making unproven drugs available is counterproductive public policy is that, if unproven remedies are made easily available it will be impossible to do scientifically valid trials of new drugs. Those suffering from AIDS will be unwilling to participate in randomized clinical trials, and those who are randomized to an arm of the study they do not like will take the drugs they "believe in" on the sly, making any valid finding from the study impossible.[20]

In 1988, for example, in what gay rights activists described as a "political ploy" in the midst of a presidential campaign, the FDA developed rules designed to permit the collapsing of phases II and III for certain drugs that "are intended to treat life-threatening or severely-debilitating illnesses."[21] In announcing the new rules, then FDA Commissioner Frank Young said: "I've seen a lot of folks who are suffering, and I want those people who have either cancer or AIDS to know that this agency has a heart as well as a mind."[22] These new rules, however, do little more than formalize procedures the FDA has always been able to use upon the request of the manufacturer. As the FDA noted in the comments to the rules, they essentially track the way the FDA actually went about approving zidovudine (AZT), the first, and for years the only, drug the FDA approved for the treatment of AIDS.

By mid-1992 even ACT-UP activists seemed to agree that the FDA (and its research rules) was not the real problem in drug development. One of their members, Mark Harrington, said at the Amsterdam AIDS Conference, "What is the point of streamlining access and approval when the result is merely to replace AZT with mediocre, toxic and expensive drugs?"[23] He argued that others should be encouraged to follow his example and volunteer for "experiments involving basic science." This will almost always require the painstaking work of randomized clinical trials.

SHOULD THE RULES FOR RESEARCH BE CHANGED WHEN THE DISEASE IS FATAL?

Randomized clinical trials (RCTs) are the "gold standard" upon which experimental treatments are judged useful, worthless, or dangerous. John McKinlay has demonstrated that in the absence of an initial well-controlled clinical trial the typical innovation in modern medicine goes through seven stages: (1) promising report; (2) professional adoption; (3) public acceptance and third-party payment; (4) standard procedure; (5) randomized clinical trial; (6) professional denunciation; and (7) discreditation.[24] He has argued forcefully that to avoid the first four and the last two stages, and the expense in terms of money and human misery that they generate, we must evaluate all newly proposed therapies at stage 5, the randomized clinical trial, before making the therapy generally available. This view is widely accepted as correct in the scientific community, and the trend has been to try to develop methods to evaluate surgery and other therapies by RCT as well, in an effort to improve the quality of care by eliminating costly therapies that provide no benefit. Although there are proposals for "community clinical trials" and to make "adjustments" in the current management of RCTs, there is no dispute that the RCT is the method most likely to produce valid results.

When Commissioner Young asserts that the FDA "has a heart as well as a mind," it is fair to ask whether the FDA's role is to provide emotional support or scientific protection to the public. The FDA may see it as compassionate to provide access to unproven remedies, but fifteen years ago it saw it as exploitative. Was it right then, or is it right today?

I think the FDA was correct on laetrile and should continue to insist on a scientifically valid randomized clinical trial before certifying drugs safe and effective. All consumer protection legislation is to some degree paternalistic, but in this case it is also realistic. FDA certification of the safety and the efficacy of drugs recognizes that the public is in no position to judge the value or usefulness of many medications, and that many drugs are dangerous and have serious side effects (which is one reason we also license physicians and require some drugs be available only with a physician's prescription). Drug manufacturers have a distinct social role: to create and sell products. Their role is not consumer protection. Libertarians and those with extreme views of individual autonomy, and even some free marketers, object to FDA regulation, equating "pursuit of quackery" with "life, liberty, and the pursuit of happiness." True autonomy requires adequate and accurate information upon which to base decisions. This is simply impossible in the absence of responsible scientific study and properly designed clinical trials. It is appropriate to concentrate energies and resources in the time of an epidemic. It is also appropriate to assign AIDS drug testing a very high priority and to approve adequate government funding to develop and test drugs that might be effective. NIH and FDA should work together more closely and develop better dispute resolution systems when disagreements persist. But it is not ultimately helpful to AIDS sufferers to rush inadequately tested drugs to market. The thalidomide episode taught us all that lesson, and our brief fascination with suramin should have reinforced it.

The good news is that even with the "faith, hope, and charity" rhetoric of the former FDA Commissioner, with the exception of permitting the importation of quack remedies for personal use, the FDA actually stuck with its consumer protection mission. And although Commissioner David Kessler endorsed quick actions on AIDS drugs, he insisted on good science as well. The FDA's two major rule innovations are designed primarily to speed up the bureaucratic aspects of drug testing, rather than to substantively change the rules for evaluating drugs. This is perfectly consistent with sound public policy. What would not be in the public interest is for the FDA to adopt the antiregulation agenda of the drug companies by relaxing its safety and efficacy standards.

The rhetoric has been turned up, but it is simply a repeat of the laetrile debate. A *Wall Street Journal* editorial, for example, accused the FDA of killing people with its testing procedures. It called on the FDA to accede to the demands of dying patients, rather than to insist on scientific soundness in experimentation, and to let the "patients and their families" be involved in revamping the current system for drug approval:

> Let defenders of the status quo explain to people with cancer, Alzheimer's or AIDS why redundant efficacy testing, in which half the patients get a placebo, doesn't constitute 'killing' in the name of FDA-mandated medical statistics. . . . AIDS patients have driven home to the U.S. medical and political establishment what enormous risks human beings in death's grip will take to gain relief or respite.[25]

What the *Journal* does not seem to realize is that it has identified the problem — desperation — not the solution. Deregulation of the drug approval process cannot produce new drugs that don't exist. Of course, money can be made by exploiting the fear of death and desperation, and perhaps this is what the *Journal* would like to see. The profiteering pricing policy of Burroughs Wellcome in making AZT available for years only to those who could pay approximately $8,000 a year for its use, and long after the original justification for this extraordinarily high price (to recoup development costs) had been met, is a useful example of such financial exploitation.[26] No wonder that the American Public Health Association petitioned the U.S. Department of Health and Human Services to require that mechanisms be put into place to ensure that if and when a more effective drug is developed at government institutions or with federal funding to combat AIDS that it will be made available at the lowest possible price. The quest for profit also threatens to inhibit scientific research and sharing of data concerning experimental AIDS drugs, as well as to increase the likelihood that useless drugs will be hyped in press conferences rather than evaluated at scientific meetings. This trend is much more likely to adversely affect AIDS sufferers than any FDA rule regarding clinical trials.

As a cover story in *Fortune* magazine has noted, "for the past 30 years the drug makers of the Fortune 500 have enjoyed the fattest profits in big business."[27] In the 1990 recession year, for example, drug makers "rewarded shareholders with returns on equity 50% higher than the median for Fortune's 500 industrial companies." The major reason for these profits is the lack of price competition and the marketing "muscle" of the large drug makers. In this context their pathetic cries that the FDA is somehow threatening their existence have no more credibility than a Paul Bunyon tale, and should be taken no more seriously.

Drug companies are nonetheless likely to continue to lobby Congress and the public to limit their liability for harm caused by dangerous drugs by eliminating the possibility of recovery for punitive damages when FDA standards have been followed, or by limiting liability for harm caused by vaccines. AIDS activists may be tempted to join the drug companies and the free marketers on these moves as well, at least if the drug companies promise more work on AIDS drugs and vaccines in return. But just as drug approval standards should not be driven solely by the AIDS epidemic, so policies for compensating the victims of drug injuries should not be driven by the AIDS epidemic. We should not forget why we have rules for drug safety.

The distinction between experimentation and therapy is a powerfully useful and protective one that should not be undermined. The fact that there is no cure for a fatal disease does not make experimental drugs designed for it "therapeutic," any more than a mechanical or baboon heart is therapeutic for someone with end stage heart disease. Experimental drugs are not a consumer good appropriately governed by the free market. If consumer choice was the only relevant issue, even if it was limited to terminally ill consumers, the drug of choice among most dying intravenous drug users with AIDS would likely be heroin (or other opiate derivatives such as morphine). These drugs are effective in relieving pain and anxiety in this population, and if they are delivered with clean needles in a medical setting, they can also be safe. If we really wanted to make drugs a consumer good for the terminally ill, we should begin here. The fact that we don't indicates that the political agenda at work in the AIDS context is not patient-centered.

Perhaps the fact that we don't make heroin available to terminally ill intravenous drug users is a way we have of punishing them for their illegal behavior.[28] It is equally plausible that we care so little for the victims of AIDS that we don't care if they get hurt by quack remedies imported from abroad. It has also been suggested that although we do not accept active euthanasia and look with disapproval on even terminally ill patients who want physicians to end their lives, we nonetheless believe that it is perfectly acceptable for individuals to volunteer for medical experiments that could hasten their deaths:

> Our quest for a formula that will banish death seems to make it acceptable to try questionable regimens on the aged and terminally ill. . . . Those who insist on using the dying as experimental subjects . . . see death as abnormal and dying patients as subhuman. We cast the terminally ill in modern rites of sacrifice, putting patients through experiments like the Jarvik heart that one might see as torture in the hope of postponing the inevitable.[29]

By making experimental drugs available to AIDS patients outside of organized clinical trials we are doing little, if anything, for AIDS patients. We really seem to be treating ourselves, giving ourselves the illusion that something is being done to combat death — an illusion that is more satisfying because it does not call for any additional government funding. But we will pay a high price for this comfortable illusion if it is used as an excuse to abandon the distinction between experimentation and therapy and to transform the FDA from a consumer protection agency into a drug promotion agency.

The FDA has been the focus of much criticism for not discovering a cure for AIDS. But this is not the FDA's responsibility. The FDA does not do research on, manufacture, or test new drugs; it approves drugs as "safe and effective" that are made and tested by others who seek to market them in the United States. As Commissioner Kessler has so well articulated, its role is not to further the interests of food or drug companies, but to protect the public. It does this, among other ways, by insisting on strict standards in drug testing. Shortcuts that undermine these standards risk the health of all who later use a drug that has been too hastily approved.

The excuse that patients are dying without treatment and have "nothing to lose" will not do. Terminally ill patients can be harmed, abused, and exploited. Realistic discussion of death and accurate education about the status of unproven AIDS drugs and the reason randomized clinical trials are needed is in order. It is not "compassionate" to make quack remedies easily available to those who can pay for them. Real compassion demands that we allocate the money and staff necessary to do real scientific research, and that when valid clinical trials demonstrate that a therapy is "safe and effective," we make it available to all who need it, regardless of their ability to pay. Compassion does not counsel us to supply dying patients with fabulous promises and faddish drugs.

11

Mapping the Human Genome and the Meaning of Monster Mythology

Precolumbian cartographers drew their maps to the extent of their knowledge and then wrote in the margins: "Beyond this point there are dragons." With the voyage of Columbus, we lost both our fear of the geographic frontier and our innocence. We accept that knowledge can generally overpower fear, but we have also learned that the application of new knowledge often has a dark side that can lead to brutality and disaster. The discovery of America, for example, led to unforeseen value conflicts of justice and fairness involving native Americans that were "resolved" only by their merciless subjugation and genocidal destruction. The Columbus metaphor is a powerful one, one that emphasizes both the need to confront mythical dragons with knowledge and the need to anticipate and plan for the real monsters, the value conflicts that new knowledge produces. Perhaps nowhere is the promise of benefit and the risk of harm so great as in genetic research. The plan to map and sequence the 3 billion base pairs that make up the genetic blueprint of a human being — the Human Genome Project — provides an opportunity to examine the relationship between science and society.[1] Can scientists and social policy makers work together to maximize the benefits of this project while minimizing its dangers?

MONSTER MYTHOLOGY

Since at least Elizabethan times, English literature has reflected a fascination with stories of scientists and physicians who have attempted to change the attributes of humankind, and the monsters their attempts have created. Shakespeare set the tone and provided the language and the setting for much of this cautionary literature. *The Tempest*, which is set on an island, forces us to confront the meaning of the natural. The lowly and grotesque Caliban is often seen as a monster, as when Trinculo says of him: "That a monster should be such a natural!" If we see nature as orderly, then the disorderly and deformed Caliban must be a monster.

When Prospero's daughter Miranda, who has grown up with Caliban and the spirits but has seen no other humans, sees the shipwrecked party from Italy she exclaims of them:

> O, wonder!
> How many goodly creatures are there here!
> How beauteous mankind is! O brave new world
> That has such people in't! (V.i.)

At the end of the play, as Prospero prepares to return to the real world and reclaim his place as Duke of Milan, he breaks his magic wand. This gesture has properly been seen as the author's commentary on the relationship between art and life: art, or at least enchanted islands, is no place for man to live, "but rather a place through which we pass in order to renew and strengthen our sense of reality."[2]

Aldous Huxley took the title of his most famous work on the social implications of the new genetics, *Brave New World*, from Miranda's description. Between Shakespeare and Huxley are at least three other writers that have altered our collective consciousness so that the creatures they created trouble our minds when we contemplate modifying modern man: Mary Shelley, H.G. Wells, and Robert Louis Stevenson.

Mary Shelley's masterpiece, *Frankenstein*, has become the metaphor for all scientific attempts to create life. Victor Frankenstein is obsessed with creating life from a construction of dead body parts. Shelley does not explain how Victor was able to "infuse a spark of being into the lifeless thing," but she does describe Victor's emotions upon seeing "the dull yellow eye of the creature open": "His limbs were in proportion, and I had selected his features as beautiful. Beautiful! Great God! His yellow skin scarcely covered the work of muscles and arteries beneath; his hair was of a lustrous black, and flowing; his teeth of a pearly whiteness." Victor's burst of emotion at achieving his goal quickly changes to horror, however, as he gazes at the creature's "watery eyes . . . his shrivelled complexion and straight black lips": "now that I had finished, the beauty of the dream vanished, and breathless horror and disgust filled my heart."

Victor leaves his laboratory and sleeps, and the creature escapes. The remainder of the novel deals with the creature, which is never given a name but simply referred to as "the monster," and its relationship to Victor. Indeed, it seems most reasonable to consider the monster either as Victor's alter ego or as a projection of his inner thoughts made flesh. Perhaps this is why we often think of the monster, instead of its creator, as Frankenstein. Victor's creation eventually kills his young nephew William, his friend Clerval, his wife Elizabeth, and, indirectly, Victor himself.

At one point in the story, the monster convinces Victor to create a wife for him. In this scene Victor is seen as God the creator and the monster as his Adam, or, alternatively, as Lucifer, the fallen angel. But having constructed the monster's would-be mate, Victor decides he cannot give her life for fear that she and the monster might propagate a "race of devils" that would "make the very existence of the species of man a condition precarious and full of terror." Victor consequently tears the female's body apart while the monster looks on, letting out a "howl of devilish despair and revenge." This scene, as much as any other, focuses the theme of the novel: the scientist's simultaneous capacity for creation and destruction.

In *The Tempest*, Shakespeare sees the chaos of nature as a constructive force that helps renew social order. Mary Shelley's vision seems different: the orderliness of scientific research produces chaos and ultimately death. As one critic has put it, a "fitting epigraph" for *Frankenstein* may be the taunt of a Fury to Percy Shelley's Prometheus: "And all best things are thus confused to ill."[3]

The dark side of an individual's personality also takes on its own life in Robert Louis Stevenson's *Dr. Jekyll and Mr. Hyde*. Jekyll determined to discover what divided good and evil in human nature, and he compounded a drug to suppress his good nature and let his evil side (Hyde) dominate. Jekyll assures us that though his nature was split, he was not:

> Though so profound a double-dealer, I was in no sense a hypocrite; both sides of me were in dead earnest; I was no more myself when I laid aside restraint and plunged in shame, than when I laboured, in the eye of day, at the furtherance of knowledge or the relief of sorrow and suffering. . . . With every day, and from both sides of my intelligence, the moral and the intellectual, I thus drew steadily nearer to that truth, by whose partial discovery I have been doomed to such a dreadful shipwreck: that man is not truly one, but truly two.

For our purposes, the murderous Hyde can be thought of as a monster in the lineage of Frankenstein's monster. Like that monster (and Caliban) he is a misshapen creature, "hardly human," who gives "an impression of deformity without any nameable malformation."[4] Although the stages are different in length, Jekyll goes through the same stages as Victor Frankenstein with his monster: he "creates" Hyde, openly admires him, flees from him, and ultimately does what he can to bring about his destruction. Neither creator can control his "monster."

Written ten years after *Dr. Jekyll and Mr. Hyde*, and another ten years before the word "gene" was coined, H.G. Wells's *The Island of Dr. Moreau* brings us into the 20th century. Like Prospero before him, Moreau is depicted as a god, if not as God himself, and rules over his island. And like Victor Frankenstein, the story involves the making of human beings by nonnatural means. Moreau has discovered how to combine transplant surgery and drugs to transform animals into creatures with a human-like shape and a human-like brain. His animal-humans talk and reject their animal (natural) ways. But they are grotesque in appearance, and their transformation is not permanent. When the shipwrecked Charles Prendick, the narrator of the tale, accuses Moreau of creating "an abomination," Moreau replies simply: "To this day I have never troubled about the ethics of the matter. The study of Nature makes a man at least as remorseless as Nature. I have gone on, not heeding anything but the question I was pursuing."

Eventually the creatures turn on Moreau and kill him, and the remainder of the tale relates the "slow and inevitable" reversion of the creatures from human to animal:

> Of course these creatures did not decline into such beasts as the reader has seen in zoological gardens—into ordinary bears, wolves, tigers, oxen, swine, and apes. There was something strange about each; in each Moreau had blended this animal with that; one perhaps was ursine chiefly, another feline chiefly, another bovine chiefly, but each was tainted with other creatures—a kind of generalized animalism appeared through the specific dispositions. And the dwindling shreds of the humanity still startled me every now and then, a momentary recrudescence of speech perhaps, an unexpected dexterity of the forefeet, a pitiful attempt to walk erect.

Their loss of speech was the ultimate sign of their loss of humanity. The story, of course, has many modern parallels. As Brian Aldiss put it in 1988: "The spirit of Dr. Moreau is alive and well and living in these United States. These days, he would be state-funded."[5]

Huxley's *Brave New World* is not about scientific research and discovery, but about the application of knowledge to enhance government control of its citizens. Huxley's work presaged the Nazi eugenics program, with its rigid biologically based class system. In his *Brave New World* natural human reproduction has been abolished; all reproduction is done artificially in state hatcheries and conditioning centers. The key to social control is the "Bokanovsky Process" in which a single embryo is stimulated to divide into ninety-six identical copies. These ninety-six embryos (or all the survivors, seventy-two was the average) are artificially gestated together under identical conditions designed to produce four basic classes of workers: gammas, deltas, epsilons, and alphas. Specific "batches" are conditioned to perform specific tasks and to love performing them. As the Director of the Hatcheries put it, conditioning "is the secret of happiness and virtue—liking what you've *got* to do. All conditioning aims at that: making people like their unescapable social destiny."

The resulting society is compactly described by Mustapha Mond, the Resident World Controller for Western Europe, to a man who had been brought back to "civilization" from the reservation and who is known as "the Savage." He explains to the Savage why it would be impossible to write *Romeo and Juliet* or *Othello* now:

Because our world is not the same as Othello's world you can't make flivvers [inexpensive autos] without steel—and you can't make tragedies without social instability. The world's stable now. People are happy; they get what they want, and they never want what they can't get. They're well off; they're safe; they're never ill; they're not afraid of death; they're blissfully ignorant of passion and old age; they're plagued with no mothers or fathers; they've got no wives, or children, or lovers to feel strongly about; they're so conditioned that they practically can't help behaving as they ought to behave. And if anything should go wrong, there's *soma*.

Huxley rejects Shakespeare's view of art and order being in harmony and suggests that at least some disorder is necessary to produce real art—order itself produces only sterile contentment.

These five works of art from three different centuries help frame the emotional and intellectual debate about the ends of genetic research today. They keep us centered on the critical issues: What does it mean to be human? and, How can human life be enhanced? Some scientists continue to insist that these questions are none of science's concern. They insist that their job is simply to explore the world in search of new knowledge; society's job is to use, misuse, apply, and misapply that knowledge. The Human Genome Project provides us with a contemporary megaproject that can be used as a vehicle to explore the proper relationship between science and society as science seeks to understand the genetic basis of human characteristics.

THE HUMAN GENOME PROJECT

The Human Genome Project is the effort to map and sequence the approximately 3 billion base pairs of nucleotides that make up the twenty-three different human chromosomes that compose the haploid human genome. The biology of DNA is well described elsewhere.[6] For the purposes of a preliminary exploration of the social policy issues raised by the project, it is only necessary to know a few basic definitions and facts. The first is that the term genome refers to the entire complement of genetic material in the set of chromosomes of a particular organism. Chromosomes are composed of genes (50,000 to 100,000 in a human being), which in turn are composed on deoxyribonucleic acid (DNA), the chemical carrier of genetic information. DNA is made of nucleotides, which are found in two linear strands wrapped around each other in the form of a double helix. The DNA strands are themselves composed of four nucleotides: adenosine (A), guanosine (G), cytidine (C), and thymidine (T). The two strands of DNA are bound together by weak bonds between base pairs of the nucleotide: A's only bind with T's, and G's only bind with C's. The size of the genome is usually expressed as the total number of such base pairs; approximately 3 billion in the twenty-three chromosome (haploid) human genome.

Genetic mapping is the process of assigning genes to specific chromosomes; genetic linkage maps determine where one genetic locus is relative
to another on the basis of how often they are inherited together. A genetic
locus is an identifiable area, or "marker," on a chromosome, the presence
of which indicates that a specific trait (such as eye color or blood type) will
be expressed by the gene. The physical map of greatest interest to scientists
is one that has the highest possible resolution. This is the complete nucleotide sequence of the human genome, and is why the project is often referred
to as "mapping and sequencing" the human genome. Current methods of
sequencing remain laborious, and the complete sequencing of the human
genome will almost certainly require major innovations in sequencing technology.

In the United States there is no single human genome project. Three
major groups are funding various aspects of genome mapping: the National
Institutes of Health (NIH), the U.S. Department of Energy (DOE), and the
Howard Hughes Medical Institute. Other organizations are doing work on
the genome in other countries, and a private organization—the Human
Genome Organization (HUGO)—has so far unsuccessfully proposed that it
act as an international coordinator among countries pursuing this project.

Of course a map is useful in getting you where you want to go, but it
doesn't tell you anything about what it will be like when you get there. For
example, a map of Boston will tell you where streets are located, but it will
not tell you who lives on them or what types of activities occur on various
streets. Likewise, a map of the human genome will tell you where genes are
located on chromosomes, but it will not disclose their functions. Analyzing
the information on the map of the human genome will be yet another,
more complex, project. And as the recent discovery of the gene for cystic
fibrosis has demonstrated, much progress can be made in identifying specific genes without having the map of the genome itself.

The complexity of putting the map itself together, however, should not
be underestimated. MIT geneticist Eric Lander has described it by using a
book reconstruction analogy:

> It's as if I took six sets of *Encyclopaedia Britannica* and shredded them, and
> spread the pieces all over the floor, and asked you to reconstruct the books.
> How do you do that? You look for the pages that overlap so you need multiple
> copies of the books. You would spend a year or two or three just gluing these
> copies together in the correct order. And then you have to read the thing. *That's*
> the genome project.[7]

The Office of Technology Assessment of the U.S. Congress summarized
five arguments which scientists give to support sequencing entire genomes,
which can also be applied to the human genome:

> The information in a genome is the fundamental description of a living
> system . . . and so is of fundamental concern to biologists.

Genome sequences provide a conceptual framework within which much future research in biology will be structured [such as] . . . control of gene expression.

Nearly 90 percent of total DNA content [is likely to have no function]. . . . Without a complete DNA sequence of several genomes, it will be impossible to determine whether such sequences have meaning or are ancestral "junk" sequences.

Genome sequences are important for addressing questions concerning evolutionary biology. The reconstruction of the history of life on this planet, the definition of gene families . . . and the search for a universal ancestor all require an understanding of the organization of genomes.

Genomes are natural information storage and processing systems; unraveling them may be of general interest to computer and physical scientists.[8]

James Watson, the codiscoverer of DNA, headed the NIH Human Genome Center until a dispute over gene fragment patenting led to his resignation in mid-1992. Watson is enthusiastic, stating that he expects that "when finally interpreted the genetic messages encoded within our DNA molecules will prove the ultimate answers to the chemical underpinnings of human existence." He has described the Human Genome Project as consisting of four phases:

One, we map all the genes; two, we sequence all the genes, or break them down into their chemical components, which is the ultimate map; three, we distribute this information to scientists around the world through "in-formatics" that are easily understood and useful; and, fourth, we build in ethical safeguards so that the information is properly used and not exploited to discriminate against anyone.[9]

The uniqueness of the Human Genome Project is not its quest for knowledge. The history of science is filled with little else. What is unique is an understanding at the outset that serious social policy and ethical issues are raised by the research, and that steps ought to be taken now to try to assure that the benefits of the project are maximized and the potential dark side is minimized.

THE LEGAL AND ETHICAL ISSUES RAISED
BY THE HUMAN GENOME PROJECT

To oversimplify somewhat, there are three levels of issues that the Human Genome Project raises: individual/family, society, and species. Almost all of our work on genetics to date has involved the individual/family level, where questions of genetic screening and counseling have center stage. Negligence in failing to offer or to properly perform these tests has resulted in lawsuits for wrongful birth and wrongful life, and standards for genetic screening and counseling have been set by professional organizations.

Issues at the second level implicate society more directly. In the Human Genome Project there are three major societal issues: population-based genetic screening, resource allocation and commercialization, and eugenics. More specifically: To what uses should the fruits of the project be put in screening groups of people, such as applicants for the military, government workers, immigrants, and others? What priority should the genome project have for federal funding, and what role should patenting laws play? Should we attempt to use the new genetics to improve our citizens, either by trying to eliminate specific genetic diseases or by enhancing desirable traits?

Issues at the third level are somewhat more speculative and involve how a genetic view of ourselves could change the way we think about ourselves. This level raises recurrent philosophical questions involving determinism, reductionism, normalcy, and the meaning of health and disease.

This brief cataloging of the major issues raised on each level suggests that there probably are no unique issues raised by the Human Genome Project. On the other hand, this project raises all of the issues in a much more focused manner (certainly a difference in degree if not in kind), and the fact that all of these issues are implicated in the genome project may itself make the project societally unique.

Individual/Family Issues

Genetic screening and counseling are techniques that have been in widespread use in the United States for more than two decades. Stated concisely: "Genetic counseling is the process whereby an individual or family obtains information about a real or possible genetic problem."[10] Counseling is usually primarily directed toward couples deciding whether or not to have children based on their risk of having a child with a genetic handicap, counseling pregnant women about the existence of genetic tests to determine the status of the fetus, and counseling parents of newborns about the genetic condition of their child.

Genetic screening bridges level one and level two issues because it is primarily a public health endeavor that actively seeks out asymptomatic people, many of whom would not otherwise seek medical care or discover their condition. It is primarily a "search in a population for persons possessing certain genotypes that (1) are already associated with disease or predisposed to disease, (2) may lead to disease in their descendants, or (3) may produce other variations not known to be associated with disease."[11] Individuals in the first category are identified for treatment, the second can receive counseling about their reproductive options, and the third are primarily identified for research purposes to help determine the genetic makeup of populations. Screening may target specific groups, such as married couples planning to have children, pregnant women, or newborns.

Since we have had a number of large-scale genetic screening and counseling programs (including Tay-Sachs, sickle cell disease, PKU, and neural tube defects) it might be supposed that we have solved the major social policy issues raised by such screening. This would be incorrect. Partly this is due to the fact that each genetic disease has unique characteristics, and thus each poses some unique issues. For example, some diseases occur most frequently in specific racial or ethnic groups, raising potential issues of discrimination and stigmatization. Other screening tests, such as those for neural tube defects, can only be done on pregnant women, and abortion is the only "treatment." Still others can only be performed on newborns, and screening for conditions, such as PKU, that require immediate treatment to prevent harm, has been made mandatory by almost all states in this context.

Although we have not solved any of the major issues raised by past genetic screening and counseling cases, we have been able to identify the major factors to be considered before initiating a screening program: (1) the frequency and severity of the condition, (2) the availability of treatment of documented efficacy, (3) the extent to which detection by screening improves the outcome, (4) the validity and safety of the screening test, (5) the adequacy of resources to assure effective screening and counseling follow-up, (6) the costs of the program, and (7) the acceptance of the screening program by the community, including both physicians and the public.[12]

This list primarily relates to the scientific validity and a cost/benefit analysis of the testing procedure. In addition, two major legal issues are implicit in all genetic screening programs: autonomy and confidentiality. Autonomy requires that all screening programs be voluntary, and that consent to them is sought only after full information concerning the implications of a positive finding is disclosed and understood. Confidentiality requires that the finding not be disclosed to anyone else without the individual's consent. While not a genetic disease, HIV infection has provided us with an opportunity to see how widespread discrimination against individuals with a particular condition demands that testing be voluntary and that the results be kept confidential to protect the rights of individuals.

Provided that testing remains voluntary, and that the results are only disclosed with the individual's permission, genetic testing based on one's genome raises questions only of degree rather than kind. The degree is that instead of one or even hundreds of conditions that can be screened for, there may be thousands. Perhaps even more important, we may find that certain genes predispose a person to specific illnesses, such as breast cancer or Alzheimer disease. This information may be very troubling to individuals, but it will be of great interest to health insurance companies and employers.

In the employment setting, for example, it has already been suggested that five principles should guide legislators, regulators, and professional groups in setting guidelines for medical screening: (1) medical inquiries of employees should be limited to job-related information; (2) only tests that are safe and of proven efficacy should be used; (3) applicants and employees should be informed of all medical tests in advance, given the results, and told when any employment decision will be based on test results; (4) intracompany and extracompany disclosure of medical records must be controlled and confidentiality assured; and (5) comprehensive, consistent, and predictable handicap discrimination legislation should be enacted.[13] These worthy principles should be supplemented with three others directed at employers: (1) ethical issues involving screening should be fully explored *before* a screening program commences; (2) screening should only be done on an individual with the individual's informed consent; and (3) counseling should be available both before and after screening, and the resources for any reasonable intervention that can benefit the individuals screened should be in place and available to him or her before screening is offered.

We have so far managed to develop genetic screening and counseling as tools that we have permitted individuals and families to use or not use as they see fit. This has followed the medical model of the beneficent doctor-patient relationship: a model of mutuality in which decisions are made for the benefit of the patient. This model has served us well to date in expanding the reproductive options of individuals. Level two concerns move us away from concern with the individual to concern with society itself.

Societal Issues

Societal issues involved in the genome cluster in three areas: population-based screening, resource allocation and commercialism, and eugenics. Of these the first overlaps level one concerns (since population screening can be used to identify individuals to help them), and the last is the most unique and troubling. All merit discussion.

Population-based screening has already been discussed in level one. It can be aimed at the attempted elimination of a genetic condition, at simply identifying the incidence of a genetic condition in a population, or at identifying the presence of a genetic condition in an applicant for a particular benefit (such as employment, insurance, and immigration). As previously discussed, autonomy and confidentiality are the major legal issues involved, and this type of screening becomes problematic primarily when it is mandatory and the results are made known to others without consent. The other two areas are more uniquely societal.

The issue of resource allocation itself has its own three aspects. The first is the obvious one: What percentage of the nation's research budget should be devoted to the Human Genome Project? Answering this question requires us to consider how research priorities are set in science and who should set them. With the federal government making a major commitment to this program (currently approximately $100 million annually each to

NIH and DOE), should Congress appropriate funds directly to the genome project (as it is currently doing) or should the program compete directly with other proposed research projects, and be peer-reviewed?

The second aspect involves making the fruits of the genome project available to all those who want them. This involves at least two questions. The first is the issue of commercialism, and who "owns" and can patent the products that are produced by the genome project. Should the fact that much of this research is federally funded mean that its fruits should be in the public domain? Or should individual companies and scientists be able to patent or copyright maps and sequences of specific areas of the human genome in order to encourage them to become involved in mapping research? Patent issues have proven the most controversial at the outset of the project, and an international agreement on patenting (or not patenting) genes and gene fragments (cDNA) may be a prerequisite to effective international cooperation. The other issue can be summed up in three words: national health financing. Specifically, should the genetic tests and their follow-up procedures be made part of a "minimum benefit package" under a national health financing program (or some other scheme for universal access), or should they only be available to those who can pay for them privately? This, of course, is also not a question unique to the genome project, but one that society must confront with every new medical technology.

The third aspect of the resource allocation issue is probably the most intrinsically interesting. It involves determining the balance of resource priorities between how much we should spend on identifying and treating genetic diseases, as opposed to how much we should spend directly on *other* conditions that cause disease, such as poverty, drug and alcohol addiction, lack of housing, poor education, and lack of access to reasonable medical care. In a country like the United States, is it ethical or rational to develop medical technologies that large segments of the population would not have access to today if they were available, or to develop technologies that even if universally available, would only be useful to a few individuals?

What is the social impact of putting the spotlight on an endeavor like the Human Genome Project? Could the fact that we are vigorously pursuing this project lead us to downplay environmental pollution, worksite hazards, and other major social problems that cause disease based on the hope that we will someday find a "genetic fix" to permit humans to "cope" with these unhealthy conditions? It has been unpersuasively and bizarrely suggested, for example, that the fruits of the Human Genome Project may help solve society's homelessness problem on the basis that many of the homeless are mentally ill, and their condition may be genetically determined and genetically treatable.[14] Finally, what role does or should international economic competition play in deciding how much federal funding should go to the genome project?

The third societal issue, and the most important one, is the issue of eugenics. This issue is perhaps the most difficult to address because of the highly emotional reaction many individuals have to even mentioning the racist genocide of the Nazis, which was based on a eugenic program founded on a theory of "racial hygiene." Although repugnant, the Nazi experience and legacy demands careful study to determine what led to it, why scientists and physicians supported it and collaborated on developing its theory and making possible its execution, and how it was implemented by a totalitarian state. In this regard our own national experience with racism, sterilization, and immigration quotas will have to be reexamined. In so doing, we are likely to rediscover the powerful role of economics in driving our own views of evolution (in the form of social Darwinism) and who should propagate.

The U.S. Supreme Court, for example, wrote in 1927, with clear reference to World War I, that eugenics by involuntary sterilization of the mentally retarded was constitutionally acceptable based on utilitarianism:

> We have seen more than once that the public welfare may call upon the best citizens for their lives. It would be strange if it could not call upon those who already sap the strength of the State for these lesser sacrifices often not felt to be such by those concerned, in order to prevent our being swamped with incompetence. It is better for all the world, if instead of waiting to execute degenerate offspring for crime, or to let them starve for their imbecility, society can prevent those who are manifestly unfit from continuing their kind.[15]

That may seem ancient history, but in 1988 the U.S. Congress's Office of Technology Assessment (OTA) in discussing the "Social and Ethical Considerations" raised by the Human Genome Project, developed a similar theme:

> Human mating that proceeds without the use of genetic data about the risks of transmitting diseases will produce greater mortality and medical costs than if carriers of potentially deleterious genes are alerted to their status and encouraged to mate with noncarriers or to use artificial insemination or other reproductive strategies.[16]

The likely primary reproductive strategy, mentioned only in passing in the report, will be genetic screening of human embryos, already technically feasible, but not nearly to the extent possible once the genome is understood. Such screening need not be governmentally-imposed; people will want it, even insist on it as their right. As OTA notes: "New technologies for identifying traits and altering genes make it *possible for eugenic goals to be achieved through technological as opposed to social control.*" (emphasis added) Huxley's *Brave New World*, rather than George Orwell's *1984*, seems to be in our future.

Much excellent work is under way on the history of medicine and its linkage to the eugenics movement. This scholarship should be made an integral part of any effort to understand the eugenics movement in the 20th century. It will also be necessary to decide whether or not to use genetics to *improve* the species, and to articulate the philosophical and moral concerns that a change in the direction of genetics from prevention and treatment to enhancement and improvement would entail.

So far most writers have insisted that it is at least premature to follow the example of Moreau and try to improve upon the species, either by enhancing certain genetic characteristics, such as height, or by altering sex cells so that characteristics modified in an individual can be passed on to future generations. Just as population-based screening provided a bridge between levels one and two, enhancing genetic traits provides a bridge between levels two and three.

Species Issues

Species issues relate to the fact that powerful new technologies do not just change what human beings can do, they change the way we think, especially about ourselves. In this respect, maps may become particularly powerful thought transformers. Maps model reality to help us understand it. Columbus changed the shape of the world's map forever—from a flat chart to a spherical globe. Monsters could no longer either prowl or guard the edge of the world because there was no edge of the world. Copernicus and Vesalius published their great works in the same year, 1543. *On the Motions of Heavenly Bodies* made it clear that the earth rotated around the sun, not the other way around. The earth could no longer be seen as the "center" of the universe.

Vesalius' "maps" of the human anatomy may have been even more important metaphors for us, for in dissecting the human body, Vesalius insisted that human beings could nonetheless only be understood as whole beings: *human* beings rather than as parts that can be fitted together to manufacture life forms. For Vesalius, who shows twenty-one of seventy-three drawings in his *Fabrica* as full-figured humans, and ten of twelve drawings in his *Epitome* as full-figured humans, the emphasis is firmly on the person, even though the treatise is concerned with the person's body parts. This is in stark contrast to the bar graph illustrations used by contemporary geneticists in mapping the genome, which are totally devoid of human reference, almost life without life. A similar lifeless reductionist phenomena can be seen in the "maps" of areas of the human brain, which are said to correspond to various human emotions and the ability to think and to conceptualize. Does this reconceptualization of the human via a new map encourage us to travel into areas that could lead us to simultaneously misunderstood and demean what it is to be human?

What new human perspectives, or what new perspectives on humans, will a sequential map of the 3 billion base pairs of the human genome bring? The most obvious is that breaking "human beings" down into 6 billion "parts" is the ultimate in reductionism. James Watson himself has used such reductionist language in promoting the Human Genome Project.

In his words, the project will provide "the ultimate tool for understanding ourselves at the molecular level."[17] Just what this means is unclear, but Watson continues: "How can we not do it? We used to think our fate is in our stars. Now we know, in large measure, our fate is in our genes." Seeing our fate in our genes, of course, resonates with level two concerns: if genes determine our fate, then we can alter our fate by altering our genes. Maybe we really will come to believe the unlikely prospect that we can look forward to the day that mental illness, and therefore at least some homelessness, can be prevented by genetic manipulation. Such a view suggests most of the species concerns.

The first is the consequence of viewing humans as an assemblage of molecules, arranged in a certain way. The almost inevitable tendency in such a view is that expressed in *Brave New World*. People could view themselves and each other as products that can be manufactured, and thus subject to quality control measures. People could be "made to measure," both literally and figuratively. If people are so seen, we might not only try to manipulate them as embryos and fetuses, but we might also see the resulting children as products themselves. This raises the current stakes in the debates about frozen embryos and surrogate mothers to a new height: if children are seen as products, the purchase and sale of the resulting children themselves, not only embryos, may be seen as reasonable.

The second concern is that, to the extent that genes are seen as more important than environment, our actions may be viewed as genetically determined, rather than as a result of free will. We have already witnessed an early example with this type of reasoning in the use of the "XYY defense." Those possessing the 47,XYY karyotype were thought to be more prone to commit crime. Individuals accused of crime who also had an extra Y chromosome consequently argued that their genetic composition predisposed them to crime and therefore they should not be held criminally responsible for their actions. This defense was generally rejected, and in the few cases where it was accepted, the defendant was confined to a mental institution until "cured." Of course, since it is impossible to remove the extra Y chromosome from any cell, let alone every cell, in one's body, a cure is not possible.

In addition to use by the criminal law, perhaps in the form of genetic screening followed by monitoring or "predelinquency detention," such genetic predispositions are likely to be used in education, and perhaps job placement and military assignments. For example, if intelligence in mathematics is found to be genetic, should schools use this information to track, grade, and promote the genetically gifted in math classes?

Finally, we know that most diseases and abnormalities are social constructs, not facts of nature. Myopia, for example, is well accepted, whereas obesity is not. We won't discover a "normal" or "standard" human genome, but we may invent one. If we do, what variation will society view as permissible before an individual's genome is labeled substandard or abnormal? And what impact will such a construct of genetic normalcy have on society and on substandard individuals? For example, what variation in a fetus should prompt a couple to opt for abortion, or a genetic counselor to suggest abortion? What variation should prompt a counselor to suggest sterilization? What interventions will society deem acceptable in an individual's life based on his or her genetic composition? Should health care insurance companies, for example, be able to disclaim financial responsibility for the medical needs of a child whose parents knew prior to conception or birth that the child would be born with a seriously abnormal genome? Should employers be able to screen out workers on the basis of their genomes? These and many other similar issues exist today based on screening for single genes. But the magnitude of the screening possibilities that may result from analysis of the map of the human genome will raise these issues to new heights and will almost inevitably change the way we think about ourselves and what it means to be human.

What options exist for policymakers who would like to have the benefits of the Human Genome Project and minimize or control the potential harms?

STRATEGIES TO REGULATE GENETIC TECHNOLOGY

The good news about the Human Genome Project is that its proponents have at least some recognition of the many social, ethical, and legal issues this research raises. NIH's National Center for Human Genome Research, for example, has pledged to spend 3 to 5 percent (and perhaps more) of its research budget for the study of the ethical, social, and legal issues that may arise from the application of knowledge gained from the Human Genome Project. The center also formed an "ethics committee" and hired its own philosopher to help them formulate and deal with the ethical issues. Likewise, the international Human Genome Organization (HUGO), made up of scientists from around the world, has formed its own ethics committee.

The issues that these groups, and others like them, will identify have been outlined. But what strategies exist to deal with them? As we have seen, English literature provides us with a rich backdrop from which to begin our consideration, but actual examples of successful regulatory intervention into either scientific research or technological application are much less plentiful. Nor have scientists and policymakers worked together well in the past. As C. P. Snow has noted: "Non-scientists tend to think of scientists as brash and boastful."[18] This attitude is certainly exemplified in the literature herein summarized, as is the view that scientists underestimate the danger of their work and vastly overestimate its importance. Scientists, on the other hand, tend to think of social policy and ethics as fields that lag behind science and cannot keep up with scientific progress and advance. It is almost as if they believe that morality is a field of knowledge "in the charge of unidentified, but presumably rather incompetent experts."[19] Experts in both fields have little experience with each other, and they generally meet only in courtrooms or in congressional hearing rooms. Scientists then often revert to the old slogan, "What's good for General Motors is good for the country," or, more precisely, as James Watson has put it, "Science is good for society."[20]

The challenge is to get beyond the literary archetypes, the stereotypes, and the clichés, and to work together to develop a coherent set of goals against which we can judge scientific priorities and actions. Once these goals are agreed on in an open and public forum, it will be easier to devise methods to attempt to accomplish them. A few such methods merit further discussion because they are the ones most likely to be used: moratoriums and bans, regulatory agencies, advisory groups, and private lawsuits.

Moratoriums and Bans

Science has had almost no experience with moratoriums, but one of the few that has actually been implemented was in the area of genetic research, specifically recombinant DNA (rDNA) research. It occurred in 1974, when, following approximately three years of discussion, a group of prominent genetic researchers called for a voluntary international moratorium on certain types of recombinant DNA research. The moratorium, which has been termed "a rare, perhaps unique, event in the history of basic science research"[21] was honored internationally from July 1974 to February 1975, when an international meeting of rDNA researchers was convened at Asilomar, California, to consider the future of the moratorium. The result of the Asilomar meeting was agreement that "most of the work on the construction of recombinant DNA molecules should proceed," but that adequate biological and physical containment measures should be taken to prevent the creation and escape of potentially dangerous "newly created organisms."

At a Workshop on International Cooperation for the Human Genome Project held in Valencia, Spain, in October 1988, French researcher Jean Dausset suggested that the genome project posed great potential hazards that could open the door to Nazi-like atrocities. To attempt to avoid such results, he suggested that the conferees agree on a moratorium on genetic manipulation of germ line cells, and a ban on gene transfer experiments in early embryos. Reportedly, the proposal won wide agreement among the participants and was watered down to a resolution calling for "international cooperation" only after American participant Norton Zinder successfully argued that the group had no authority to make such a resolution stick.[22]

Zinder was correct. A moratorium and ban on research that no one wants to do at this point would have only symbolic value—and negative symbolic value at that. It would signal that the scientists could handle the ethical issues alone, and could monitor their own work. It would tend to quiet the discussion of both germ line research and gene transfers in early embryos, both subjects that deserve wide public debate. But Dausset also had a point. The Nazi atrocities grew out of the combination of a public health ethic that saw the abnormal as disposable and a tyrannical dictatorship that was able to give physicians and public health authorities unlimited authority to put their bestial program into practice.

Regulations

It was a combination of the Asilomar call for ending the moratorium, and its simultaneous call for biological and physical containment, that led the federal government to develop specific guidelines governing the conduct of rDNA research by facilities receiving federal funds. These guidelines primarily relied on a series of biological and physical containment measures that increased as the risk of the rDNA experiment increased. Compliance was to be supervised locally by an Institutional Biosafety Committee (IBC), which was requested, but not required, to open its meetings "to the public whenever possible, consistent with protection of privacy and proprietary interests."[23]

A few cities and states were not content to rely on the federal guidelines, so they developed their own. In Cambridge, Massachusetts, the home of Harvard and MIT, as well as many private biotechnology firms, Mayor Al Vellucci said in 1976: "They may come up with a disease that can't be cured—even a monster. Is this the answer to Dr. Frankenstein's dream?"[24] Recombinant DNA research is not, of course, the answer to Frankenstein's dream of animating dead tissue; it is more the answer to Moreau's dream of combining various species into a new, unique creature. Nonetheless, as Lewis Thomas observed, having man don the mantle of creator of life raises the fundamental questions that the Frankenstein myth exemplifies:

> The recombinant DNA line of research is upsetting . . . because it is disturbing in a fundamental way, to face the fact that the genetic machinery in control of the plant's life can be fooled around with so easily. We do not like the idea that anything so fixed and stable as a species line can be changed. The notion that genes can be taken out of one genome and inserted in another is unnerving.[25]

The Frankenstein myth resonated because of rDNA's ability to create new life forms that the creator could not control, and also because of the public's concern that scientists were doing this work for their own enjoyment rather than society's betterment. As Mayor Vellucci put it: "I don't think these scientists are thinking about mankind at all. I think that they're getting the thrills and excitement and the passion to dig in and keep digging to see what the hell they can do." The Mayor here encompasses not only the driving force behind Frankenstein, but that behind Jekyll and Moreau as well. The President's Commission on Bioethics summarized the "Frankenstein factor" in rDNA research as follows: "The fear was that for researchers creating a new life form—even a monster—would be a matter of curiosity; for the public, it would be an assault on traditional values." As a result of their concern, the city of Cambridge developed regulations that called for laboratory inspections by a publicly appointed committee.

Oversight Committees

Closely related to regulation is the establishment of oversight committees. The most prominent of these in the genetics research field has been the Recombinant DNA Advisory Committee (the "RAC") and its subcommittee on genetic engineering. The RAC is a National Institutes of Health committee that advises the secretary of the U.S. Department of Health and Human Services on all matters relating to rDNA research and reviews certain genetic experiments, approving them before they can be carried out. The three specific areas over which the RAC has retained oversight, even in private facilities, are (1) cloning toxin-producing genes, (2) introducing drug resistance into an organism, and (3) deliberately releasing genetically engineered organisms into the environment.[26]

Another type of oversight committee is one that studies an area and makes recommendations as to how it should be regulated. Perhaps the most successful such entity to date has been the President's Commission for the Study of Ethical Problems in Medicine and Biomedical and Behavioral Research, usually called simply "The President's Bioethics Commission" (1978–84). This Commission issued a number of very influential reports, including one on genetic engineering entitled *Splicing Life*. Among the commission's recommendations was that the RAC broaden its areas of scrutiny "to include issues raised by the intended uses of the technique rather than solely the unintended exposure from laboratory experiments."[27] The commission also sensibly suggested that the "next generation" RAC should be financially independent of federal funding agencies like NIH, to avoid any real or perceived conflict of interest. Although the RAC did later broaden its agenda to include prior review of all proposed research on genetic modification of human beings, it is still part of NIH. When it is appropriate to begin human experiments with gene therapy remains controversial. As early as 1980 it was suggested that human trials should not begin until three conditions are met in animal trials: (1) the new gene should be put into target cells and remain there; (2) the new gene should be regulated appropriately; and (3) the presence of the new gene should not harm the cell.[28]

Self-Regulation and Private Tort Suits

The RAC was heavily lobbied to transform its guidelines into voluntary "laboratory standards" in the early 1980s, but it refused. Most scientists would prefer to police themselves and not have nonscientists involved in monitoring or regulating their work. On the other hand, they are often horrified at the notion that they might be held personally responsible for the harm that their research causes others. The final formal speaker at the Asilomar conference, for example, Professor Roger Dworkin, suggested that current law already imposes heavy obligations on scientists to be careful and to have a laboratory workplace that is "free of hazard." He got the scientists' immediate attention by suggesting that a multimillon-dollar lawsuit "may sneak up on you" if you're not careful. But he also made the equally important point that courts traditionally look to the industry to set its own standards, and they almost always rely on industry standards in determining the relevant standard of care.[29]

The fact is that in most areas, even those heavily regulated, the professionals themselves will have much, if not everything, to say about the standards applied to their work. Under almost any standards, Frankenstein and Moreau would be guilty of gross negligence and cruelty in abandoning their creations and inflicting suffering upon them. Jekyll might properly argue that he was experimenting on himself, but, of course, he would still be criminally responsible for the murders committed by Hyde.

Future lawsuits are likely to be of three kinds. The first will involve the accidental or purposeful release of a dangerous organism into the environment. This is the type of harm Mayor Velluci worried about, and which could give rise to traditional tort suits alleging nuisance, trespass, battery, and/or negligent failure to contain the organism. The second kind of suit will involve those tho apply the new knowledge gained by the genome project to the clinical setting: cases involving wrongful birth (for failure to counsel about existing technology that results in a couple having a child they would not otherwise have had, and who is genetically handicapped) and cases involving wrongful life (suits by a child alleging that it would have been better off not having been born, and would not have been born if the physician had properly counseled its parents or properly performed agreed to screening tests). The third type of lawsuit will be one for breach of confidentiality leading to a loss on the basis of discrimination. For example, a physician may be sued for improperly disclosing a genetic diagnosis to an employer who then fires the employee on the basis of the genetic information. As can be seen from this listing, tort suits will be most useful *after* genetic screening tests have been developed and will likely have little impact on their ultimate development itself. In this regard it is at least of some interest that many physicians already consider the legal profession to be Frankenstein's monster incarnate, and the actions of malpractice attorneys every bit as destructive as the creatures on Moreau's island.

WHERE DO WE GO FROM HERE?

It seems reasonable to conclude from the various methods that have been employed to review genetic research and the clinical applications of that research that individual/family concerns (level one) will be dealt with by a combination of oversight committees, regulation, self-regulation, and private lawsuits. Societal concerns (level two) are not readily approached by private lawsuit, and so they will likely require congressionally mandated regulation, most likely based on suggestions by advisory committees with broad public input. Species concerns (level three) are not subject to legal regulation at all, except insofar as specific practices, such as the purchase and sale of "high grade embryos," can be outlawed altogether. But this may be the area that has the most long term impact on us, and the one about which we therefore need the most careful and creative thinking.

It is on the species level concerns that the cautionary tales with which this chapter opened focus. Mary Shelley's tale, for example, teaches us a lesson that we find hard to deal with seriously: as difficult as it is to create a monster, it is even more difficult to control it or to restore order after the creation has spawned chaos. In seeking to control our world, we may in fact lessen our control over it. Robert Oppenheimer unwittingly made this point in reference to the Manhattan Project to a Congressional Committee in 1945. He was testifying on the role of science in the development of the atomic bomb:

> When you come right down to it, the reason that we did this job is because it was an organic necessity. If you are a scientist, you cannot stop such a thing. If you are a scientist, you believe that it is good to find out how the world works; that it is good to find what the realities are; that it is good to turn over to mankind at large the greatest possible power to control the world.[30]

The striking thing in Oppenheimer's testimony is his emphasis on the notion that science is unstoppable, with the simultaneous insistence that its goal is control over nature—irreconcilable concepts that seem equally at the heart of the Human Genome Project. Of course, with the atomic bomb, control quickly became illusory. The bomb, which carries with it the promise of the total annihilation of mankind, has made the nation state ultimately unstable and put it at the mercy of every other nation with the bomb. Necessity has forced all nuclear powers to move, however slowly, toward a transnational community.

In view of the way scientists have thought about their pursuits and projects in the past, it is informative to review the goals of the Human Genome Project set forth above, with the list of the legal, ethical, and social policy issues raised by the project. There is almost no overlap. Scientists are working on an interesting scientific question to gain new knowledge and insight into what genes do, and what we can learn about man's origins and relationship to other species. If we take the scientists at face value, they have given no more thought to the potential social applications of genome mapping and sequencing than Frankenstein had given to the consequences of creating his monster, or than Moreau had given to the consequences of his experiments in modifying life forms. Our own "brave new world" will not be ruled by scientists, any more than scientists decided whether or not to use the atomic bomb or whether to send a man to the moon. Social policy will ultimately be set by elected politicians and their advisers. It is already past time to begin to involve the electorate in a national debate about the appropriate uses (and the misuses) of the products of the Human Genome Project.

In this discussion, the focus should be on two central questions: what does it mean to be human, and, how can human life on this planet be enhanced? To even begin to address these issues in the genome context, the public and policymakers need to understand the Human Genome Project, and the cartographers of the human genome need to be able to recognize and deal with the *real* monsters lurking outside their laboratories.

With both real and psychological walls crumbling around the world, the time may be at hand for meaningful international dialogue and cooperation on the Human Genome Project. It may also be possible, although perhaps this is wishful thinking, to engage the world in a responsible debate about all of our futures, and to do so in a manner that strives to enhance the dignity of all human beings. Playwright, former political prisoner, and former president of Czechoslovakia, Vaclav Havel expressed it well in a 1984 speech on "Politics and Conscience":

> To me, personally, the smokestack soiling the heavens is . . . the symbol of an age which seeks to transcend the boundaries of the natural world and its norms and to make the matter merely a private concern, a matter of subjective preference and private feeling. The process of anonymisation and depersonalization of power, and its reduction to a mere technology of rule and manipulation, has a thousand masks. . . . States grow ever more machine-like, men are transformed into casts of extras, as voters, producers, consumers, patients, tourists or soldiers. . . .
>
> The question . . . is . . . whether we shall, by whatever means, succeed in rehabilitating the personal experience of human beings as the measure of things, placing morality above politics and responsibility above our desires, in making human community meaningful, in returning content to human speaking, in reconstituting, as the focus of all social activity, the autonomous, integral and dignified human "I," responsible for himself because he is bound to something higher. . . . If we can defend our humanity, then, perhaps, there is a hope of sorts that we shall also find some more meaningful ways of balancing our natural claims to shared economic control, to dignified social status. . . . As long, however, as our humanity remains defenseless, we will not be saved by any better economic functioning, just as no filter on a factory smokestack will prevent the general dehumanization. To what purpose a system functions is, after all, more important than how it does so; might it not function quite smoothly, after all, in the service of total destruction?[31]

Havel's image of the smokestack is striking: the inanimate destroyer has replaced the animate monster in industrial society. Governments grow more machine-like and, in consequence, treat their citizens as interchangeable parts of that machine. The machine-men become alienated even from themselves; and technology cannot save them from artificiality. Only their "natural" humanness and their ability to distinguish good from evil can save humanity.

Havel obviously did not have the Human Genome Project in mind when he wrote his 1984 speech, nor when he delivered a speech to a joint session of the U.S. Congress in February 1990. Nonetheless, his 1984 words aptly summarize the challenge we face, and his 1990 words to the Congress properly insist that we all take personal responsibility for our own actions and the future of our world: "Without a global revolution in the sphere of human consciousness, nothing will change for the better in the sphere of our being."[32]

In 1992, after more than two years as president of Czechoslovakia, Havel reaffirmed his belief in the ability of postmodernist politicians to rediscover the "soul, individual spirituality, [and] first-hand personal insight into things" and to have "the courage to be himself and go the way his conscience points." Although Havel was speaking specifically about the need to fill the void left by the death of worldwide communism with a new humanism, his words seem directly applicable to the Human Genome Project:

The end of Communism is, first and foremost, a message to the human race. It is a message we have not yet fully deciphered and comprehended. In its deepest sense, the end of Communism has brought a major era in human history to an end. It has brought an end not just to the 19th and 20th centuries, but to the modern age as a whole.[33]

In Havel's vision, and in the visions of the authors we have reviewed, "the modern era has been dominated by the culminating belief, expressed in different forms, that the world—and Being as such—is a wholly knowable system governed by a finite number of universal laws that man can grasp and rationally direct for his own benefit." This view, both Havel and history suggest, is well wide of the mark, and the very survival of our species depends on the adoption of a paradigm based not on further collection of information but on "such forces as a natural, unique and unrepeatable experience of the world, an elementary sense of justice, the ability to see things as others do, a sense of transcendental responsibility, archetypal wisdom, good taste, courage, compassion and faith in the importance of particular measures that do not aspire to be a universal key to salvation."[34]

Can the "new world" United States learn from the old? Can "new science" learn to take its social responsibilities seriously? Can we use our species consciousness to help us confront not only the promise but also the perils of the new genetics? It will not happen easily in a country where new is still seen as better, and where the future is still seen as limitless. It is, after all, not Mary Shelley's but Gatsby's view of our future that prevails:

Gatsby believed in the green light, the orgiastic future that year by year recedes before us. It eluded us then, but that's no matter—tomorrow we will run faster, stretch our arms further. . . . And one fine morning—
So we beat on, boats against the current, borne back ceaselessly into the past.[35]

12

Outrageous Fortune:
Selling Other People's Cells

Biotechnology has come to mean mining for biological gold. Perhaps the most emblematic bioethics-biotechnology case is the case of John Moore. California courts decided who could reap profits from a cell line developed from his spleen, and in the process gave "insider trading" a whole new meaning.[1]

In 1976 John Moore, then a surveyor with the Alaskan pipeline, sought medical treatment for hairy cell leukemia from hematologist-oncologist David W. Golde at the University of California at Los Angeles (UCLA). As is standard procedure in this disease, Golde recommended that Moore's spleen, which had enlarged from about a half pound to more than fourteen pounds, be removed. Moore quickly improved after the surgery. Golde took a sample from the spleen and isolated and cultured an immortal cell line capable of producing a variety of products, including the lymphokine GM-CSF (granulocyte-macrophage colony stimulating factor). In 1979, Golde filed a report of possible patentability with the University of California. In 1983 the University applied for a patent on the cell line naming Golde, and his research assistant Shirley Quan, as inventors. The patent was granted in 1984.

Moore, who had since moved to Seattle, had been returning to California to see Golde about every six months. He told an interviewer that he never would have known about the existence of the cell line had Golde not called him in September 1983 and told him he had "missigned the consent form" (circling I "do not" instead of I "do" grant the University all rights in "any cell line"). Moore then decided to consult attorney Sanford Gage.[2]

In September 1984, Moore filed suit against the University of California, Golde, Quan, and two corporations, alleging eleven types of wrongdoing (including conversion, lack of informed consent, and breach of fiduciary duty) and seeking an accounting and other relief. The trial court essentially decided that Moore had no right to bring suit. Moore appealed, and in July 1988 a California Court of Appeals, in a 2 to 1 decision, determined that Moore had stated a proper cause of action for conversion.[3]

THE APPEALS COURT DECISION

Judge David Rothman, writing for the majority, concentrated on just one issue: Did Moore state a cause of action for conversion? Conversion is a strict liability tort that under California law is committed against a person if the person can prove (1) ownership or right to possession of property at the time of the conversion, (2) the wrongful conversion or disposal of the property, and (3) damages. As a strict liability tort, conversion requires neither knowledge or intent of the defendant, but instead "rests upon the unwarranted interference by the defendant with the dominion over the property of the plaintiff from which injury to the latter results." For example, in one case the defendant bought a building in which the plaintiff was a subtenant who had used the basement to store numerous barrels of wine. The defendant, thinking the barrels were junk, sold them. He was liable for conversion in spite of his lack of knowledge of their value or intent to wrongfully profit from their sale.

Thus the Moore case raises three questions regarding conversion: Were the spleen cells Moore's property? Did Golde wrongfully take them? And did Moore suffer damages as a result?

ARE CELLS PROPERTY?

By California statute: "The ownership of a thing is the right of one or more persons to possess and use it to the exclusion of others. . . . The thing of which there may be ownership is called property." We are unaccustomed to think of the human body as property and have put many controls over the disposition of organs and deceased bodies, including a prohibition on the sale of organs and tissue for transplantation. Nonetheless, we do have the exclusive right to our organs and tissues, at least while they are in our bodies, and the court seems correct in concluding: "The essence of property interest—the ultimate right of control . . . exists with regard to one's own body."

The court saw this as debatable, but it had no sympathy at all with the defendants' position that researchers, doctors, universities, and private companies can own human cells, but individuals cannot. Similarly, the defendants' contention that a diseased spleen is a thing of no value was negated by the fact that the cells from the spleen were the foundation of a multimillion-dollar industry.

The court was equally unimpressed with the argument that permitting the plaintiff to participate in the economic gain from his cells would inhibit scientific progress:

> Biotechnology is no longer a purely research oriented field in which the primary incentives are academic or for the betterment of humanity. Biological materials no longer pass freely to all scientists. As here, the rush to patent for exclusive use is rampant. The links being established between academics and industry to profitize biological specimens are a subject of great concern. If this science has become science for profit, then we fail to see any justification for excluding the patient from participation in those profits.

ABANDONMENT AND CONSENT

Wasn't Moore's surgically removed spleen just "medical waste" that he abandoned for the physicians to dispose of as they saw fit? This has certainly been the traditional view. For example, when another patient sued a physician and hospital for cremating his amputated leg, the knowledge of which he said caused him to have nightmares, the Kentucky Supreme Court was unsympathetic. It ruled that, at least in the absence of "any specific reservation, demand, or objection to some normal procedure," the patient accepts the standard method the hospital uses to dispose of amputated body parts when he consents to surgery.[4] And the American Medical Association's legal office has recommended use of the following clause in standard surgical consent forms: "I consent to the disposal by hospital authorities of any tissues or body parts that may be removed."[5] Such disposal has always meant incineration or burial and does not envision, for example, burial at sea.

Although not relying on the Kentucky case, Judge Rothman reached a similar conclusion. He asserted that "internment or incineration" would have been proper disposal methods about which Moore could not have complained. But "any use . . . which is not within the accepted understanding of the patient is a conversion. It cannot be seriously asserted that a patient abandons a severed organ to the first person who takes it, nor can it be presumed that the patient is indifferent to whatever use might be made of it." The conclusion follows naturally: "commercial exploitation" of human tissue is improper "without the consent of the living patient." As to damages, the court concluded that this was an issue properly for the jury.

Dissenting, Judge Ronald George would have dismissed the case because he thought Moore's claim trivial. He said, for example, that he was "not prepared to extend the constitutionally sanctified right of property . . . to the refuse found on the floor of the barbershop or nail salon, in the hospital bedpan, or in the operating room receptacle." Moore's contribution to the value of the cell line was minimal, "like unformed clay or stone transformed by the hands of a master sculptor into a valuable work of art." Finally, as a matter of public policy, Judge George thought that permitting patients to sell or profit from their organs and tissues would impede medical progress because patients might refuse to cooperate or try to sell to the highest bidder. Therefore, he thought it proper for the legislature, not the courts, to decide what should be done in a case like this.

THE CORRECT ANALOGY?

Is the fact that Moore's spleen was diseased and removed for therapeutic reasons sufficient to conclude that it was of no value to him? Judge Rothman said no and suggested the following analogy. Suppose crude oil is ruining a farmer's corn crop, and suppose that the farmer may even be willing to pay an oil refinery to take it off his land. Even though the farmer cannot make any use of the oil without the aid of the refinery, he is still entitled to a share in the refinery's profits from the product of his land.[6]

Other agricultural analogies have been suggested. For example, under Roman law, as long as crops remain in the ground, they are generally owned by the person who owns the ground. If they are removed, ownership depends on whether they are *fructus naturales* (perennials such as trees and grasses) or *fructus industriales* (annuals such as corn): Severed vegetables belonged to the gardener, whereas severed trees belonged to the landowner. The distinction was based on the amount of human input: the more effort expended, the more likely ownership was to reside in the gardener. This analogy favors the physician. So does a similar Roman law doctrine, "specification," that holds that when an entirely new product is fashioned out of products belonging to another, the person who performs the transformation owns the final product.[7]

Neither of these doctrines, however, settles the question of damages. Even if the physician-researcher now owns the cell line, he may still owe the patient something. Judge George thought that something would be the value of the portion of the spleen that was taken at the time—that is, nothing or almost nothing. But, since the cells are living and reproduce, a more apt agricultural analogy may be one stemming from farm animals. The progeny of animals are the property of the mother's owner under the maxim *partus sequitur ventrem* ("the birth comes from the womb"). In addition, an owner wrongfully deprived of livestock can get the value of the eggs from converted chickens and milk from converted cows. These cases support a claim that the patient would have for the value of the output of the cell line resulting from wrongly taken tissues or cells.[8]

This suggests what may be the proper analogy. Suppose a farmer's cow is dying and threatens to infect the rest of his herd. His neighbor agrees to care for the cow on the neighbor's farm, both of them believing the cow's illness is fatal. Under the neighbor's care, the cow recovers. Instead of returning the cow, he keeps it. Over the years, it has a dozen calves before the farmer discovers what the neighbor has done. Under animal progeny cases the farmer should be able to recover not only the value of the cow, but also the value of the calves as well (perhaps deducting the cost of food and medicine).

The problem with treating Moore's spleen like garbage is that Moore did not abandon it (his physician removed it to do with it whatever is customarily done with removed organs), nor, had he known his spleen was valuable, would he have abandoned it after removal. Indeed, it is primarily because of what researchers fear patients will do (that is, not voluntarily relinquish their rights in commercial products resulting from manipulation of their cells) that researchers oppose even discussing the potential value of cells with patients. Perhaps a more apt analogy involving garbage is that a person is usually happy to have their garbage removed; if there are two competing garbage companies, however, and one will pay to take the garbage away (or will do it cheaper than the other), people will usually let the company that will pay have the garbage. If yet a third company discovers a way to turn garbage into gold, most people would want to charge that company even more, and, if their garbage is unique, they might well hold out for a share of the profits.

THE CALIFORNIA SUPREME COURT

The California Supreme Court ignored all of these interesting and useful analogies and examined only two questions: Can Moore sue Golde for failure to disclose his pecuniary interest in producing a cell line from Moore's spleen as a breach of his fiduciary duty to the patient? And can Moore sue the research companies and others who have used the cell line for a share in their profits from it? In a 5 to 2 opinion, Justice Edward Panelli, writing for the California Supreme Court, answered the first question affirmatively but refused to grant the patient any ownership interest in his cells after they had been removed from his body.[9]

The California Supreme Court has been the nation's leader in the area of informed consent, deciding in 1972 that a physician had a "fiduciary" responsibility to the patient to disclose the nature of the proposed treatment, its alternative, risks, and problems of recuperation.[10] Past cases have all concentrated on the patient's choice, enhancing that choice by providing "material" information to the patient, information that might cause the patient to accept or reject the proposed treatment. Remarkably, the California Supreme Court ruled that the doctrine of informed consent requires a full financial disclosure by a physician because failure to make a financial disclosure is a violation of trust that undermines patient autonomy.

The goal is to protect patients from physicians whose judgment might be influenced by profit and who might thus be in a conflict-of-interest position with their own patients. In the court's words:

A physician who treats a patient in whom he also has a research interest has potentially conflicting loyalties. . . . The possibility that an interest extraneous to the patient's health has affected the physician's judgment is something a reasonable patient would want to know in deciding whether to consent to a proposed course of treatment. It is material to the patient's decision and, thus, a prerequisite to informed consent.

This is not to say that physician-researchers are evil-minded or intentionally advocate procedures not in their patients' best interests, only that "consciously or unconsciously . . . the physician's extraneous motivation may affect his judgment."

Selling Cells

The remaining defendants—the Regents of the University of California, a researcher, and two corporations—were not physicians and thus had no independent fiduciary duty to the patient. The appeals court had found them potentially liable for conversion of Moore's property interest in his cells. The California Supreme Court, however, reversed this holding. It gave three reasons: no previous court had ever decided that a patient had a continuing property interest in excised cells; California statutes drastically limit the patient's interest in excised cells; and the patented Mo cell line is "both factually and legally distinct from the cells taken from Moore's body."

Probably because none of these reasons is terribly persuasive, the court went on at length to discuss the public policy reasons that it believed supported the denial of Moore's property claim. Again there were three: a fair balancing of interests counsels against recognizing the claim; the legislature should solve this problem; and Moore's rights can be protected by a suit against the physician. Of these three, the centerpiece of the opinion is the first. The court essentially concluded that the biotechnology industry is both wonderful and fragile. Since it is wonderful, we must all do our part to foster it; since it is fragile, we must protect it from harm:

> Research on human cells plays a critical role in medical research. . . . Products developed through biotechnology that have already been approved for marketing in this country include treatments and tests for leukemia, cancer, diabetes, dwarfism, hepatitis-B, kidney transplant rejection, emphysema, osteoporosis, ulcers, anemia, infertility, and gynecological tumors, to name but a few. . . . The extension of conversion law into this area will hinder research by restricting access to the necessary raw materials.

In the court's flowery words, recognizing conversion would threaten "to destroy the economic incentive to conduct important medical research . . . . With every cell sample a researcher would purchase a ticket in the litigation lottery." On the other hand, denying Moore's property claim "will only make it more difficult for Moore to recover a highly theoretical windfall."

Justice Armand Arabian concurred because he thought a market in human flesh would "commingle the sacred with the profane." On the other hand, he favored a legislatively created licensing scheme that would establish a fixed rate of profit sharing between researcher and subject.[11] He seemed to genuinely regret the lack of compensation to Moore, but concluded his opinion with a quotation from *Hamlet*, noting that "Courts cannot and should not fashion a remedy for every 'heartache and the thousand natural shocks that flesh is heir to.'"

The Dissenting Opinions

Justice Allen Broussard argued that the majority confused the right to control one's body parts *after* removal with the right to control them prior to removal. More important, Broussard also noted persuasively that the majority's conclusion cannot rest on the proposition that there is no ownership or right of possession in removed body parts because if another drug company or medical center now stole the cells from UCLA, "there would be no question but that a cause of action for conversion would properly lie against the thief." He here captures the irony of the conclusion that everyone *except* the patient can own the patient's removed cells and treat them as property. Finally, he argued that, unlike traditional informed consent cases where the plaintiff must prove that a reasonable person would not have consented to the procedure if the required material information had been provided, in an economic damages case like this, the plaintiff should only have to prove that "the doctor's wrongful failure to disclose information proximately caused the plaintiff some type of compensable damage." Although the majority did not discuss it, Broussard opined that "in appropriate circumstances, punitive as well as compensatory damages would clearly be recoverable in such an action."

Justice Stanley Mosk's dissent made it painfully clear that the majority had virtually no rational basis for its opinion other than its view that upholding Moore's claim would be bad for business. For example, the majority relied on statutes that permit the "scientific" use of body parts after donation or autopsy. But Mosk argued that this does not extend to commerce. In his words, the question is not between not-for-profit science and for-profit science (as the majority accused him of), "but the concept of *science*: the distinction I draw . . . is between a truly *scientific* use and the blatant *commercial* exploitation of Moore's tissue." Whatever the statutes on the disposition of human tissues, Mosk concludes, "at the time of its excision he [Moore] had at least *the right to do with his own tissue whatever the defendants did with it*." (emphasis added)

THE BIOTECH INDUSTRY

The core of the dissent, like the core of the opinion, is the public policy discussion of the nature and the future of the for-profit biotechnology industry. The majority saw it as a congenial enterprise in which cell lines are freely shared for the good of scientific progress. Mosk is not so kind, noting that the "rush to patent for exclusive use has been rampant," and with it has come "a drastic reduction in the formerly free access of researchers to new cell lines and their products."

The biotechnology and pharmaceutical companies have also "demanded and received exclusive rights in the scientist's discoveries, and frequently placed those discoveries under trade secret protection. . . . Secrecy as a normal business practice is also taking hold in university research laboratories." As for the burdens of upholding Moore's strict liability conversion claim, Mosk is not persuaded. Researchers usually keep records in any event, and by such record keeping any researcher "can be assured that the source of the material has consented to his proposed use of it, and hence that use is not a conversion."

Mosk argued that public policy actually requires an acceptance of Moore's claim because of the deep respect we accord to the human body "as the physical and temporal expression of the unique human persona" and principles of equity and fairness. According to Mosk, our traditional respect for the individual's body has been demonstrated by laws against torture and slavery, and these laws are directly implicated "whenever scientists or industrialists claim . . . the right to appropriate and exploit a patient's tissue for their sole economic benefit — the right, in other words, to freely mine or harvest valuable physical properties of the patient's body."

The second policy concern is fairness: "Our society values fundamental fairness in dealings between its members, and condemns the unjust enrichment of any member at the expense of another." Justice Mosk terms such unjust enrichment both "inequitable and immoral," quoting Thomas Murray as saying, "If biotechnologists fail to make provisions for a just sharing of profits with the person whose gift made it possible, the public's sense of justice will be offended and no one will be the winner."

The precise contours of the informed consent holding are unclear, but Mosk argued that it is a "paper tiger" because few patients would actually refuse to consent based solely on economic considerations. In his view such a cause of action would only give patients "a veto over their own exploitation." A recognition of their continuing property interest in their own tissue, however, "would give patients an affirmative right of participation" in the role of equal partners in commercial biotechnology research.

Finally, in an unusual conclusion, Justice Mosk disassociated himself completely from the "amateur biology lecture that the majority imposes on us throughout their opinion." He did this because there was no evidence at all about molecular biology in the record before the court (all the scientific material was in an appendix in the Golde brief), the material was irrelevant to the law, in technological jargon, and "no member of this court is a trained molecular biologist or even a physician." Thus, he concluded, it is not surprising that "some of their explanations appear either mistaken, confused, or incomplete."

BLINDED BY SCIENCE

There are many ways to look at this case. As is clear from its text, the majority simply accepts the "chicken little" argument that if John Moore's property interest in his cells is upheld, the biotechnology industry's sky will fall on them and medical progress will suffer a major setback. In this regard the justices seem to have been blinded by science and unable or unwilling to distinguish it from commerce. They are blinded in another way as well, as Justice Mosk notes, when they adopt complex molecular biology terms which they proceed to use in ways that are at the very least unclear, and often either incorrect or irrelevant. Since the court will not permit these issues to even be heard, there will be no occasion for any fair presentation of the science actually involved in creating and maintaining cell lines. Even a "law and economics" approach would have required giving some value to Moore's cells, and would have insisted that it be taken into account as a cost of doing business in the biotechnology arena.

It is not necessarily wrong for courts to base their ultimate conclusions on their interpretation of public policy. On the other hand, courts have an obligation to analyze and struggle with novel questions of law as part of our common law tradition. It is thus very disappointing to see the majority simply ignore the insightful and powerful analysis of the appeals court on the issue of conversion. Instead of searching for possible analogies in the law that might illuminate the conflict, the court summarily dismissed the conversion claim with the unhelpful statement that Moore was invoking "a tort theory originally used to determine whether the loser or the finder of a horse had the better title."

Even though commentators on this case have concentrated on the conversion/property aspects of it, and have correctly argued that it is a major victory for the biotechnology industry, the most important aspect of the opinion deals with the expansion of the informed consent requirements based on the fiduciary nature of the doctor–patient relationship. The court had no problem with a biotechnology industry that breathlessly pursues profits: This is the way American business operates. But physicians are another matter altogether: when physicians are in a position to personally profit from their own treatment recommendations, the court believes they must disclose this financial or research aspect to their patient as part of informed consent. Of course this applies to Golde and Moore. But their rationale would also apply to physicians who recommend a procedure or treatment that will pay them more than an alternative treatment or procedure. Incentives need not be just financial; any "interest extraneous to the patient's health" that might affect the recommendation must be disclosed. Should informed consent now concentrate as much on the financial motives of the physician as on the nature of the proposed procedure? Should the physician's tax returns and percentage of income derived from the recommended procedure be part of informed consent? Must the physician disclose marital problems, kids in college, a loss in the stock market, or other personal or financial troubles that might affect her judgment?

The expansion of the informed consent doctrine in this manner requires much more analysis than the court presented. When, for example, does the physician's personal interest in the treatment recommendation or personal problems become so overwhelming as to *disqualify* the physician altogether as a potential advisor to the patient? Under what circumstances might a second, neutral, opinion be required? In the organ and tissue business we already have two examples where ethical standards, although not law, counsel that even the appearance of a conflict of interest should disqualify the physician from making certain decisions. The first is that transplant surgeons should not be involved in the determination of death of a potential donor, and the second (as discussed in the following chapter) is that physicians who perform abortions should not get any reward, financial or academic, from fetal tissue research.

MINING FOR BIOLOGICAL GOLD

Garbage companies have no obligation to tell their clients what is being done with their garbage—but physicians do. The doctor–patient relationship is a fiduciary relationship, and part of that trust is the assumption that anything not disclosed to the patient is withheld because the information could not affect the patient's decision, or the withheld information concerns something done for the patient's benefit. This is hardly the case when a patient's organ is mined for biological gold. Here, information is withheld for the benefit of the physician or researcher, and the justification offered is that the patient might not agree to donate the tissue, but might instead expect some compensation in the event it is transformed into a commercial product.

To paraphrase Leona Helmsley, the majority opinion concludes that "only the little people can't sell cells." This result will seem unfair to almost everyone. Legislation thus seems both reasonable and likely. What should such legislation contain? Judge Rothman seems correct. If human cells are to be sources of profit, patented, or both, the person from whom these cells derive should have at least as much standing to own and profit from their commercial exploitation as the physician and the biotechnology company. This leaves essentially two choices. My preference is to discourage increasing commercialization of the body and its tissues by amending the Patent Act explicitly to prohibit the patenting of human cells (including genes and gene fragments), and the Organ Transplant Act to include a prohibition on the sale of human tissue and cells for any purpose (not just when they are intended for transplantation).

Until we can overcome our appetite for profit, however, we will need to deal with the world as we find it. Fairness and respect for persons require that we explicitly inform patients that their organs, tissues, and cells may be used for commercial purposes when this is intended. Patients should have a right to accept or reject this use, and they should be offered reasonable compensation if they agree to it. This compensation could be in the form of a small payment for exclusive rights or an agreement that a small percentage of profits (or gross sales) would accrue to the patient in the unlikely event that a commercially successful product were developed.

Since most removed tissues will not turn out to be valuable, however, and since paying even a small price for all of them may simply be a waste of money, perhaps the most reasonable thing to do is to provide that compensation shall be paid based on a standard fee schedule (such as 1 percent of gross sales), payment to be made either to the individual or to a nonprofit cell line storage facility, the election to be made by the patient at the time of consent to the removal. A clause in a standard consent form requiring the patient to simply waive all property rights in tissues and cells should be legally ineffective as a coercive "adhesion" contract.

This or some similar scheme will have to be adopted if we want to prevent physicians and researchers from being seen as simply opportunistic profit seekers. The law cannot remedy every "heartache and the thousand natural shocks that flesh is heir to," but it can serve quite adequately to craft reasonable commercial agreements that protect against "the slings and arrows of outrageous fortune" and are fair to all parties.

III

PUBLIC SECTOR
BIOETHICS

13

The Politics of Fetal Tissue Transplants

Research involving human fetal tissue has been the subject of intense political debate in the United States for two decades, and the use of fetal tissue for transplant continues this controversy in another forum.[1] Since *Roe v. Wade*,[2] the federal government has focused public attention on fetal research by creating panels of experts. For example, in 1974 Congress created the National Commission for the Protection of Human Subjects of Biomedical and Behavioral Research and put the formulation of regulations on fetal research first on its agenda. The resulting regulations were reasonable, but no federally funded research on either fetuses or in vitro fertilization has been done in the United States, primarily because of the Reagan and Bush administrations' view on the moral status of the human embryo. In this regard, the "right to life" groups may be viewed as the most effective political lobbying "bioethics" groups of the 1980s.

The law approves of fetal tissue transplants. Current federal regulations, for example, permit the use of tissue from deceased fetuses for experimental transplants when conducted in accordance with state law.[3] Virtually all states permit such experiments.[4] Nonetheless, ethical concerns remain, and there has been continued political resistance to using public money to fund research with fetal tissues. Ethical issues cannot be resolved by a vote of experts, but experts can help to publicly define and clarify issues and build consensus. Expert panels can take the political heat off elected officials on controversial issues, and politics is inherent in public funding. The most recent series of disputes began in October 1987, when the National Institutes of Health (NIH) submitted a request to the Assistant Secretary for Health asking approval to transplant human fetal tissue into the brain of a patient suffering from Parkinson disease.

In March 1988, Assistant Secretary Robert Windom asked the NIH to establish a special advisory panel to answer ten questions regarding fetal tissue transplant research. And in May 1988, a moratorium on federally funded transplant research using fetuses from elective abortions was announced.

HUMAN FETAL TISSUE PANEL

NIH's twenty-one–member Human Tissue Fetal Transplant Research Panel invited more than fifty individuals, including representatives of sixteen groups, to present their views in public sessions. On December 5, 1988, the panel finalized its report,[5] and on December 14 the advisory committee to the NIH Director unanimously adopted it. The panel wisely separated the transplantation of fetal tissue from issues involving abortion. This is legally and ethically appropriate, but politically untenable. For example, before President Bush's nominee for Secretary of Health and Human Services (HHS), Louis Sullivan, was confirmed, he had to agree with administration policy on only two issues: abortion and the fetal tissue transplant ban.

The panel's task was somewhat simplified by limiting discussion to the use of tissue from *dead* fetuses (excluding live but nonviable fetuses), by rejecting any payment for fetal tissue (consistent with an October 1988 amendment to The National Organ Transplant Act), and by rejecting intrafamilial donations. The panel concluded that, although it is of "moral relevance" that the fetal tissue is obtained from an induced abortion (rather than a spontaneous abortion or an interrupted ectopic pregnancy), use of the tissue in research is "acceptable public policy" because "abortion is legal and . . . the research in question is intended to achieve significant medical goals." This conclusion was accepted on a vote of 15 to 2; it included recommendations that the abortion decision be kept independent from the decision to retrieve and use fetal tissue, that recipients be informed of the fetal source of the tissue, and that fetal tissue be accorded the same respect given other cadaveric human tissue. In answering the remaining questions, the panel adopted the following recommendations: the abortion decision must be made before any discussion of use of the tissue; anonymity between donor and recipient should be maintained; the timing and method of abortion should not be influenced by the potential uses of fetal tissue; and consent of the pregnant woman is necessary and sufficient for use of tissue unless the father objects.

The panel also concluded: "There is sufficient evidence from animal experimentation to justify proceeding with human clinical trials in Parkinson disease and juvenile diabetes." Many of these recommendations were adopted unanimously, and no more than two panel members dissented from any of them. The most illuminating part of the report, however, is not its bland prose, but the dissent and the response to it, because these exchanges capsulize the national debate.

Dissenting Voices

Dissenters James Bopp and James Burtchaell argued that research using electively aborted fetuses is "ethically compromised" by the absence of authentic informed consent, by incentives it will offer for more abortions, and by complicity with the abortion. The consent issue is the standard argument that a woman who decides to abort her fetus thereby forfeits all rights and interests in the fetus and its remains.[6] The incentive argument posits that many women are ambivalent about abortion and that this ambivalence might be tipped in favor of abortion if they were informed that some good might come out of it.[7] The complicity argument, as stated by the dissenters, is primarily an emotional appeal based on the Nazi analogy.

John Robertson's persuasive response was joined by nine other panel members. He noted that a woman does not lose or forfeit all interests in an aborted fetus simply by choosing abortion. If she did, this "would lead to a policy of using fetal remains without parental consent or to a total ban on fetal transplants." The assertion that abortions will increase was characterized as "highly speculative." It was also argued that even if there was "some" increase in the number of abortions, it would not follow that fetal transplants would be unacceptable, because this assumes "that even a marginal increase in abortion should bar fetal tissue transplant research." Robertson rightly rejected the complicity argument completely, noting first that just because society is willing to use the organs of individuals killed in automobile accidents or murdered, this does not mean society or transplant surgeons are accomplices in automobile accidents or murder. The Nazi analogy fails because those experiments were on live, unconsenting prisoners, who suffered greatly from them, whereas fetal tissue research will be on dead fetuses that cannot be harmed and have been aborted and used with voluntary and informed consent.

The dissenters' central argument was that federal funding of fetal research would "institutionalize" government complicity with the "abortion industry." This is a powerful argument, as *Rust v. Sullivan*, discussed in Chapter 1, illustrates. But the federal government already profits directly from those who perform abortion by taxing their earnings, and since only dead fetuses are used, it is more correct to say that it is transplantation itself that would be "institutionalized." Those with serious misgivings about using dead fetal tissue are surely correct that dead fetuses are not the same as dead hamsters or even kidneys. Nonetheless, it is difficult to justify the use of organs and tissue for transplant from dead children, and not permit the transplantation of tissue from dead fetuses. Some who object to such use may be reacting not to the fetus, but to the role of the not-to-be-mother, and this role was arguably inadequately addressed by the panel. Kathleen Nolan, for example, has argued that the image of the "devouring mother" is an especially powerful and destructive one for our view of women as mothers. In her words: "By allowing tissue retrieval, [these women] seem to 'fail to protect' the dead fetus, letting it fall prey to the needs of others. Subliminally, this threatens unconscious beliefs about the role of women as mothers. . . . No matter that the fetus is dead—mothers should still fend off the scavengers."[8]

Images of research physicians as scavengers, and mothers as indifferent to the use of their deceased children, disturb many. But the fetus does not have the status of a child,[9] and after it is dead, it does not have any protectable interests of its own. On the other hand, the dead fetus, like the dead adult, is not abandoned property, and because of what it is and what it symbolizes it should be treated with respect. The mother's real role (like that of any surviving relative) is *not* to consent to burial or use of body parts for transplantation. Rather, as the next of kin, she has the legal authority to dispose of the body in the customary manner (usually burial or cremation) and to object to any use of the body not consistent with such custom because of the mental anguish such nontraditional or nonrespectful use of the body might cause her.[10] Treating fetal remains with respect may require us not to put the fetus on public display, but when the choice is burial, incineration, or use in legitimate research, the latter can be as respectful of the remains as the former.

OTHER ISSUES

An independent report from Stanford University was fundamentally consistent with the NIH panel,[11] and together these reports indicate wide agreement in the medical community on the major issues in fetal tissue use. One troubling difference, however, must be noted. The Stanford report attempted to sidestep the elective abortion issue, recommending, "If tissue from spontaneous abortions can satisfy the medical demands for both quantity and quality of tissue, it would be preferable to avoid the ethical problems of using induced abortions." Use of tissues from spontaneous abortuses is particularly problematic. It is now well established that about 50 percent of first trimester spontaneous abortuses and 20 percent of second trimester spontaneous abortuses are chromosomally abnormal.[12] Moreover, many microorganisms have been associated with spontaneous abortions, including cytomegalovirus, herpes type I and II, rubella, toxoplasmosis, and *Ureaplasma urealyticum*.[13] It would be indefensible to transplant abnormal or infected fetal tissue that would increase both the risk of transplant failure and the risk of infection for the recipient. Tissue from spontaneously aborted fetuses should not be used for transplantation into a human subject.

This is why the Bush administration's 1992 proposal to develop a tissue bank of fetuses from spontaneous abortions and ectopic pregnancies was impractical. Although administration officials lauded this compromise approach in public, in private they were well aware of NIH estimates that the total number of fetuses likely to be procured annually by this method was about 25 (not the 1,500 to 2,000 figure they were using).[14] Only the election of Bill Clinton ended the dominance of abortion politics in this area.

The primary objection to use of fetal tissues from elective abortions remains political: if therapeutically successful, such use would create a new constituency (sick people who could benefit from such transplants and their families) that would be opposed to outlawing elective abortions.[15] Of course, as both a scientific and ethical matter, the central issue is whether or not it is reasonable to do transplant experiments with fetal tissue at this time. Neither panel attempted to examine this question in any depth, and it remains the central issue in the early 1990s. The politics of abortion has thus led us to focus on the tangential question of the source of the tissue, rather than on the real question of whether it is scientifically reasonable to think that it can benefit sick people. The subjects of the proposed transplant research are not the fetuses (which are dead), but the recipients of the fetal tissue.

Initial transplants for Parkinson disease using the patient's own adrenal tissue sparked tremendous press coverage, and approximately 100 such transplants were done in the United States on the basis of initial reports of success in Mexico.[16] This experience indicates that local institutional review boards are inadequate to protect subjects of such research, just as they failed to protect the subjects of recent high-profile experiments with artificial hearts and xenografts (see Chapter 15). Adrenal tissue transplants have had very disappointing results,[17] and serious questions have been voiced concerning the original Mexican cases.

Fetal tissue is thought to have unique properties, and its use for Parkinson disease also subjects the patient to one less surgical procedure. Fetal tissue transplants for Parkinson disease were initially done in Mexico and Sweden, the Swedish researchers initially reporting "no improvement of therapeutic value" in their two patients.[18] The American Academy of Neurology urged "great caution in expanding the current human experience except as research conducted in highly-specialized centers."[19] Nonetheless, at least two U.S. centers went ahead with fetal tissue transplants for Parkinson disease (using private funds) before the NIH panel issued its report. These two centers, Yale University and the University of Colorado, have continued their work and reported some success in February 1992.[20] To his credit, Hans Sollinger, who already had an NIH grant to do fetal pancreatic tissue transplants for juvenile diabetes, voluntarily decided not to proceed until after the panel reported. Obviously, the use of national expert panels can only be effective in setting guidelines if privately funded researchers voluntarily refrain from conducting their own experiments while deliberations are proceeding.

REGULATING NEW SURGICAL PROCEDURES

There is no current method to regulate clinical trials of new surgical procedures (as there is to regulate such trials with new drugs), and no effective way to regulate experiments financed with private funds. Irresponsible proliferation of fetal tissue transplants, however, may persuade Congress and the public that such regulation is needed. It would be most beneficial to science and the public if such experimentation could be confined to a few centers with demonstrated excellence, where careful research could be pursued until safety and efficacy are demonstrated. The NIH panel provided an excellent beginning. But it is only a beginning and should not be taken as a signal for proceeding with human trials using fetal tissue for transplant. We have more scientific work to do, including work with animals to help determine such things as cell survival, growth curves, and graft-host immunology.[21]

Both panels also skipped lightly over some practical issues, including how the abortion is performed. As my colleague Sherman Elias has noted, it is, in fact, feasible to remove the fetus whole by concurrent use of ultrasound to aid in directing instruments within the uterine cavity. If fetal tissue proves therapeutic, there will be women willing to consent to such a procedure. If the abortion could be performed in a way that would enhance the potential usefulness of the fetal tissue, without additional risk to the woman, there will also be tremendous pressure to adopt this technique. More discussion of what choices a woman should be given about the abortion procedure itself, as well as its timing, is needed.

The relationship between the physician performing the abortion and the researcher also requires additional discussion. Sherman Elias and I believe that the woman should be asked about the use of her fetus as a tissue source after she has decided to have an abortion, but before she has had it. After the abortion, she should be given an opportunity to withdraw her consent (since no use can actually be made of the tissue until the fetus is dead). After she has been given an opportunity to change her mind, and the physician has performed the standard inspection of the tissue to make sure that the abortion is complete, the tissue should be taken out of the operating room and turned over to the researcher. Dissection of the tissues should be performed in a restricted facility that optimizes the success of the procedure (for example, sterile environment and proper dissecting instruments). To avoid any conflict of interest, there should be no academic (for example, coauthorship in publications or grant support) or other incentive for the physician performing the abortion, nor anyone else involved in the woman's care, to obtain her agreement for use of the fetal tissue.

Transplantation challenges our ethical precepts, and ethics has traditionally taken a backseat to the temptations and incentives to do first-of-their-kind transplants. Despite this, the public has generally applauded these transplants, at least where they have been seen as an attempt to save a life that would otherwise certainly have been lost. Fetal tissue transplants are much more problematic, and the public may be less forgiving of ethical shortcuts. Saving a life is not at issue, and the source of the tissue, although not forbidden, is troublesome to many. The world *is* watching, and this opportunity to demonstrate good science, good ethics, and compassionate patient care should not be wasted.

14

From Canada with Love:
Death and Organ Donation

Brain death is so closely linked to organ transplantation that it sometimes seems that you can't have one without the other. This is true when it comes to organ transplantation itself, which usually requires a brain dead corpse whose circulation is maintained by mechanical ventilation to preserve the organs. But the converse, of course, is not true: transplantation need not be contemplated to determine death on the basis of cessation of all brain function. This chapter examines two approaches to transplantation that have been effectively discredited: postponing the determination of death to put pressure on relatives to "donate" organs, and using live, anencephalic newborns as organ donors.[1]

THE JEFFREY STRACHAN CASE[2]

What recourse, if any, do the parents of a dead child have if a hospital refuses to release the body of their child to them unless they agree to organ donation? On Friday, April 25, 1980, 20-year-old Jeffrey Strachan committed suicide by shooting himself in the head. He was rushed to the emergency room of New Jersey's John F. Kennedy Memorial Hospital. By 5:25 p.m. there was no spontaneous respiration. The emergency room physician placed the young man on a mechanical ventilator, advised his parents that their son was "brain dead," and asked them to consider donating his organs for transplant. At 8:10 p.m. that same evening, a neurologist confirmed that Jeffrey was dead, and again asked the parents if they would donate their son's organs. The parents could not decide, and the neurologist suggested that they think about it and return in the morning. The neurologist wrote in Jeffrey's chart:

This patient is brain dead. At present we are working with parents trying to obtain permission to harvest kidneys and corneas and possibly heart. Our staff is working with transplant team personnel in this effort. If they get permission to harvest, proceed.

Jeffrey was transferred to the intensive care unit, and a representative of the Delaware Valley Transplant Program advised the parents that a decision would have to be made by 11:00 a.m. the next day because thereafter the organs would deteriorate. On Saturday morning, Jeffrey's father advised the attending physician (a new physician) that he and his wife did not wish to donate their son's organs and that they wanted him removed from "life support" systems. The physician asked them to think it over some more. Nonetheless, he wrote in the chart: "The family has decided not to permit the harvesting of any organs [the neurologist] . . . is informed; the case is dismissed."

The phrase "case dismissed" apparently meant that the organ procurement agency would no longer consider using the organs for transplant. Jeffrey's father returned Saturday evening to reaffirm the decision. He spoke with another neurologist who confirmed (again) that Jeffrey was dead. The new neurologist told him that his son would be taken off mechanical support systems "as soon as the hospital administrator tells us the procedure."

The hospital administrator called the hospital lawyer, who advised him to "run EEGs until we have a clear understanding of what the boy's condition is and on Monday discuss further what to do and if necessary call the Prognosis Committee together." He also advised the administrator that if the family wanted the body before Monday, they would have to obtain a court order. The Strachans were so advised at 2:00 a.m. Sunday morning.

EEGs were performed on Sunday and Monday. At 9:40 a.m. on Monday morning, yet another physician examined Jeffrey and again concluded that he was dead. At 2:00 p.m. he noted in the chart, "patient officially brain dead." At 2:30 p.m. the parents were told that the respirator would be removed if they would sign a release prepared by the hospital's lawyer. The release read:

We have been advised by the attending physicians of our son, Jeffrey Strachan, that he has been declared "brain death." (sic) It is therefore requested that all life support — life-support-death devices be discontinued as soon as possible.

In making this request we are fully aware of our legal responsibilities and further hold harmless John F. Kennedy Memorial Hospital and the attending physicians with regard to discontinuance of life support devices.

At 4:05 p.m. all support systems were discontinued. Shortly thereafter another physician, who had not been previously involved, pronounced Jeffrey dead and signed a death certificate. The parents claimed his body almost immediately.

Jeffrey's parents sued the physicians, the organ procurement agency, the hospital, and its administrator for, among other things, the emotional harm they suffered as a result of the hospital's negligence for (1) not having proper forms or procedures for turning off a respirator and (2) improperly withholding the body of their son from them. The suits against the physicians and the transplant program were voluntarily dismissed prior to trial. The jury awarded the parents $70,000 on each count, for a total of $140,000. The hospital appealed.

In a 2 to 1 opinion, the Appellate Division reversed the decision, holding that the hospital had no duty to provide consent forms or procedures (since all decisions involved were medical, not business decisions) and that there was no duty to release a dead body until it had actually been pronounced dead by a physician, a death certificate signed (or a notation made in the chart), and support systems removed. The majority determined as well that there would be no recovery for emotional distress because the parents were merely "bystanders" who did not suffer any physical injury themselves. In a powerful and persuasive dissent, Justice Virginia A. Long demonstrated that the majority had misstated the real issues involved and thus had arrived at a faulty conclusion. She reasoned that Jeffrey was determined dead days before he was pronounced dead and that the parents were not bystanders at all, but direct victims of the hospital's negligence. Because of her dissent, the parents had a right to have the appeal heard by the New Jersey Supreme Court.

The New Jersey Supreme Court's Opinion[3]

The court ruled that it was improper for the trial court to *ask* the jury to decide if a hospital had a duty to have procedures in place to deal with brain death. Duty is a question of law that must be decided by judges, not juries. Nor was the court willing to fashion and impose a specific procedural duty on hospitals:

> The imposition of a paperwork duty does little to advance either the mission of health-care providers or the needs of society. If "procedures" are to be viewed as more than mere "paperwork" and considered indispensable in this area—in the nature of a standard that governs the medical community—then those *procedures should be designed and imposed by those most directly involved, the physicians and the hospitals themselves.*
>
> *That is the business of the medical community itself, not of this court.* (emphasis added)

As to withholding the body itself, the court began its analysis by noting that while the law has always recognized that the next-of-kin has a "right to bury the dead," the traditional characterization of this as a "quasi-right in property" to the body is "somewhat dubious." The court quoted *Prosser & Keeton on Torts*, which concluded that the property notion was fashioned "out of thin air" and that "in reality *the personal feelings of the survivors are being protected*, under a fiction likely to deceive no one but a lawyer." (emphasis added)

The real wrong in failure to release a body is not withholding the survivor's property but, rather, "the wrongful infliction of mental distress." Since this tort can only be committed *after* the individual has died, the court needed to determine when Jeffrey died to determine if the body was wrongfully withheld from his parents. The court concluded that Jeffrey "was pronounced brain dead by the emergency room physician at 5:25 p.m. on Friday" and that at least after the neurologist confirmed brain death Friday evening "there can be no doubt that on deeming Jeffrey brain dead, the doctors considered Jeffrey 'dead.'" Thereafter, the failure to release the body to the parents on request "posed a plain affront to their dignity and autonomy and exposed them to unnecessary distress at a time of profound grief." The majority of the Appellate Division simply could not see that the parents were harmed. The New Jersey Supreme Court, however, had no such difficulty:

> Although plaintiffs were told that their son was brain dead and nothing further could be done for him, for three days after requesting that their son be disconnected from the respirator plaintiffs continued to see him lying in bed, with tubes in his body, his eyes taped shut, and foam in his mouth. His body remained warm to the touch . . . a scene fraught with grief and heartache.

The court agreed with Judge Long that this was not a bystander case because, since Jeffrey "was no longer alive," he could suffer "no harm" at the hands of the defendants. Instead, the parents' distress flowed directly from the hospital's failure to perform their duty to release their child's body for burial. The court thus recognized the "longstanding" exception to the rule that emotional damages will not be awarded to someone who has not been physically injured: the negligent handling of a corpse. However, because the court was uncertain that the jury would have awarded $70,000 for improperly withholding the corpse had it not also found the hospital negligent for not having proper forms and procedures, the case was sent back for a new trial solely on the issue of damages for failure to release the dead body.

Lessons

A major problem in medical practice over the past two decades has been the trend for physicians to abdicate their responsibility for *medical* decisions to hospital administrators, lawyers, and courts. This has resulted in the increasing bureaucratization of medicine to the detriment of both physicians and patients. In this case none of the physicians seemed willing to pronounce death until the hospital administration approved it. The hospital administration, in turn (instead of insisting that the physicians do their job), was also unwilling to take responsibility and so consulted the lawyer.

The lawyer, in turn, advised three alternative procedures, including consulting a judge, all of which could only serve to further frustrate and alienate physicians from the practice of their profession.

The good news is that the New Jersey Supreme Court, in spite of its history of inventing procedural mechanisms for physicians to limit their liability and help them feel more comfortable, refused to further reinforce the bureaucratization of medical practice. Instead it said firmly what courts should say more often: procedures should be designed by the medical community itself. The courts may ultimately be called on to rule on the propriety of medical procedures, but courts should not set them initially, just as courts should not routinely permit themselves to be used by doctors, hospital administrators, and their lawyers to avoid taking professional responsibility for their decisions. This case provides an instructive example of how hospital administrators and hospital lawyers often forge "solutions" to medical practice "problems" that are disconnected from biological reality and compassionate medical practice, and serve primarily to bureaucratize medicine in a destructive way.

Since the cause of action is based on the suffering of the family of a *deceased* individual, the ruling has no application to lawsuits brought by the families of living patients (while the patient is still alive, the hospital's duty is to the patient, not the family who remain traditional "bystanders.") On the other hand, the ruling might apply to one narrow class of "living" patients: individuals in persistent vegetative states. This same court has previously argued that such individuals "do not experience . . . any benefits or burdens" and that decisions about their care are appropriately made by their families (see Chapter 8). If this language is taken at face value, and if a family reasonably demands that their relative in a persistent vegetative state be removed from support systems, and if the hospital negligently refuses to comply, causing the family emotional distress, it is possible that this court might permit the relatives to sue the hospital in this case as well. This would be reasonable since, if we conclude that a patient in a persistent vegetative state has no interest in whether his body is maintained on support systems or not, and if the individual's family is very emotionally involved and for good reason wants the support systems removed, and if the hospital refuses for some arbitrary reason, the family is predictably and severely injured by having to continue to see their loved one in an arguably degrading state in which they could suffer all the "grief and heartache" Jeffrey's parents suffered in this case, and over a much longer period of time.[4]

Even though this case occurred long before the "required request" laws and regulations, the physicians initially involved in Jeffrey's care were extremely aggressive about organ donation. The organ procurement agency itself seems to have acted properly and professionally, but the physician and hospital had no clear idea what to do. Indeed, the hospital administrator and the hospital lawyer seemed to have had little knowledge about brain death at all, since the suggestion that the case be decided by a "prognosis committee" or a judge is ludicrous.[5] In our era of required request, no request should be made until after the patient is pronounced dead; and if the request is refused, the body should immediately be released to the family. Making requests prior to the pronouncement of death leads not only to real conflicts of interest (between treating the patient as a person and as an organ source for someone else), but also to the type of suffering and confusion apparent in a case like this.[6] It could also reinforce the two primary reasons the public gives for not signing organ donor cards: fear that doctors "might do something to me before I'm really dead" and fear that "doctors might hasten my death."[7]

Even though we have been over this ground many times before, great discomfort and uncertainty about brain death remains. Surveys consistently show that administrators are uncertain about brain death, and this attitude and lack of knowledge translates to inappropriate actions. Release forms, for example, are totally unnecessary and inappropriate to making a decision not to treat a corpse. It is time to stop using the phrase "brain dead" and simply use the term "dead," since this single word more precisely and accurately describes reality. This confusion, between the dead and the near dead or dying, probably made experimentation with use of anencephalic newborns as organ sources inevitable.

THE CASE OF BABY GABRIEL

The international case of heart-donor Baby Gabriel provided an early opportunity to examine the law and ethics of using anencephalic newborns as organ sources. Baby Gabriel's mother, Karen, like her husband Fred, a Catholic, had rejected maternal serum alpha-fetoprotein testing that would have helped determine the status of her fetus because she would not have an abortion. In her eighth month of pregnancy, however, she became concerned because her fetus had stopped kicking. Ultrasound discerned that her fetus was anencephalic. She was presented with three options: induced labor, cesarean section, or carrying the fetus to term. The parents decided to continue with their plans for natural childbirth and to offer the child's organs for transplantation. They carried through this plan at Soldier's Hospital in Orillia, Ontario. The parents and child, who was baptized and named Gabriel after the archangel who guards the gates of heaven, spent the night together at the community hospital. The couple had been married two years, and this was their first child. It seems clear from their statements that they cared for her very much. As Karen said: "I immediately fell in love with her the first time I touched her."

Baby Gabriel breathed without assistance throughout her first night of life, but the following day she was transferred to Children's Hospital in Western Ontario, where she was placed on a mechanical ventilator and preparations were made for organ donation. There appear to have been no infants, in either the United States or Canada, who were on the waiting list for organs. Thus this was not a case of a dying child in search of an organ, but of a dying organ in search of a child. Leonard Bailey of Loma Linda, California, had a pregnant patient whose fetus had been diagnosed *in utero* as suffering from hypoplastic left heart, but she was not due to deliver for some weeks. A decision was made to deliver that child by cesarean section to take advantage of the available organ. Baby Gabriel was pronounced dead in Canada, then flown to Loma Linda, where death was confirmed. The heart transplant to another Canadian, named Paul, was performed and was successful.

Press commentary and some physicians treated the Baby Gabriel case as new even though anencephalic infants had been a major, albeit controversial, heart source for infant transplants in this country more than two decades ago. In June 1966, almost eighteen months before Christiaan Barnard performed the world's first human-to-human heart transplant, Adrian Kantrowitz was set to perform what would have been the world's first such transplant from an anencephalic newborn to a 2-month-old infant. He waited for the heart to stop beating to declare death, but the procedure had to be abandoned when resuscitation efforts proved futile. On the basis of this experience, however, he concluded that use of an anencephalic infant as a heart donor was a "realistic possibility." Three days after Barnard's historic operation, Kantrowitz performed the first human-to-human heart transplant in the United States. Once again the donor was an anencephalic newborn. To locate the donor, Kantrowitz had sent telegrams to some 500 U.S. hospitals seeking an anencephalic infant for organ donation. This time the infant was cooled by immersion in ice water, and the heart was removed immediately after it ceased beating spontaneously. The recipient died six and one-half hours later. Kantrowitz described the operation as "technically successful."[8]

Determination of Death

The central issue in the ensuing debate about using anencephalic infants as organ sources was whether they must be dead or not, and if they must be dead, how death could be determined. Some argued that since anencephalic newborns lack higher brain function, they should not be considered as living human beings, and thus their organs should be available for immediate use. Although almost all agree that anencephalic infants, unlike almost every other handicapped newborn, need not be treated to prolong their lives, it is almost as universally agreed that they are live human beings and that killing them would be murder.

In January 1987, transplant surgeon Calvin Stiller had called an international group to London, Ontario to discuss this issue. Leonard Bailey attended. The group concluded that anencephalic infants could be used as organ donors, but only after pronouncement of death using classic brain death criteria. To utilize such criteria, it would be necessary to put the child on a mechanical ventilator, because simply permitting the child to stop breathing naturally would usually result in unusable organs that deteriorate as the child's breathing becomes more compromised. This intervention would likely prolong the child's life, and, in the most extreme (possible, but unlikely) scenario, the child's brain stem might become strong enough to sustain independent breathing for weeks, or even months or years. Research on the effect of fully supporting an anencephalic infant on the infant itself seemed in order.

Alexander Capron agreed with the conclusion of the Canadian group: breathing anencephalic newborns are dying, not dead, and it would be misguided and destructive to amend either our brain death laws or the Uniform Anatomical Gift Act to permit the harvesting of organs from live anencephalic newborns. In his review of the subject, he concluded that rather than sacrificing live patients for transplants, "medical ingenuity should be directed toward finding ways to care for dying anencephalic (and other) babies so that when they become brain-dead, they can be organ donors."[9]

Arthur Caplan (who presented his position to the London meeting) disagreed. He argued that anencephalic infants should be considered a separate category of human ("living but brain absent") and their parents should be able to donate their organs prior to their death. He justified this position on the basis that the anencephalic child can never develop even a "semblance of personhood," that "the need for these organs is real," that successful transplantation "seems promising," and that (most convincing for Caplan), "many parents are eager to have their dead or anencephalic child used as a donor in the hope that something good might come of a tragic situation."[10] All of these arguments apply with equal force to other severe genetic disorders, and this approach seems to ignore the interests of the newborn anencephalic completely.

Since the country's first human heart transplant, great strides have been made in setting forth the criteria for the determination of death. There is now general medical, legal, and ethical agreement that an individual is dead either when the individual has irreversible cessation of circulation and respiration or when there is irreversible cessation "of all functions of the entire brain, including the brain stem." The medical consultants to the President's Commission concluded in 1981 that, because of the "increased resistance to damage" of their brains, "physicians should be particularly cautious in applying neurologic criteria to determine death in children younger than five years."[11]

Responding to that challenge, a Task Force for the Determination of Brain Death in Children was established to develop guidelines for children under five. After years of study and deliberation, the group's report, which has been widely endorsed, was published in June 1987.[12] The guidelines provide accepted clinical criteria for the determination of brain death in three categories of children: those over 1 year of age, those aged 2 months to 1 year, and those aged 7 days to 2 months. The criteria are inapplicable to infants under 7 days of age. For infants less than 2 months, in addition to meeting strict clinical criteria, two electroencephalograms separated by at least forty-eight hours are recommended. The guidelines are recommendations only and are not meant as universal requirements. The group did not specifically deal with anencephalic infants, but the underlying assumption with regard to infants was that the insult to the brain was "irreversible." Since anencephalic newborns have no higher brain, different clinical criteria could be used to determine brain death for them.

New Clinical Criteria for Anencephalics?

This left two policy choices: abandon attempts to justify use of anencephalic infants as organ donors on the basis that there is no current clinically accepted manner in which to declare brain death in these infants; or do the research necessary to establish a clinically valid procedure for declaring brain death in these infants. The Canadian group decided to take the second route and experiment on methods to use anencephalic newborns as organ donors who can be validly declared brain dead on classic criteria. The group developed a basic protocol that calls for the parents to agree, prior to birth, that (1) the infant will be resuscitated, (2) periodic testing will be done to determine brain death (removal from the ventilator at six- to twelve-hour intervals for a ten-minute period to determine ability to breathe spontaneously), (3) organ donation is acceptable, and (4) there will be a definite end period (to be determined by the parents, but not more than fourteen days), after which the infant will be removed from the ventilator and permitted to die. Low dose morphine is administered to prevent potential suffering on the part of the infant, although whether or not anencephalic newborns can suffer is unknown.

This is a true experiment in the sense that there has never been a clinical trial to determine how anencephalic infants do with full ventilator support. This, in turn, is because anencephalic infants have almost never been so supported, primarily because the condition is quickly and universally fatal. As one pediatric ICU specialist put it, it would be "futile and inhumane" to artificially support respiration in these infants. How can we determine if such research is legally and ethically proper?

Like all provinces except Manitoba, Ontario has no brain death law. Canadian physicians follow the common law rule that "you're dead when the doctor says you're dead," at least as long as the doctor makes the determination of death in accordance with accepted medical standards. This is perfectly reasonable, as is the Canadian insistence that both a pediatric neurologist and a neonatologist agree on the determination of death.

First, we must determine if it is proper in this instance to use dying newborns as means to helping other newborns rather than as ends in themselves. What makes anencephalic infants different from all other organ donors is that they are not placed on life-support systems initially for their own sake, but solely for the sake of others. Specifically, since anencephalic newborns are not routinely resuscitated, intubated, or placed on ventilators and given other support, we cannot justify these interventions as "treatment" for the anencephalic newborn. Rather, these interventions can only be seen as treatment for the benefit of the ultimate organ recipient, and perhaps as treatment for the parents. If it is never ethically appropriate to prolong an unconsenting person's dying process for the sake of another, then our inquiry is at an end. Only if we conclude that it may be appropriate (e.g., if the harm to the dying child is trivial, and the benefit to others is enormous) do we go to the second step.

The second step entails research to determine (1) how long anencephalic infants can survive with the support available in an intensive care unit, (2) whether anencephalic infants feel pain or have other sensations, (3) the state of the kidneys, liver, and heart of anencephalic infants (which will determine their general usefulness for transplant), and (4) whether it is true that the condition of anencephaly can be easily and accurately distinguished from all other abnormalities of infants.

Under existing federal research regulations such research would be difficult to do in the United States. Since the pregnant woman's consent is contemplated prior to birth, and since her decision to carry the pregnancy to term is necessary to begin the research, compliance with the federal (and applicable state) rules regarding research on fetuses *in utero* is necessary. At the least, this requires that risk to the fetus be "minimal" (true while the fetus is a fetus, but not after birth) and consent of both parents. In addition, after birth the regulations regarding protecting children would come into force. This type of research would arguably fall under section 46.407, research not otherwise approvable, which presents an opportunity to understand, prevent, or alleviate a serious problem affecting the health or welfare of children. The IRB would initially have to make this determination, and then the secretary of HHS would have to consult with an expert panel who agrees with this assessment and makes other conclusions, including that "the research will be conducted in accordance with sound ethical principles." Nonetheless, a research protocol was ultimately developed and implemented at Loma Linda, resulting in the conclusion that it was not practicable to use anencephalic newborns as donors if one had to wait until they died to take their organs.[13]

How important this research would be to the potential recipients of these organs depends on two other critical facts. The first is the success of infant organ transplants. It is premature to begin a quest for novel organ sources until there is reasonable clinical data on the efficacy of infant organ transplants. The second relates to the usefulness of anencephalic newborns as a source of organs in the future. With the widespread, even routine, use of maternal serum alpha-fetoprotein (MSAFP) screening, and the common use of ultrasound, almost all anencephalic fetuses will be identified prior to the end of the second trimester of pregnancy. The vast majority of women will opt to terminate the pregnancy, at least unless organ donation is actively advocated by obstetricians. Obstetricians have not been involved in organ procurement historically, and what role they will play remains uncertain. In Baby Gabriel's case the diagnosis of anencephaly was made unusually late (in the 32nd week of pregnancy). Nonetheless, a second anencephalic infant was offered for organ donation in Ontario within two weeks of the Baby Gabriel case, and, since some women will reject pregnancy termination, some anencephalic infants will continue to be born.

In counseling pregnant women, obstetricians must consider that since the majority of anencephalic fetuses are stillborn, the majority of women who do opt to carry their anencephalic fetus to term so that its organs can be used will do so in vain. Their attempt to "redeem" the tragedy by organ donation will fail, and tragedy will thus be compounded, not softened. Compassion for these parents may therefore dictate counseling pregnancy termination rather than holding out organ donation as an option.

Baby Gabriel did not herald new approaches to using anencephalic infants as organ donors, and the fact that the first try at such an approach was successful probably led to overly optimistic predictions of the utility of using such infants as donors. In 1992 the question of using anencephalic infants made headlines around the country when the parents of Baby Theresa of Florida offered their child's organs for transplant. The discussions that followed the Baby Gabriel case were ignored, and the press responded to the drama of parents trying to "redeem" the birth of their child through organ donation as if the issue was entirely novel. The Florida Supreme Court, however, was not beguiled. It ruled in late 1992 that there was "no basis to expand the common law to equate anencephaly with death."[14] The real lessons we learned (again) were about law and ethics in organ transplantation: changes in the law were neither necessary nor desirable. We must continue to focus on determining death in the donor and on obtaining uncoerced consent from the next of kin for organ donation.

15

Death and the Magic Machine: Consent to the Artificial Heart

Artificial heart implants represent the most public and publicized human experiments in the history of the world, and as such can be used to illustrate generic legal and ethical issues in human experimentation.[1] In Solzhenitsyn's *Cancer Ward*, Oleg Kostoglotov is confronted by his doctor, Ludmilla Afanasyevna. The doctor wants to use an experimental hormone treatment, but the patient refuses. Psychiatrist Jay Katz argues in his *Silent World of Doctor and Patient* that what makes conversation impossible between them is the patient's undisclosed intention of leaving the hospital to treat himself with "a secret medicine, a mandrake root from Issyk Kul." Oleg could not trust the doctor with this information because the doctor would disagree and make the treatment decision for him regardless of his wishes, because the doctor believed "doctors *are* entitled to that right. . . . Without that right there'd be no such thing as medicine."[2]

Katz objects to this notion, pointing out that "if doctors are 'entitled to that right,' then patients must continue to trust them silently." But he also chastises "proponents of informed consent and patient self-determination" (among whom I number myself), who "have insufficiently appreciated that trusting oneself and others to become aware of the certainties and uncertainties that surround the practice of medicine, and to integrate them with one's hopes, fears, and realistic expectations, are inordinately difficult tasks."

Using the application of informed consent to artificial heart experimentation, I will argue in this chapter that Katz is certainly correct in proposing more in-depth, informed, and trusting conversation between doctor-researcher and patient-subject. But much more than conversation is required to promote and protect the rights and welfare of individual subjects.

Solzhenitsyn's fictional patient, Oleg, knows about his folk remedy and so satisfies the informational requirements of informed consent:

> When I get back to Ush-Terek I'll use the issyk-kul root to keep the tumor from producing metastases. There is something noble in curing with strong poison. Poison doesn't pretend to be innocent medicine. *It says plainly: I am poison. Watch out! Or else. And we know what risk we're taking.* (emphasis added)

Suppose that it was not Oleg, but Afanasyevana who was proposing to use the issyk-kul root, and suppose doctor and patient had discussed this "experimental treatment" at length and that Oleg understood the risks perfectly. Under these conditions would we or should we conclude that it is perfectly acceptable for the issyk-kul root to be administered to Oleg? This commentary will argue that while such informed consent is a necessary precondition to lawful human experimentation, it is not a sufficient one. Prior to the conversation and offer of an experimental intervention, an independent judgment must be made that the intervention, be it surgery, radiation, or an issyk-kul root, is a reasonable medical experiment from both a scientific and public policy perspective. This is necessary to protect the patient's welfare—to prevent patients from being demeaned and dehumanized by accepting offers they are in no position to refuse.

Medical ethicist John Fletcher, for example, correctly argues that "the major ethical question in research is whether the experiment ought to be done at all."[3] The law, as embodied in the Nuremberg Code and current NIH regulations, is consistent with this view. The Nuremberg Code (formulated by U.S. judges sitting in the Nazi War Crimes Trials on the basis of international criminal law) sets forth ten prerequisites for legal human experimentation. The first principle deals with the informed consent of the research subject, or what may be termed the subject's rights. The other principles have primarily to do with protecting the subject's welfare (see Chapter 11).

These principles have been codified by NIH and FDA regulations, and local committees, called institutional review boards (IRBs), are mandated to review research protocols prior to subject recruitment, to see to it that these preconditions have been observed. Our initial experience with heart transplantation and our current experience with the artificial heart illustrate how informed consent can be improperly used as an excuse to justify massive assaults on the welfare of human subjects, even though the quality of the consent is highly questionable, and the quality of the experiment itself does not meet the welfare requirements of the Nuremberg Code.

INFORMED CONSENT TO HEART TRANSPLANTATION

Using Philip Blaiberg's *Looking at My Heart*, Jay Katz persuasively demonstrates that Blaiberg (the recipient of the world's second human-to-human heart transplant) regressed when in the presence of Christiaan Barnard. He saw him as an "omnipotent parent and hero. . . . Barnard became General Smuts, under whom Blaiberg had served and admired greatly. . . . Barnard also became Christ, the powerful protector." But in identifying Barnard as Christ, Blaiberg may have "confused his own identity with that of the surgeon." He actually said he wanted to go through with the operation "not only for my sake but for you [Barnard] and your team who put so much into your effort to save Louis Washkansky." Barnard himself seemed unaware of this confusion on the part of his patient, and of his own conflict of interest (between wanting to perform the world's second human heart transplant for himself and attempting to convince Blaiberg that the operation was in Blaiberg's best interests). Indeed, Barnard even began talking about the operation as fulfilling not his own goals, but "Washkansky's dream." This, as Katz notes, "is startling and suggests that he was as confused about his identity as Blaiberg was about his own."

Louis Washkansky (the recipient of the world's first human-to-human heart transplant) was also not particularly interested in discussing the details of heart transplantation. Barnard did not press the issue, deciding "no words were needed." But were they? Katz argues that more words (conversation) may not have changed the ultimate decision, but could have improved "the nature and quality of Barnard's and Washkansky's thinking about available choices."

> Both, at best, had reflected on the forthcoming operation in isolation, and neither had any idea what had transpired in the other's mind. At the least, respect for Washkansky's psychological autonomy required Barnard to challenge his patient's silent acquiescence. . . . *If Washkansky wanted a new heart, he also had to have the heart to learn more about the operation.* (emphasis added)

Katz continues by noting that since the first heart transplant operations were "extraordinary" procedures, candidates should have been required to learn about them and not permitted to waive disclosure and consent: "Barnard should have insisted they talk for a while." Katz concludes his discussion of this case by noting the common clinical controversy over whether to respect the patient's "rights" or "needs"; I shall restate this "conflict" by attempting to construct a system that protects both the rights and welfare of subjects of extraordinary human experimentation.

Katz presents a psychoanalytic explanation of the dynamics of the doctor–patient relationship in the dramatic human experimentation context, and suggests conversation to help elucidate issues of transference and countertransference. He argues powerfully that "magical and hopeful expectations exist side-by-side with expectations of cruel disappointment." Later he notes that when medical knowledge and skill prove impotent against the claims of nature, "all kinds of senseless interventions are tried in an unconscious effort to cure the incurable magically through a 'wonder drug'

a novel surgical procedure, or a penetrating psychological interpretation."
He hopes that through education,

> at least medical students can learn to appreciate that *it may be their magical
> hopes that cause them to intervene*, rather than believing that they are responding
> to the *magical expectations of their patients*. Thus doctors' heroic attempts to
> try anything may not necessarily be responsive to patients' needs but may turn
> out to be a *projection of their own needs onto patients*. (emphasis added)

This powerful insight is descriptive not only of the behavior of human
heart transplant pioneers, but also seems to have set the standard for the
behavior of surgeons involved in artificial heart experimentation. In his
autobiography, *One Life*, Christiaan Barnard has a conversation with himself in which he tries to explain why he did not have further discussions
with Louis Washkansky about the risks and likely outcomes of the first
human-to-human heart transplant:

> I offered a chance, and he grabbed it, without asking any questions. *At the
> South Pole, the wind can blow in one direction only—north. At the point of
> death, any promise of help can go in one direction only—toward hope.* So I
> offered him hope, believing this was my duty. To have refused it would be a
> betrayal of myself and my profession. In a way, *we share the same hope.* We're
> in this together.[4] (emphasis added)

This rationalization, of course, is consistent with Katz's notion that Barnard had confused himself with his patient. It is also consistent with Afanasyevna's view that "doctors *are* entitled." It takes this view even further,
however, by arguing that doctors have a duty: "to have refused it would be
a betrayal of myself and my profession." But it also indicates that Barnard
believed that for Washkansky there really was no choice; that since he was
dying he *must* accept a heart transplant: it is his only hope, and some hope
is always better than none. Later, Barnard refined the analogy, and the
rationale for action in the absence of full discussion, by arguing that for
Washkansky the alternatives were so obvious that the choice was trivial:

> For a dying man, it is not a difficult decision because he knows he is at the end.
> If a lion chases you to the bank of a river filled with crocodiles, you will leap
> into the water convinced you have a chance to swim to the other side. But you
> would never accept such odds if there were no lion.

This "lion and the crocodiles" analogy has become the standard by which
artificial heart experimenters discuss the decisions of their patient-subjects.
For example, when Denton Cooley implanted the world's first totally *artificial* heart into the chest of Haskell Karp in 1969, he initially argued that his
own skill and the patient's consent were the only justifications needed:

I have done more heart surgery than anyone else in the world. . . . Based on this experience, I believe I am qualified to judge what is right and proper for my patients. *The permission I receive to do what I do, I receive from my patients.* It is not received from a government agency or from one of my seniors.[5] (emphasis added)

Later, however, he restated the issue of the patient's consent in "lion and crocodile" terms: "He was a drowning man. A drowning man can't be too particular what he's going to use as a possible life preserver. It was a desperate thing, and he knew it."[6]

A decade and a half later we witnessed the advent of the permanent artificial heart and the use of artificial hearts on a temporary basis as a bridge (or "tollgate") to a human heart transplant. The informed consent issues remained relegated to secondary concern and unaddressed in any but a crude and primitive manner.

PERMANENT ARTIFICIAL HEARTS AND INFORMED CONSENT

Prior to performing the world's first permanent artificial heart implant, William DeVries, like Cooley, underlined his view of the importance of informed consent as the primary justification for performing the procedure. The major problem was that the only power source available was an approximately 400-pound drive cart (which had to be attached to both a power source and a source of compressed air) that made ambulation almost impossible. Many, including one of the device's designers, Robert Jarvik, believed the device shouldn't be used on humans until it was easily portable and entirely implantable. DeVries disagreed:

Many people have asked us the question as to—it's not fully implantable, why then would you do it? Why don't you wait ten years, when it's implantable, and then do it. *But the key is informed consent. Why should I let people die,* when I can give them a chance to live—if they're willing to accept the limitations of the external pumping system?[7] (emphasis added)

DeVries is certainly correct insofar as he asserts that the informed consent of his subject is a necessary prerequisite to acceptable human experimentation: if the subject's competent, voluntary, informed, and understanding consent cannot be obtained, the experiment cannot be lawfully or ethically performed. Even in this regard, however, it can be persuasively argued that although the consent form and process used by DeVries in the Barney Clark case is a vast improvement over the consent process used by Barnard, and a considerable improvement over the consent form and process used by Cooley, it was still seriously deficient.

Specifically, Clark signed an eleven-page consent form more notable for its length than its content. It was incomplete, internally inconsistent, and confusing. It assumed, as his physicians then believed, that Clark would either die on the operating table or go home in about ten days and continue to be mentally competent for the rest of his life. It took no account at all of a "halfway success"—survival coupled with severe confusion, mental incompetence, or coma. No provisions were made for proxy consent to additional procedures or experiments in the event of incompetence, for a mechanism to terminate the experiment, or for how Clark would die. These, and other shortcomings, are serious and evidence a lack of clear thinking and planning on the part of DeVries and the Utah IRB.[8] But one can argue that it is easy to be critical of *any* initial attempt and that no local IRB could have done better. As Al Jonsen has put it, the Utah IRB (in devising a consent form and process with DeVries) was asked "to build a Boeing 747 with Wright Brothers parts." What about changes that were made during the next five years in the consent form and process?

Disturbingly, there were very few changes, and most were for the worse. After DeVries moved to Humana Audubon in Louisville, Kentucky, to conduct his permanent artificial heart implants, he did three more. In May 1985, after completing all of these implants, he discussed the issue of informed consent to the artificial heart with *New York Times* medical writer, Lawrence K. Altman. Altman reports:

> Dr. DeVries has repeatedly said that the four men in whom he has implanted artificial hearts were so coerced by their disease that they felt that death was their only alternative. In signing the 17-page [double-spaced] consent form, each recipient, Dr. DeVries has said, "told me in their own way that they didn't care" if they read it or not, and had signed it primarily because they had to [in order] to get the device.[9]

This is a devastating admission from a surgeon who used informed consent as *the* primary justification for permanent artificial implants in humans. Was it the patient or DeVries who believed in every case that "death was their only alternative"? And what would it take to persuade DeVries either that there were other alternatives or that death could be preferable to the "magic machine"? Katz's concern with requiring conversation, and exploring what myths or beliefs the surgeon and his patient are harboring that permit them to accept silence, seems especially critical when dealing with the most highly publicized experiment in the history of the world. The primary rationale for accepting silence seems to be the same one that comforted Barnard and Cooley: the patient was dying and so had no choice. In DeVries' words, concerning Barney Clark: "He was too old for a transplant, there were no drugs that would help; the only thing that he could look forward to was dying."[10]

These experiences raise the question of whether we can ever justify experimentation on very sick, terminally ill patients. Doesn't their disease, Solzhenitsyn's story of Oleg notwithstanding, inevitably coerce them into "volunteering" for something they will necessarily see as hopeful? And won't parents inevitably volunteer their children for even bizarre and unprecedented experiments, like xenografts, if they are led to believe the experiment might prevent death? Here Katz helps us again, by insisting on explicit recognition of the limits of interventions at the end of life. Of course, we can only justify experimentation on such individuals if we can obtain their voluntary and informed consent.

But informed consent alone is an insufficient justification for radical human experimentation. Proper attention to the other precepts of the Nuremberg Code, for example, would have required us to address the questions of whether there isn't an *a priori* reason to believe that "death or disabling injury" will necessarily follow from this experiment, whether such a "halfway success" of continued life in a severely compromised state doesn't amount to "unnecessary physical and mental suffering and injury," and whether the "anticipated results" justify the performance of this experiment. The welfare of the subject of this experiment does not seem to have been adequately addressed, and, until it was, consent for the experiment should not have been sought.

DeVries sometimes seemed to justify this experimental shortcoming by acting as if he believed he was engaged in therapy, not experimentation at all. At times, for example, he suggested that his goal was to get his patient to go home or to "play a round of golf." In fact, this scenario never seems to have been realistic. Clark realized, shortly before his death, that, although he had also hoped for some therapeutic gain, he had become involved in pure non-therapeutic experimentation for others. Asked by DeVries in his only publicly shown videotaped interview, "It's been hard for you, hasn't it, Barney?" Clark replied, "Yes, it's been hard, but the heart itself is pumping right along, and I think it's doing well."[11] Clark, it seems, fully realized what DeVries could not openly admit: the subject, who at the outset was a patient seen as an end with the artificial heart used as a means to sustain him, had become simply a means to the end of sustaining the artificial heart. Clark might nonetheless have agreed to this experiment in advance even if he had known that he would spend most of his 112 remaining days on earth in an intensive care unit, extremely debilitated and depressed, and mentally incompetent at most times. But if this had been known, the experiment should not have been approved by the IRB since it would have violated most of the basic precepts of subject protection set forth in the Nuremberg Code.

Consent, even informed consent, cannot convert an otherwise unacceptable experiment into an acceptable one. Before patients are asked to consent to experimental procedures, the procedure itself must be independently judged to be a reasonable one to perform on a human being. Using informed consent in a vacuum, without such independent review, makes desperate, dying patients targets for quackery, because an offer of "life" from a physician (who patients are likely to mistake and misidentify as Christ or God) is an offer dying patients are in no reasonable position to refuse. Use of informed consent in this context converts it from a shield designed to protect the patient into a sword designed to attack the patient's vulnerability. There is an element of paternalism in this suggestion, of course, but no more than that involved in licensing physicians (including these experimenters) and regulating prescription drugs. But we are unlikely to succeed at protecting subject welfare unless we provide terminally ill patients with more procedural protections than we provide healthy volunteers. Much more imaginative work needs to be done on informed consent to permanent implants (and more experimentation with animal models as well) before additional implants can be justified. IRBs have been unable to contribute much to protecting patients in this setting, and, although their prior review is legally and ethically required, it has been superficial to date and remains insufficient to adequately protect potential subjects.[12]

ARTIFICIAL HEARTS FOR "TEMPORARY" USE

The first two mechanical hearts implanted in the world were implanted by Cooley for temporary use in 1969 and 1981.[13] After these two implants, five permanent implants were performed, four by DeVries, and one in Sweden by Bjarne Semb. Since these seven implants, the field has been dominated by "temporary" mechanical implants, used to sustain the patient until a human heart for transplant becomes available. This use is controversial for many reasons, not the least of which is that as long as there is a shortage of human hearts for transplant, temporary artificial hearts are unlikely to save any net lives; they will only change the identity of those who actually obtain the human hearts.[14] Moreover, the way these devices change the recipient's identity is an inherently unfair one, by permitting those with "temporary" artificial hearts to "jump the queue" and become first in line for the next available matching human heart.

But my quarry here is informed consent. Initially it should be noted that temporary artificial hearts *always* have the possibility of becoming de facto permanent (e.g., if the patient suffers a complication, like stroke, that makes him or her ineligible for a human heart transplant). Since this risk is real, we should require informed consent procedures at least as rigorous as those for permanent implantation.

The historical record, unfortunately, is one of almost indifference to informed consent. This highly experimental intervention has been consistently justified primarily on the basis that it is a therapeutic modality in an emergency setting. The third use of such a temporary device (after Denton Cooley's two) was perhaps the most clumsy and embarrassing since it involved a device that was not even designed or approved for use in human beings. The case is described in some detail because it has set the tone for a rash of "me-too" experiments similar to those that followed Christiaan Barnard's first human-to-human heart transplant[15] and has directly caused the FDA to take a laissez faire attitude toward "temporary" implants that seems to be an abdication of the agency's responsibility to protect the public from unproven and untested medical devices.

THE CASE OF THE PHOENIX HEART

On Tuesday morning, March 5, 1985, Jack Copeland, Chief of University Medical Center's Heart Transplant Team in Tucson, Arizona, performed a human heart transplant on Thomas Creighton, a 33-year-old, divorced father of two. The procedure was not a success, as Creighton's body rejected the heart. At 3:00 a.m. Wednesday morning a search for another human heart began, and Creighton was placed on a heart-lung machine. At 5:30 a.m. a call was placed to Cecil Vaughn of Phoenix, asking if he had an artificial heart ready for human use. Vaughn was scheduled to implant an experimental model developed by dentist Kevin Cheng into a calf later that day and had never considered use of the device in a human. Nonetheless, he called Cheng. Cheng told him: "It's designed for a calf and not ready for a human yet." Asked to think about it for ten minutes, Cheng recalls, "I knelt and prayed." When Vaughn called him back he said: "The pump is sterile, ready to go."[16] The two helicoptered from the hospital to the airport, chartered a jet to Tucson, and then took another helicopter to the Tucson hospital. They arrived at 9:30 a.m. Wednesday morning. The implant procedure began at noon. Designed for a calf, it was too large, and the chest could not be closed around the device. The implant maintained circulation until 11:00 p.m. that night when, in preparation for a second heart transplant, it was turned off, and Creighton was put back on the heart-lung machine. By 3:00 a.m. Thursday, a second human heart transplant was completed. The next day Creighton died.

The press treated the story like a modern American melodrama. *USA Today* called the implantation of Cheng's heart "the fulfillment of an American dream." The *New York Times* editorialized that "the artificial heart has at last proved it has a useful role." *Time* headlined the event as a "bold gamble," and *Newsweek* faulted the FDA, noting, "It's hardly fair to doctors, or their patients, to make them break the law to save a life." The FDA initially termed the unauthorized experiment a violation of the law, but by week's end it did an about-face and was flailing itself as "part of the problem."[17]

Copeland relied on the same two basic excuses his predecessors had used to justify the implant in the absence of the patient's consent: (1) the "only other option was just to let him die" so "we had nothing to lose" and (2) in an emergency, a physician can do anything to save the patient's life.[18] Neither of these assertions can stand scrutiny. The physician may have "nothing to lose," but the patient certainly does. The choice is not, as the five permanent implant patients have all demonstrated, simply one between "life and death." The much more likely scenario is life in a severely disabled and debilitated state—a risk to which *only the patient* should be able to consent. The rationale, that for a dying patient anything is justified, is an illustration of what Katz has termed "magical thinking": that the doctor actually has the power to conquer death and that prolonging life (or prolonging the dying process) is always a reasonable medical goal.

Likewise, the emergency argument is misplaced. All heart-diseased patients will encounter such an "emergency" before they die, and to use this as an excuse to experiment dehumanizes them, making them "fair game" for any experiment no matter how bizarre or extreme. This, of course, is not the law. "Emergencies" like this are anticipatable and must be planned for, with the patient's consent, if risky and extreme experimental interventions are to be offered.

The FDA collapsed when Copeland asserted he was only trying to "save a life" and did not notify the agency of his plans because he did "not want to make the government his [Mr. Creighton's] executioner."[19] Katz would probably see this assertion as another example of identity confusion on the part of the surgeon: Copeland seems to be projecting the role of "executioner" on himself and took objectively useless steps to try to prevent the death of his patient, which he had (albeit in an attempt to save him) directly caused by his own interventions. Conversation with the patient might clarify this confusion, but more than conversation is required to prevent a recurrence of such well-intentioned but pointless "experimentation."

Instead of attempting to curtail and contain experimental temporary use, the FDA actually took steps that served to encourage and spread it, and did so in a way that almost guaranteed that nothing scientifically useful would be learned from temporary implants. In October 1985 the FDA released proposed guidelines that permit *any* surgeon to use any artificial heart in an "emergency" like the one just described.[20] By February 1986 the FDA had also given four centers approval to do ten such implants each, and by the end of 1986 at least fifteen additional "temporary" implants had been performed.[21] There was no master protocol, no uniform patient selection criteria, and no improvements in the area of informed consent.

Moreover, the informed consent forms and processes devised by these first four centers to use the artificial heart as a planned temporary measure were all different and all defective, suffering from all or almost all of the shortcomings involved in obtaining consent for permanent use. It seems likely that the reason consent has not been taken seriously in the temporary setting is because the primary justification for use of the temporary artificial heart is its alleged "emergency" nature. In fact, in at least two of the first five such implants, the patients themselves did not personally participate in any meaningful way in the consent process. And in Europe's first temporary use, the patient was not even told of the planned procedure "because we wanted to prevent him from being disturbed."[22] This is unacceptable. No patient who does not personally consent to its implantation should be seen as an appropriate subject for experimentation with the artificial heart since this is a profoundly radical experiment that can have predictable, devastating effects on the subject.

Indeed, Copeland's third bridge patient (his second was a spectacular success) endured perhaps the most brutal course of any of the permanent or temporary recipients, and it is impossible to reasonably argue that her personal consent should not have been required for each step of her experimental course. Bernadette Chayrez became the second woman in the world to receive an artificial heart on February 3, 1986.[23] Four days later it was removed and replaced with a human heart. The transplant was unsuccessful, and, without the patient's consent but with that of her family, she became the first person in the world to receive a second artificial heart on February 9. The implant turned out to be permanent, and Chayrez spent the rest of her life, 212 days, in the hospital on her "temporary" artificial heart. She died on October 11, 1986, shortly after an attempt to transplant another human heart into her body.

In commenting on the experience, Copeland has been unable to recognize the ethical issues or to properly separate his own identity from that of his patient. He has said, for example: "It was almost like we were married to her; we all felt so close to her after all these months." In this role (i.e., as her spouse) he could not envision terminating the experiment even when it was a clear failure. In his words: "If you cannot transplant a patient, *the only option* is to maintain them the best you can on a total artificial heart." He could not face the patient's death and suggests that perhaps "a committee of bioethicists and critics who want to save a few bucks" could "turn the pump off. . . . Let them turn the *damned thing* off." The "damned thing" Copeland was referring to was, of course, the artificial heart, but he may just as well have been describing his patient. As for ethical problems, Copeland is clear:

> "I don't see any ethical problems at all in what happened with Bernadette. . . . I see the work that we are doing here in the same light as . . . sending up the spacecraft into outer space. Now what possible benefit can we derive from that? A tremendous benefit. *Our endeavors are the same.*"[24] (emphasis added)

With such a fantasyland view of one's activities, it should probably not be surprising that informed consent is a relatively trivial matter to the heart implanters. They should, however, recall that even at the height of our competition with Russia to put the first man on the moon, the United States rejected a proposal to send a man to the moon before we could ensure his safe return. Even though volunteers could be obtained, it was thought to be *a priori* wrong to send a man to his death even for something clearly seen as in the national interest. Informed consent was simply an inadequate justification for taking a human life. It is also an inadequate justification for artificial heart experimentation.

Even if it was sufficient, however, we are not taking it seriously at all in the temporary setting. And informed consent must be taken seriously, at least seriously enough to establish uniform minimal standards that all U.S. centers using "temporary" artificial hearts must meet regarding informed consent. Of course, these should be developed in conjunction with a uniform master protocol and patient selection criteria, so that some useful scientific information can be obtained from multicenter use.

CONCLUSION

Artificial hearts did not create all the problems they have exposed in our informed consent and IRB review procedures. Nonetheless, these problems are real, and the advent of the artificial heart provides us with an opportunity to take meaningful action. This action should not only protect the rights and welfare of potential recipients of the artificial heart but also help set high standards for other controversial human experiments and develop fair and equitable allocation schemes for human organs. Work on informed consent is necessary, but not sufficient to permit artificial heart experimentation.

Because the issues of patient consent and quality medical research in the area of artificial heart have not received sufficient attention and concern to adequately protect subjects of these experiments, there should be a moratorium on all total artificial heart research in humans. This moratorium should continue until the scientific reasonableness, proper use, clear patient selection criteria, adequate informed consent procedures, and clear rules on stopping individual experiments have been developed and approved by a joint review and oversight committee of the FDA and NIH. The de facto moratorium on permanent artificial heart implants should be continued because of the devastating results they have had on subjects and their families, because their original justifications are no longer valid, and because the consent process used is too primitive to protect human subjects. Temporary artificial heart implants should be suspended for the same reasons, and additionally because as long as there is a shortage of human hearts for transplant, temporary artificial hearts can save no net lives and are therefore useless.[25]

Human experimentation is a public enterprise, and the uses to which we put humans, as well as the mandatory minimum procedures we use to protect their rights and welfare, are matters of serious public concern. As illustrated by the most public experiments in history, these issues are taking a back seat to the hype and glitz of what currently passes for scientific medicine. It is imperative that we reassert the importance of human values implicit in the Nuremberg Code before the code is quietly rewritten by magical inventors and researchers.

The following thoughts of another patient in *Cancer Ward* provide a fitting conclusion to a discussion of "death-defying" magical heart implants and informed consent:

> Of course he knew that since all people are mortal, some day he too would have to turn in his check. But *some day*, not now! It was not frightening to die *sometime*, it was frightening to die right now. Why? Because: How would it be? Afterwards, what? And how would it be not to exist, how would it be without me? . . . *He could not even think about it, he could not decide or say anything.* (emphasis added)

16

Rationing Medical Care

Harris Wofford summed up the feelings of many Americans in his success-ful 1991 senatorial campaign when he said: "If criminals have a right to a lawyer, I think working Americans should have the right to a doctor." Our health care system is sick and more than tinkering is required to fix it. Although we spend more money as both a percentage of gross national product and per capita on medical care than any other country in the world, we continue to have a nonsystem. Almost 40 million citizens, one-third of them children, are completely uninsured and are effectively rationed right out of the system. This inequity is no longer socially or ethically tolerable. Almost 90 percent of Americans agree that our health care system needs "fundamental change"; when compared to countries like Canada and En-gland, our system has been accurately described as the most expensive, least well-liked, least equitable, and perhaps least efficient system of health care delivery in the world. It is wasteful, technologically-driven, death-denying, legalistic, and individualistic.

The three major issues are how to control cost, maintain quality, and improve access. The policy problem we have consistently refused to ac-knowledge is that all three of these issues must be dealt with *simultaneously*. Dealing with only one at a time will ultimately be self-defeating. There is virtually unanimous agreement that every American should have access to "an adequate level of care." This package should be developed publicly with wide input. This level of care should also be a floor, not a ceiling; in-dividuals with private insurance or other resources should be permitted to purchase additional coverage. Although this would undercut equity some-what, outlawing self-pay would be an impossible political departure from traditional American individualism and is unnecessary to meet the goal of providing basic health care to all. The inability to develop a minimum benefit package has led to private approaches to decrease the "maximum" benefit package by defining "futility," and to numerous public approaches.

PUBLIC APPROACHES

There are at least four basic public approaches to provide medical care to the currently uninsured. Two federal programs are in place, and two state programs are developing. Medicare pays for almost all hospital-based care for those over age 65, and could form the basis for 2 single-payor model similar to the Canadian system. Medicaid, the federal-state welfare program, requires only that states pay for ten specifically mandated services, but most of its budget winds up paying for nursing home care, and state budgetary limits make expansion improbable. The two stop gap state approaches illustrated by Massachusetts and Oregon may be prototypes for a national plan.

In 1988 Massachusetts took the national lead in attempting to provide universal access to medical care for its citizens by requiring all employers to provide health insurance or pay into a state fund ("pay or play"), and by having the state provide insurance for all those who are not employed. But the recession killed the program in 1992. The problem was that without simultaneously introducing cost and quality control measures, the state and employers could not afford to provide access to what is already the most expensive state medical system in the United States. The astronomical costs of this program ultimately destroyed it.

Oregon's proposal is that the money now spent on Medicaid should be reallocated to cover both the state's Medicaid population and its uninsured. The elderly and disabled would be exempt, making the plan politically possible but fiscally useless. Because *no* plan can provide sufficient funds to cover everyone for everything medicine has to offer, Oregon has proposed that physician and citizen groups prioritize all medical procedures, from antibiotics to heart transplants. This ordering is roughly based on a cost/benefit analysis that is heavily weighted toward giving highest priority to those treatments that are inexpensive and provide the most additional years of quality life, and giving low priority to expensive treatments that provide few added years of quality life. What medical procedures would be available each year would depend on the amount of money allocated by the legislature.

This method of "lengthening the line and thinning the soup" has the very important advantages of being public and explicit. But by limiting rationing to only some segments of the poor, it is unfair; and by ignoring quality control, it fails to address one of the three major issues we confront. The medical care debate in both Oregon and the nation is often framed in terms of rationing. And, whereas during World War II rationing was common and meant simply a "fair allocation of scarce resources," rationing now has an exclusively negative connotation and is a code word for denial of care. Although I think the Oregon plan is unfair, it should be acknowledged that unfairness is always "compared to what?" For currently uninsured Oregonians, for example, the plan is an improvement; were it now in place, and if Oregon tried to alter it to the system that now exists, the unfairness claim would be even more valid.

Another way to ration is to make people wait for services. The American Medical Association has countered that Americans "would rather sue than queue," apparently without realizing that Americans in most large cities must already wait five to seven years to get a jury trial in a civil suit. Americans, in fact, recognize and accept shortages and waits in virtually every sphere of life. On the other hand, given the amount of money we now spend, the Canadian system could be adopted without accepting their elective surgery shortages. We must nonetheless address the issue of what makes Americans think medical care is different from all other goods and services. Many already believe that we must ration medical care more systematically and drastically than we do now. Others believe that further rationing is premature until we stop forcing unwanted treatment and stop performing useless and unnecessary treatment. This seems reasonable, but it will be medicine's successes, not its failures, that will continue to drive up tomorrow's health care bill. Accordingly, we may have to move on both fronts simultaneously.

There is, for example, wide agreement among commentators that we should institute a meaningful program of technology assessment that emphasizes cost effectiveness and support it with a financing mechanism that pays only for the most cost-effective medical interventions for various medical problems. Our confusion over implementation stems from inexact and conflicting goals: increasing length of life, alleviating suffering, and improving quality of life. We will need to examine the basic values behind our health care system, and change them, before the system bankrupts us fiscally and culturally.

THE BRITISH APPROACH

Other countries, of course, have faced the same problem. Great Britain has perhaps tackled it most directly. British commentator Rudolph Klein quotes former British Minister of Health, Enoch Powell, as saying in 1966:

> There is virtually no limit to the amount of medical care an individual is capable of absorbing. . . . There is hardly a type of condition from the most trivial to the gravest which is not susceptible of alternative treatment under conditions affording a wide range of skill, care, comfort, privacy, . . . efficiency, and so on. . . . There is the multiplier effect of successful medical treatment. Improvement in the expectation of survival results in lives that demand further medical care. The poorer (medically speaking) the quality of lives preserved by advancing medical science, the more intense are the demands they continue to make. In short, the appetite for medical treatment *vient en mangeant*.[1]

American philosopher Daniel Callahan has adopted a powerful metaphor to make Powell's point better: the "ragged edge" of medicine's frontiers. Like tearing a piece of rough cloth, "no matter how far we push the frontiers of medical progress we are always left with a ragged edge—with poor outcomes, with cases as bad as those we have succeeded in curing, with the inexorable decline of the body however much we seem to have arrested the process." And even when we do solve some problems, "there will then be others to take their place."[2]

The point is that frontiers will *always* be there as long as we persist in our desire to live as long as we can. The outcome can always potentially be improved at the margin, even though the improvement may be worthless to the patient and extraordinarily expensive to society. We cannot win "the struggle with the ragged edge. We can only move the edge somewhere else, where it will once again tear roughly, and again and again." The problem breeds another: We do not know where to stop. If these commentators are correct, and I think they are, we must devise a socially acceptable set of standards to tell us where to stop before the health care budget erodes our entire way of life by consuming resources that can and should be better spent on living life rather than extending life. Unless we change, we will spend a trillion dollars on medical care by 1995; two trillion by the year 2000.

The major engine driving our current cost inflation in medical care remains the fee for service compensation system. The more physicians do to patients, the more they get paid. And paying physicians for medical services the same way we pay automobile manufacturers for the cars they produce encourages physicians to do more and more to patients. Unlike automobile manufacturers, however, who will continue producing only until marginal cost equals marginal revenue, there is no natural point (other than death) for physicians to stop treating individual patients. As health analyst Alan Sager has noted, this leads to a system in which physicians and hospitals tend to do more and more to fewer and fewer patients at higher and higher cost; and, he might have added, with less and less benefit. Free market advocate Clark Havinghurst has put it simply:

> The current nearly unbearable cost of health care is the inevitable result of giving physicians, hospitals, and technology suppliers nearly a generation (since the enactment of Medicare and Medicaid) in which to invent and sell ever more costly goods and services in a market lacking significant price sensitivity.[3]

And to compound the bureaucratization of medicine, we have 1,600 health insurance companies, each with their own rules and forms.

What can be done? England has managed to provide universal entitlement to health and medical care to its population at half the percentage of gross national product the United States spends. Why the difference? Klein argues that the major difference is based on the concept of the "right to care": British citizens have no legal right to anything, thus what they get through the National Health Service is what they get—there is no right to demand more, and no obvious mechanism to do so. In addition, as Klein has put it elsewhere, Britain is an "original sin society" that accepts the limitations of human life, whereas America is a "perfectibility of man" society that sees the possibilities for improving and extending life here on earth as virtually limitless.

Callahan likewise thinks the solution to changing our value system is to put communitarian values in front of individual values; this would include agreeing to recognize our mortality and to curb our appetite for medical "progress" by strict, centralized technology assessment that includes the social consequences of medicine's potential "successes." We need to talk "about the relationship between good health and the good self, between good health and the good society." We need to ask "what kinds of lives we want to live, and how the quest for health should fit into that life." These are, of course, central philosophical questions.

THE DEMAND FOR MEDICINE

The real issues in American health care are how to make decisions about individual patients, and how to articulate and deliver a decent minimum benefit package for all Americans. It is commonplace to blame the victim by alleging that Americans demand the "best" as their right. Individuals do ultimately consume medical care, but they do not do so in isolation. As Klein has noted in the British context: "It was the producers — the doctors — who generated demands: indirectly by shaping the expectations of consumers, directly by their decisions as to what resources to apply to the treatment of any given patient." Advertising does not just drive the demand for clothes, cars, and breakfast food; it also drives the demand for medical care. We have been taught to demand medical technologies that are touted as "miracles" that can cure us. The amazing thing is not that many Americans want all the miracles — it is that so many reject them.

Our real problem may thus not be that we have too much self-determination, but that we have too little. Demands for added medical care are usually taken seriously only when the patient has the financial resources to pay *and* the physician believes the added care is not unreasonable. Demands to stop or not start care on insured patients are more often the occasion for a psychiatric consult than for honoring self-determination. Nancy Cruzan's problem (discussed in Chapter 7) is *our* problem because it represents a perverse communitarianism: medical treatment that considers societal interests as more important than individual interests. This is why Nancy was treated in her persistent vegetative state: the state of Missouri decided that she must be treated, regardless of her own or her family's wishes, in order to affirm and symbolize the state's interest in the preservation of life "regardless of its quality." *Cruzan* illustrates Ivan Illich's view of death in the modern health care institution: "Natural death is now that point at which the human organism refuses any further input of treatment . . . death happens [only] when the patient becomes useless not only as a producer but also as a consumer."[4] The patient is cared for not as a person, but as a natural resource to be mined until exhausted, both biologically and financially.

The health care system of every country is shaped by the country's political system and values, not the other way around. The pluralistic American political system was not founded on the idea that the government should control our daily lives, but on the notion that the government exists to enhance the "life, liberty and pursuit of happiness" of the individual, and thereby the community. With liberty as its hallmark, we once believed (and I think we still do) that life without liberty is not worth living. Thus to argue that the problem with Americans is that we put too high a value on self-determination, and should look for other values instead to live by, is to argue against our basic political system itself.

We seem to be spending much too much money and medical resources on the dying. But how can we decide how much we should be spending? For example, 30 percent of all Medicare expenditures are made for recipients in the last year of life, but the older a person is when he or she dies, the less money Medicare spends on their last year of life.[5] This doesn't mean it is cheaper to live longer; only that the older you are, the cheaper it is to die.

PROGRESS AND MORTALITY

Where are we headed with our medical system and its continuing quest for newer and more expensive ways to prolong our lives? Medicine has created its own demand and has changed the way we think about ourselves and our concept of a "natural" life span. It is possible that our thinking might evolve to accept inherent limits on life and medical progress. But it seems equally plausible that some new breakthrough or disaster in medicine could itself change the way we think about it. For example, a mutant strain of HIV that infected and ultimately killed half the population would lead us to quickly reevaluate the balance between public health (prevention) and medicine (treatment). Likewise, the development of a drug that greatly enhanced or even prolonged old age might lead us to reject current concepts of an "average life span" and to seek to live years or even decades longer. Can we, or should we, limit research into new medical technologies?

Americans may well vote to limit "halfway" technologies like artificial hearts or brain transfers into robot bodies;[6] but it seems unlikely that they will ever (or should ever) vote to limit medical research designed to discover technologies, drugs, and medical techniques that lengthen life while maintaining its quality. This is because there is no coherent argument for arbitrarily ending a life that could be prolonged with reasonable quality at a reasonable price.

On the other hand, there is no possibility of containing costs (and thus making quality medical care available to all Americans) unless we can come to grips with our mortality. George Bernard Shaw put it well to the British population in his preface to *The Doctor's Dilemma* in 1911, the year England developed its first national health insurance system: "Do not try to live forever. You will not succeed." We must confront our own deaths before we can confront the inherent limits of modern medicine. No plan is economically feasible without limits; and no limits are politically feasible without a recognition that quality of life is much more important than length of life.

Novelist John Updike, who believes Americans are victims not of limits but of dreams, could have been talking about our appetite for longevity and medical care when he said, "There is no enough [in America]. Maybe that's one of the words Americans have a very hard time learning: the word enough."[7]

17

Minerva v. National Health Agency,
53 U.S. 2d 333 (2020)

SUPREME COURT OF THE UNITED STATES

No. 111-252

<table>
<tr><td>Minerva et al.,
Petitioners,
v.
National Health
Agency</td><td>On Appeal from the United
States Court of Appeals for
the District of Columbia.</td></tr>
</table>

[Argued November 12, 2019 – Decided April 10, 2020]

Synopsis

In 2016 the National Health Agency ("the Agency") promulgated regulations which provided for the allocation of artificial hearts in the United States under the authority of the National Health Insurance Act of 1996 (P.L. 104-602). The regulations prohibited the manufacture, sale, or implantation of an artificial heart without a permit from the Agency; prohibited individual purchasers from being recipients of artificial hearts without a permit from the Agency; and provided that permits to recipients be issued only by the Agency's computer, which would pick qualified applicants at random from a master list. This regulation is challenged by P. Minerva, a thoracic surgeon, and two of her patients, Z. Themis and Z. Dike. Themis did not meet the Agency's qualification standards as he is less than fifteen years old; Dike, while meeting the standards, has not yet been chosen by the computer. The plaintiffs challenge the regulations as a violation of their right of privacy, and challenge both the qualification criteria and the random selection procedure and due process under the Fifth Amendment to the U.S. Constitution. This appeal is taken from a decision in favor of the Agency by the Court of Appeals for the District of Columbia. *Minerva v. National Health Agency*, 294 F.3d 28 (D.C. Cir. 2018). Additional relevant facts are set forth in the opinion of the Chief Justice.

CHIEF JUSTICE CLIO delivered the opinion of the Court.

When Congress passed the National Health Insurance Act it granted exceptionally broad powers to the National Health Agency ("the Agency"). One of these powers was the exclusive authority to allocate scarce and expensive medical resources. The Agency has been granted the authority to suspend and revoke medical licenses—all of which have been issued exclusively under federal authority since 1996—of individuals who violate, aid a violator, or conspire to violate the allocation regulations promulgated by the Agency. These provisions of the Act have been previously challenged and upheld by this Court in *Arusha v. National Health Agency*, 29 U.S.2d 124 (2008). In that case, which involved an agency decision to prohibit the use of kidney dialysis machines and ordered all existing kidney dialysis clinics shut down based on a cost-benefit analysis, this Court found such action permissible. Our decision was grounded on a finding of a compelling governmental interest in containing costs and properly allocating resources under the National Health Insurance Program, and a finding that no other reasonable alternative was available to the Agency with regard to this technology. The authority of the Agency to make allocation decisions and to enforce these decisions through licensing sanctions is thus no longer open to challenge.

After three decades of frustration, the implantable artificial heart, powered by a battery, was developed and widely tested in the late 1990s. By 2014 more than 10,000 of these devices were being implanted annually in the United States at a cost of approximately $200,000 each (in terms of 2000 U.S. dollars). The 2014 projections of the National Health Agency were that the annual demand for such hearts would reach approximately 100,000 by the year 2025, and that the National Health Service did not have sufficient funds, personnel, or facilities to implant and maintain such a large number of devices. For example, while the devices are serviceable, they do break down, and all are equipped with a monitoring and warning system that advises the wearer when to get to an emergency department (ED) for service and repair. Up to 20 percent of all ED visits may involve such maintenance in twenty years time. Moreover, a Social Security study found that unlimited use of this device could result in people living longer and this would have the effect of drastically increasing Social Security payments without increasing tax revenues.

Accordingly, the Agency decided, after more than a year of public hearings, to make available annually a maximum of 20,000 artificial hearts. The Agency was statutorily established as the exclusive controller of supply in an effort to ensure both adequate quality control and fairness in patient selection procedures. The allocation scheme promulgated by the Agency and challenged by the plaintiffs provides:[1]

(1) To be placed on the National Waiting List for Artificial Hearts, the candidate must meet the following criteria: He or she must
   (a) be more than 15 years old but less than 70 years old;
   (b) be capable of living at least 10 additional years if the implant procedure is successful; and
   (c) not be a chronic alcoholic or a drug addict.
(2) Individuals certified as meeting the criteria in part (1) by a physician certified by the National Health Agency as a qualified thoracic surgeon shall have their names immediately placed on the National Waiting List for Artificial Hearts. Individuals will be selected from this list at random at the rate of 400 a week. Individuals will be notified of their selection by hologram which will indicate the data and place of the implant procedure. All transportation costs will be paid by the National Health Service. Individuals shall remain on the list until they die, or until such time as they fail to meet any of the criteria set forth in part (1).

I

Plaintiff Minerva's initial argument is that these regulations have "no rational connection with a patient's needs and unduly [infringe] on the physician's right to practice." *Doe v. Bolton,* 410 U.S. 179 (1973). She argues that her patients should be permitted to purchase artificial hearts with their own funds and have her implant them without any interference from the Agency. This argument need not detain us. When the National Health Insurance Act was passed, Congress made it a national priority to provide all its citizens with unlimited access to a specified amount and type of medical care. Any other care was to be rendered at the discretion of the National Health Agency and pursuant to its regulations. So long as such regulations are consistent with the Act and are reasonable methods of rationing expensive and scarce medical resources, they will not be found by this Court to violate a physician's right to practice.

The National Health Agency has permitted a private market in many types of health care—although not in any area of thoracic surgery. This is

---

[1]21 C.F.R. 324.885 (1)–(2) (2015). The government has had similar schemes under study for more than a half century. *See, e.g.,* Dept. of Health, Education, and Welfare, Pub. No. (NIH) 74-191, The Totally Implantable Artificial Heart: A Report of the Artificial Heart Assessment Panel of the National Heart and Lung Institute (June 1973); J. Katz and A. M. Capron, *Catastrophic Diseases: Who Decides What?* 184–196 (1975); and F. Moore, *Transplant: The Give and Take of Tissue Transplantation* 107, 287 (1972). For some early thoughts on how this opinion should be written, see Annas, G. J., Allocation of Artificial Hearts in 2002: *Minerva v. National Health Agency, 3 Am. J. Law & Med.* 59 (1977).

because after the publication of numerous studies in the late 1990s demonstrating a gross oversupply of surgeons, residency positions in this specialty were sharply curtailed. As a result, by 2010 the supply of surgeons in general, and thoracic surgeons in particular, was deemed to be near optimal. The supply, however, was at a point where the shifting of a significant number of surgeons out of the National Health Service would have severely restricted the ability of the Health Service to provide adequate surgical services to the population.

Accordingly, the Health Agency prohibited private surgical practice except under very restrictive conditions. This prohibition was upheld by the court in 2014 in *American Medical Association v. National Health Agency*, 48 U.S.2d 10 (2014). The basis for this decision was that failure to restrict private surgical practice would endanger the health of the members of the public who could not afford private surgical services, since the supply of surgeons and surgical services in hospitals was not adequate to permit elective procedures to be performed on a large scale without a significant decrease in the supply of surgical services to the Health Service. The same rationale, of course, applies to the present case. If a private market in artificial hearts were permitted, a significant percentage of the one million patients a year who need such hearts would purchase this procedure. These purchases could take more than half of all existing thoracic surgeons out of the Health Service, leaving the remainder of the population without sufficient services in this vital area. These effects were felt as early as 2012 when, with fewer than 10,000 implant procedures being performed annually, the average waiting time for other thoracic surgery increased from four to six months. Justice Melpomene argues that a black market in artificial hearts will be produced by these regulations. This is sheer speculation, and in any event the potential existence of such a market should not prevent the federal government from adopting a policy it believes is right and just.

We cannot allow the avarice of a few to jeopardize the health of the many, especially in view of the fact that the many subsidized the training of all currently practicing physicians, continue to subsidize all hospital and surgical facilities, and almost completely subsidized the development of the AH777 model of the artificial heart. The private market in health care is a fiction to which this Court will not subscribe. The physician's "right to practice medicine" properly is regulated and circumscribed by the National Health Agency for the benefit of the public. The regulations properly seek to extend the lives of as many citizens as possible — within the fiscal, personnel, and facility realities of the National Health Service.

II

Plaintiffs Themis and Dike challenge the regulations as a denial of Fifth Amendment due process and equal protection of the laws. The due process argument can be disposed of easily. Plaintiffs argue that they have a right to a hearing, a right to be represented by counsel, a right to an appeal, a right to access to all of the information on file at the National Health Agency concerning each qualified candidate, and a right to challenge the qualifications or comparative qualifications of each candidate.

While the arguments put forth are interesting, they are not persuasive. The allocation scheme is not adversarial. It does not seek to pit the plaintiffs against all other candidates. Indeed, it is possible that *all* the candidates in a given year will be found to be qualified. The scheme is merely an exclusionary one, designed to deny the operation to those who would not derive a sufficient benefit from it to warrant the societal expenses involved. Moreover, the issues are not based on facts personal to the applicant, as in other cases requiring an adjudicatory hearing, but are much more in the nature of applying general policy guidelines. Davis, *Administrative Law* ¶7.03. Therefore, no procedural due process safeguards, other than the certification of the examining physician, are constitutionally required. Furthermore, such additional due process mechanisms, if utilized, could do more harm than good. By delaying the implantation process and by involving the certifying physicians in court battles, time would be lost that could more effectively be spent in screening and treating patients. All potential recipients would suffer.

The equal protection argument is stronger; but, for the reasons set forth below, we reject it. The plaintiffs correctly assert that, although the federal government has not directly created the scarcity in artificial hearts, when it attempts to regulate their distribution the government is bound by the mandate of equal protection. Under the equal protection doctrine of the United States Constitution it also "seemingly makes no difference that the threatened interest is a privilege rather than a right. Even a privilege, benefit, opportunity, or public advantage may not be granted to some but withheld from others where the basis of the classification and difference in treatment is arbitrary."[2] To deny artificial hearts to a group of citizens, the federal government must demonstrate that the classification is based on reasonable grounds in light of the purpose sought to be attained by the Congress, and is not arbitrary and does not cause invidious discrimination. Plaintiffs have urged us to declare the right to an artificial heart a "fundamental interest," or to declare the qualifications for selection "suspect" so that the federal government must demonstrate a compelling state interest to uphold the regulations. We decline to construe the issues at stake so broadly. While the right to life is certainly fundamental and worthy of constitutional protection, the individual's interest in obtaining specific scarce and expensive medical devices is not. Likewise, while the criteria do establish a certain category of qualified recipients, they are drawn narrowly and with a rational relationship to a legitimate governmental purpose. This Court has been very reluctant to expand either the list of fundamental interests or of

[2]Van Alstyne, The Demise of the Right-Privilege Distinction in Constitutional Law, 81 *Harv. L. Rev.* 1439, 1454–55 (1968), citing *Weiman v. Updegraff,* 344 U.S. 183, 192 (1952).

suspect classifications, and we find no necessity to do so in this case. We do note, however, that even if we concluded otherwise, we would find that the federal government had a compelling public well-being interest in promoting the allocation scheme outlined in the regulations, and that the scheme was reasonably related to this interest.

In general, this Court will not interfere with government-mandated allocation schemes. Thus, in *Dandridge v. Williams,* 397 U.S. 471 (1970), we upheld Maryland's AFDC program even though in setting an absolute maximum of $250 per family it discriminated against members of larger families. Likewise, in *Belle Terre v. Boraas,* 416 U.S. 1 (1974), we found a regulation which limited the number of unrelated persons living in a household to be a valid means of controlling vehicular traffic and overcrowding. However, in *Dept. of Agriculture v. Moreno,* 413 U.S. 528 (1973), we struck down a food stamp regulation requiring all members of a household to be related. Even though the federal government argued that this requirement was necessary for the prevention of fraud, we could find no rational relationship between this regulation and the purpose of the statute: to feed the poor. The distinctions between these cases are worth emphasizing. In no instance in *Dandridge* was any family completely deprived of a fundamental requirement of life, and the issues in *Belle Terre* did not involve necessities of life.

This Court will not permit the federal government to deprive its citizens of life's necessities. It will, however, permit the allocation of resources that, while important, are not commonly thought of as necessities of life, provided that the allocation scheme is based upon a valid governmental interest, is for a legitimate purpose, is reasonable, and is not invidiously discriminatory.[3] As applied to the National Health Agency, we conclude that the state cannot deprive its otherwise healthy citizens of "life's necessities" such as emergency medical services. However, when an expensive medical technology can properly be labeled a luxury, even though it does sustain life, the state need not provide it to all citizens.

We find that an artificial heart is no more necessary to an individual than a castle or dinner at Maxim's. Individuals need food, shelter, and medical care—but they may not convert the shield against starvation, exposure, and sickness that the federal government may decide to provide into a sword with which to extract luxuries that society cannot afford. Nature, not the federal government, takes the lives of those who are unsuccessful in the artificial heart lottery. The purposes of maximizing lives within resource constraints and of preventing the destruction of the National Health Service are valid, and the rationing scheme adopted is reasonably related to accomplishing these purposes.

We find that the current regulations are not constitutionally objection-

[3]*See generally* Note, Developments in the Law—Equal Protection, 82 *Harv. L. Rev.* 1065 (1969). Congress exempted allocation determinations of the National Health Agency from the Americans with Disabilities Act.

able. There seem to be only two ways to avoid rationing: universal treatment or universal nontreatment. The first option is simply not feasible. Congress has refused to vote the more than $20 billion (in terms of 2000 dollars) in funds annually required for universal treatment, and through this Congressional refusal the taxpayers have indicated that they would rather retain the money necessary for this program for their own discretionary use than to pay for the tax increase necessary to finance it. The second option, universal nontreatment, makes sense only if it is in fact impossible to make nonarbitrary distinctions among competing applicants, or impossible to devise an equitable rationing process. We find neither to be the case, and therefore conclude that the federal government has a right to enforce its rationing scheme.[4]

III

Plaintiffs have raised the following objections to the Criteria for Placement on the National Waiting List for Artificial Hearts: (1) by specifically denying treatment to most applicants, the regulations cheapen human life and undermine society's belief in the equality of life; (2) the criteria are not medical at all, but are based on "social worth," a criterion specifically denounced in the Conference Committee Report on P.L. 104-602, and a criterion which also undermines our belief in the equality of life; and (3) the artificial heart lottery provisions are unnecessarily imprecise and lead to squandering the federal government's resources since they fail to take into account the relative life expectancy of one applicant versus another or the degree to which one applicant desires the implantation as opposed to another. Thus, the scheme inherently is inequitable and irrational, and only significant modifications in it would make it constitutionally acceptable.

We shall deal with these objections in the order in which they were raised. The first is a general argument against any attempt to ration scarce medical resources, and we reject it outright. By attempting to save as many lives as possible, society does not cheapen human life. On the contrary, it attempts to the best of its ability to protect and prolong life. The fact that all will not benefit from this new technology does not mean that no one should.[5] All citizens cannot live within ten miles of an emergency department equipped to deal in the most efficient way with cardiac arrest. This does not mean we must close these facilities. It only means that they should not be permitted to discriminate arbitrarily among patients who present themselves for treatment.

Themis' argument focuses on the age limitations utilized. We find, how-

---

[4]*Cf. Ross v. Moffitt,* 417 U.S. 600 (1974) (equal protection does not require absolute equality, only freedom from unreasonable distinctions).

[5]As our predecessor Oliver Wendell Holmes so aptly stated, "the law does all that is needed when it does all it can." *Buck v. Bell,* 274 U.S. 200, 208 (1927).

ever, that they are reasonably related to the purposes of the regulation and, therefore, are proper. The fifteen year cut-off reflects both the age of majority (lowered from eighteen to fifteen in 2012) and thus of consent to medical procedures, and the fact that the thoracic cavity will not, in general, be large enough to house the standard AH777 model of the artificial heart currently in use. The rationale for not implanting the heart in anyone incapable of giving informed consent, is sufficiently dealt with in the concurring opinion of our sister Justice Melpomene.

Parenthetically, we note that the seventy-year age limit reflects the overall judgment of the Agency that individuals beyond this age are so likely to be afflicted with other conditions that could prove fatal that it makes more medical sense simply to eliminate them entirely from the process rather than to spend the resources to screen them. One may disagree with these reasons, but Themis has failed to demonstrate to the satisfaction of the Court that these age limitations are so arbitrary as to erode our belief in the equality of human life.

The second objection is more serious. Social worth criteria are properly condemned because they are so imprecise as to maximize the probability of arbitrary decisions based on personal biases of the decisionmaker. We believe, however, that the criteria formulated by the Agency are essentially medical in nature and as such are capable of precise and nonarbitrary application by qualified thoracic surgeons. All of the screening surgeons must meet the strict requirements for certification by the Agency, and we must assume that they will honestly and fairly perform their functions under the regulations. *Withrow v. Larkin,* 421 U.S. 35 (1975). Moreover, the criteria are reasonable in that they preclude from allocation those who will gain only marginally from the implant, and thus help to maximize society's benefits as compared to the costs of this program. Age, prognosis with the implant, drug addiction, and alcoholism are all characteristics that are readily ascertainable by a qualified physician and all can be considered strictly medical criteria.

The third argument is somewhat troublesome, but inasmuch as the plaintiff Dike has not suggested any way in which desire can be quantified and measured on a comparative basis, we need not deal with it.

IV

Additional support for the type of rationing scheme chosen by the Agency is found in law and custom. An 1842 case, for example, involved an American ship which was near Newfoundland, en route from Liverpool to Philadelphia, when it struck an iceberg. The crew and half the passengers escaped on two overly filled lifeboats. One contained forty-one individuals and after about twenty-four hours it became clear that unless some went overboard, all would perish. The first mate instructed his crew (eight in number) to throw fourteen passengers overboard, using the rule "not to

part man and wife, and not to throw over any women." At the trial of
one of the seamen for homicide, the court instructed the jury that under
extraordinary circumstances the "law of necessity"[6] may justify taking a
life, but that in choosing who shall live and who shall perish "there should
be consultation and some mode of selection fixed, by which those in equal
relations may have equal chance for life . . . for ourselves we can conceive
of no mode so consonant both to humanity and justice [as casting lots]."[7]

Not only was a lottery approved, but the court also concluded that the
first mate and as many of the crew as were necessary to run the boat were
not required to take part. Thus, the court sanctioned the exclusion, based
on specified criteria, of certain members of society from a lottery scheme.
While this case involved choosing individuals to die, not to live, as is the
case in allocating artificial hearts, the same standard applies in the latter
case. The traditional rule of the sea when a ship is sinking has always
been "women and children first." This principle seems to rest on the belief
that women are necessary for the survival of the species, and that children
have more years left to contribute to society than adults. Both this traditional principle and the lifeboat case sanction "social worth" criteria under
certain extreme cases, the arguments of our sister Justice Urania notwithstanding.[8]

The decision of the Court of Appeals of the District of Columbia is
accordingly

Affirmed

Calliope, Terpsichore, and Polyhymnia, JJ. join in THE CHIEF JUSTICE'S
opinion.

JUSTICE MELPOMENE, concurring in the result.

While I join my sisters in upholding these regulations as valid and constitutional exercises of authority by the National Health Agency, I feel com-
pelled to pen a separate opinion. In my view, there should be *no* allocation
scheme whatsoever mandated by the federal government: artificial hearts
should simply be outlawed in this country. I come to this conclusion even
though I myself have such a device pumping blood through my arteries. It
never gives me peace. When I am alone in my bed at night I hear it. It
reminds me both of my mortality and of my humanness—but it also taunts
me. I am no longer fully human; I am already partially dead.

Furthermore, how can one give informed consent to receive such a de-

---

[6]For a brilliant discussion of this concept, see Fuller, The Case of the Speluncean Explorers,
62 *Harv. L. Rev.* 616 (1949).

[7]*United States v. Holmes,* 26 F. Cases 360, 367 (Cir. Ct. Pa. 1842). See also *Holmes v.
N.Y. City Housing Authority,* 398 F.2d 262 (2d Cir. 1968) (the court indicated it would
approve an allocation scheme in public housing based on a first-come, first-served basis with
certain specified exceptions).

[8]*See* Dukeminier & Sanders, Legal Problems in Allocation of Scarce Medical Resources:
The Artificial Kidney, 127 *Arch. Intern. Med.* 1133, 1134 (1971).

vice? I did, or so I thought, but when faced with death, people are likely to consent to anything. We all know this. It is ancient history that Christiaan Barnard noted of the first recipient of a human heart that consent to this procedure was not heroic but to be expected:

> He was ready to accept it because he was at the end of the line. What else was there to say? . . . For a dying man, it is not a difficult decision because he knows he is at the end. If a lion chases you to the bank of a river filled with crocodiles, you will leap into the water convinced you have a chance to swim to the other side. But you would never accept such odds if there was no lion.[9]

Likewise, Denton Cooley wrote of the first human ever to receive an implanted artificial heart: "He was a drowning man. A drowning man can't be too particular what he's going to use as a possible life preserver. It was a desperate thing and he knew it."[10]

Currently, implants are no longer experimental, and the situations of patients are no longer so "desperate." Nevertheless, it is my experience that a significant number of candidates feel they *must* have an artificial heart, and will do almost anything to gain access to one.[11] This impulse may be based solely on the irrational desire to live forever.

It is my view that any attempt to ration artificial hearts, even one so carefully drawn as the regulations under consideration, will fail to prevent significant black markets in such hearts; will encourage surgeons in the National Health Service (who consider themselves grossly underpaid) to operate in this market; and will encourage patients to attempt to bribe health officials and physicians, and to commit other crimes in an effort to obtain an artificial heart.

For these reasons—because the artificial heart is fundamentally inhuman and inhumane, because informed consent can never be obtained, and because allocation will lead to many undesirable side effects in society—I would outlaw these devices altogether. Nevertheless, since I believe this is properly a legislative decision, I would uphold regulations that at least attempt to limit their distribution.

JUSTICE URANIA, with JUSTICE THALIA and JUSTICE ERATO join, dissenting.

The Supreme Court today approves an allocation scheme that is inherently inequitable and unjust, that undermines society's view of the sacredness and equality of human life, and that makes social worth the standard for longevity in our society. The majority asserts that the allocation scheme reflects the application of rational and exact medical criteria. In fact, how-

---

[9]C. Barnard & C. B. Pepper, *One Life* 311 (1969).

[10]*Quoted in* J. Thorwald, *The Patients* 402 (1972).

[11]In this regard it is my view that while a deductible of one year's income would help to measure "desire," it would not significantly reduce the number of applicants since money becomes less meaningful as the time available to spend it decreases.

ever, the regulations permit individual physicians to make arbitrary decisions based solely on their own views of social worth. Since physicians in
general, and thoracic surgeons in particular, are likely to have a white
upper-middle class male bias in this area,[12] such a classification scheme is
inherently violative of the equal protection mandate of the Fifth Amendment.

I

The true character of the regulations may be seen in a recent study of the
persons who were accepted and those who were rejected for places on the
National Waiting List for Artificial Hearts for the year 2018 (the only full
year for which statistics are available).[13] In that year more than two million
persons applied for the Waiting List. Of that number, one million, or fifty
percent, were rejected. Of these, more than ninety percent were rejected on
the basis of criteria (b) (incapable of ten additional years of life), or criteria
(c) (chronic alcoholism or drug addiction). The statistics also indicate that
at least seventy percent of each of the following categories of individuals
were rejected:

I.Q. lower than 80:	98%
History of mental illness:	80%
Criminal record:	75%
Indigency:	80%
Unemployed:	70%

The generality of the statistics does not permit further breakdown into
more specific income level, I.Q., or type of mental illness. Nonetheless, I
submit that these figures are sufficient to warrant the conclusion that the
scheme mandated by the regulations discriminates invidiously and unconsti-
tutionally against the mentally deficient, the mentally ill, those with prior
criminal records, the poor, and the unemployed. While the regulations, as
written, are difficult to attack, they are clearly *not* the criteria that surgeons
have actually been using to select patients. There is *no* rational connection
between such invidious discrimination and the state's purpose; thus, the
regulations must fail a constitutional test. Although the majority concludes
that the classification established by these regulations should not be considered suspect, these figures clearly indicated not only that it should, but that
it is. Accordingly, the state should be required to demonstrate a compelling
interest to permit these regulations to withstand an equal protection challenge. Whether the interest in maintaining the viability of the medical care
delivery system is compelling or not depends in large part on one's view

[12]The plaintiff, Minerva, is one of the few exceptions to this rule.
[13]Glantz, Patient Selection for Artificial Hearts: The First Year, 46 *Am. J. Law & Med.* 232
(2019).

of its credibility. In my view, the government has failed to demonstrate adequately that a less restrictive allocation system would lead to a total breakdown of the National Health Service. Until such evidence is forthcoming, I would rule that the compelling interest test has not been met, and therefore find the regulations constitutionally deficient.

In addition, the legislative history indicates that Congress intended that only objective medical criteria be permitted to enter the decisionmaking process. There was testimony, for example, concerning some of the initial methods used to screen patients for kidney dialysis forty years ago. One lay member of a screening committee in Seattle testified that

> the choices were hard. . . . I remember voting against a young woman who was a known prostitute. I found I couldn't vote for her, rather than another candidate, a young wife and mother. I also voted against a young man who, until he learned he had renal failure, had been a ne'er-do-well, a real playboy. He promised to reform his character, go back to school, and so on, if only he were selected for treatment. But I felt I'd lived long enough to know that a person like that won't really do what he was promising at the time.[14]

All members of the Conference Committee found these types of social worth judgments disgusting. In their final report to Congress they quoted the following language from a study of the Seattle committee of which this woman was a member:

> The descriptions of how this committee makes its decisions . . . are numbing accounts of how close to the surface lie the prejudices and mindless cliches that pollute the committee's deliberations. . . . What is meant by "public service," a phrase so difficult to define in a pluralistic society? Were the persons who got themselves jailed in the South while working for civil rights doing a 'public service'? What about working for the Antivivisection League? Why should a Sunday-school teacher be saved rather than Madalyn Murray? The [decisions] paint a disturbing picture of the bourgeoisie, of the Seattle committee measuring persons in accordance with its own middle-class values. This rules out creative nonconformists, who rub the bourgeoisie so much the wrong way but who historically have contributed so much to the making of America. The Pacific Northwest is no place for a Henry David Thoreau with bad kidneys.[15]

The regulations are so loosely drawn, especially subsections (b) and (c), that they permit physicians to exercise completely unbridled discretion in making their choices, and permit them to make these choices not on the basis of fixed medical criteria, but on the basis of their own, sometimes warped, views of social worth. The results of the study support the con-

---

[14]R. Fox & J. Swazey, *The Courage to Fail,* Chicago: U. of Chicago Press, 1974. See also R. Fox & J. Swazey, *Spare Parts,* New York: Oxford U. Press, 1992.

[15]Sanders & Dukeminier, Medical Advance and Legal Lag: Hemodialysis and Kidney Transplantation, 15 *U.C.L.A. L. Rev.* 357 (1968). *And see* Annas, The Prostitute, the Playboy, and the Poet, 75 *Am. J. Public Health* 187 (1985).

clusion that this is precisely what has been occurring. It is apparent that physicians are basing their survival estimates on such things as "cooperativeness," "rehabilitation potential," "self-esteem," "low intelligence," "impulsive, irresponsible behavior," "self-destructive wishes," "difficulty relating to authority figures," and so on. A demonstrated "connection between the favored traits severally considered and ability to survive"[16] should be demanded if such criteria are to continue in use. No such connection has been demonstrated. Accordingly, the regulations should be struck down.

II

The Agency has convinced the majority that its age limitation is reasonable, but it has not convinced me. A youth of twelve or thirteen, such as plaintiff Themis, may have a body capable of receiving the artificial heart and should not arbitrarily be denied it simply because most other children his or her age could not be fitted with the AH777. Likewise, is it reasonable to reject a seventy-one-year-old applicant with a life expectancy of twenty years, while accepting a sixty-nine-year-old with a life expectancy of ten years? Such an allocation scheme is de facto irrational. Since it could be much more fairly drawn, it cannot stand constitutional challenge. I would much prefer to have simply a first-come, first-served scheme than to set such patently arbitrary criteria. While the first-come, first-served system would also discriminate arbitrarily, such discrimination would be more in the nature of "acts of God" rather than explicit acts of government, and thus would not serve to cheapen our view of human life and the equality of man.[17]

III

Further, to characterize the artificial heart as a "luxury" — which the majority does — is playing with words. Today's luxury is tomorrow's necessity. The heroic or extraordinary treatments of the late 20th century are today commonplace in our hospitals. Artificial hearts are prolonging lives. They could prolong far more lives both now and in the future if more resources were allocated to this critical field. When, in fifteen or twenty years, all the other civilized nations of the world routinely implant such devices in their citizens, will the majority change its mind? Will artificial hearts then become "natural" or at least necessary for life? If so, why must we sacrifice the present generation for the next?

[16]Note, Patient Selection for Artificial and Transplanted Organs, 82 *Harv. L. Rev.* 1322, 1339 (1969).

[17]*See, e.g.,* Childress, Who Shall Live When Not All Can Live? 53 *Soundings* 339, 247–53 (1970). *See generally* G. B. Shaw, *The Doctor's Dilemma* (1905).

IV

The allocation scheme is a threat to our values and an insult to our intelligence. We need not be guided in our decision by the unwritten rules of sailors who prowled the sea in their sail-drawn ships almost two centuries ago. How much better to learn from the more advanced planets with whom we have recently established contact. On Zeno, for example, all are eligible for artificial organs — but must make the election by their twenty-fifth birthday and accept permanent sterility as the price. In this way, they both lengthen life and control total population size (and thus the cost of the program).[18] While I do not propose that we accept such an alternative without study or legislative mandate, I do reject the current scheme and the majority's endorsement of it.

JUSTICE THALIA, dissenting.

I join with my sister Urania in her dissent. Nonetheless, I write to argue that her analysis leads to an additional and inescapable conclusion: the regulations violate a candidate's right to due process. It is apparent that no matter what criteria are utilized, fairness is enhanced when there is more than one decisionmaker. It is inappropriate and unfair to expect a patient to dispute the findings of the examining physician to the physician herself. A procedure requiring the concurrence of two of a board of three physicians would be much fairer and presumably would lead to much more consistent and accurate decisionmaking. In addition, if the criteria specified in the regulations are to be applied, and "survivability" is defined as I believe my sister Justice Urania accurately indicates it is presently defined, then many more due process protections than currently exist are mandated by the U.S. Constitution. Contrary to the majority's view, the types of facts at issue in the screening process are extremely personal, and ones that are unique to the candidate. Due process, therefore, requires that the candidate be given a full adjudicatory hearing upon request. Davis, *Administrative Law* ¶7.03.

Additional safeguards are also necessary. The patient's life is at stake, and Congress has mandated a system that excludes social worth from consideration so that the fundamental belief of our society in the equality of human life is not destroyed. To insure that each potential patient has a fair opportunity of being included in the National Waiting List for Artificial Hearts it is essential that at the minimum he or she be permitted (1) to examine in advance all records in the hands of the decisionmaker; (2) to have an opportunity to refute their accuracy and to supplement them; (3) to have an opportunity to call and cross-examine any individual who has presented information that might disqualify the applicant from consideration; (4) to have a record of the reason for the decision; and (5) to have

---

[18]Communication from Zeno II Tracker Station, NASA Classified Document 2119652 (level of classification is classified) (quoted with permission of the Director).

an opportunity to appeal the decision to an appeals board. Unless these minimal procedural safeguards are provided (and I also favor mandatory representation by counsel upon request, but it is not constitutionally required), it is my opinion that these regulations are constitutionally deficient and must be struck down.

JUSTICE EUTERPE, dissenting.

I find the arguments of my colleagues all very interesting but, with the exception of Justice Melpomene, irrelevant. Have we progressed so much in this country that we have lost sight of our purpose as a nation? The unsubstantiated communications from Zeno notwithstanding, surely no one in their right mind will argue that we can make our citizens immortal. Even if we can produce an artificial heart that will last forever, the other tissues and organs will continue to deteriorate. While reading is not currently in fashion in our society, some will recall *Gulliver's Travels* and Swift's description of the Struldbrugs, creatures who did achieve immortality, but whose minds and bodies suffered from the decay of old age nonetheless:

> At ninety they lose their teeth and hair; they have at that age no distinction of taste, but eat and drink whatever they can get, without relish or appetite. The diseases they were subject to still continue without increasing or diminishing. In talking, they forget the common appellation of things and the names of persons, even of those who are their nearest and dearest friends and relations. For the same reason, they never can amuse themselves with reading, because their memory will not serve to carry them from the beginning of a sentence to the end; and by this defect, they are deprived of the only entertainment whereof they might otherwise be capable. . . . They are despised and hated. . . . They were the most mortifying sight I ever beheld. . . . Besides the usual deformities in extreme old age, they acquired an additional ghastliness in proportion to their number of years, which is not to be described.

The energies of the National Health Agency should be directed toward the young and the middle-aged and toward making life more enjoyable and richer. It should not be directed toward prolonging the agony of death and the miseries of old age. If we are unwilling as a society to pay for the implantation of an artificial heart into each of our citizens who can reasonably benefit medically from it, then we should have the courage to adopt a rule which says that *no one* shall have such a device implanted. Such a rule promotes equality and fairness. It is also an attempt to allocate resources toward medical and health measures that make our lives worth living, rather than ones that prolong lives that are not worth living. I would rather deprive all of the aid of the artificial heart, as did Conrad's Lord Jim and the rest of the crew who deserted the passengers of the Patna, than to arbitrarily choose who shall live, as the first mate did in the lifeboat case summarized by the Chief Justice.

Even if one were determined to implant artificial hearts in some, surely the market system is a better allocator of 20,000 hearts a year than the administratively clumsy and arbitrary scheme envisioned in the regulations. Although ability to pay is itself somewhat of a social worth criterion, when coupled with a strong desire to have an implant and a willing physician, I believe it is a proper characteristic to use for deciding who will receive a medical device which is of dubious value to either the individual or society. It might also be appropriate to create a "distinguished citizen" award, the recipients being individuals of tremendous importance to our society whose lives should be prolonged for the good of us all without respect to their financial ability or even their desire for an implant.

Finally, I do not think it purely a coincidence that all five Justices in the majority are recipients of artificial hearts, while none of the four in the minority applied for one either before or after the regulations under question went into effect. While the decision on disqualifying oneself because of a conflict of interest or bias in a particular case is for each individual Justice, I cannot help but observe that the decision would have been unanimously decided against these regulations had these Justices taken the step of disqualifying themselves from hearing this case.

18
Siamese Twins: Killing One to Save the Other

The separation of Siamese twins with conjoined hearts, while a rare event, has received some ethical and legal discussion.[1] Most of it, unfortunately, has been characterized by fuzzy thinking and flawed analogies. Perhaps this is inevitable. Siamese twins have always seemed bizarre to us. Their very name comes from history's most famous such twins, Eng and Chang Bunker. Born in Siam in 1811, they lived until 1874 and were exhibited around the world by P. T. Barnum. The second most famous are Amos and Eddie Smith, fictional Siamese twins who are the subjects of Judith Rossner's challenging novel, *Attachments*, and who, in the novel, also spent some time with Ringling Brothers Barnum & Bailey.

Siamese twins continued to be referred to in freakish, carnival sideshow terms ("double-headed monster," thoracopagus monster, *monstruo doble, Doppelmisbildungen*, and *les monstres à deux têtes*), in the medical literature well into the 20th century. Are Siamese twins "monsters" that do not merit the care we routinely provide other infants, or are they two persons, each of which merits care in its own best interests? Can one twin be sacrificed so that the other may be made "human"?

Conjoined twins are the product of a single ovum, and thus the children have the same chromosomal composition and sex. Approximately three-quarters of all such twins are joined at the chest (thoracopagus twins) and have a conjoined heart. Of this group it is believed that surgical separation is hopeless in the vast majority of cases; and, even in the others, where success is theoretically possible by sacrificing one of the twins, no twin with a conjoined heart has survived for more than a few months after separation.[2] On the other hand, unlike the Bunkers and the Smiths, no thoracopagus twins with conjoined hearts have survived longer than nine months remaining attached, apparently because their heart strength is insufficient to maintain adequate circulation for both bodies.

STRAINING FOR ANALOGIES

The case that has received the most commentary occurred in October 1977 at Children's Hospital in Philadelphia. The attending physician was former Surgeon General C. Everett Koop. Survival of both twins following separation was impossible, and survival of one very unlikely. Could one twin be "sacrificed" so that the other might have a chance to live? Because the parents were deeply religious Jews, they would not consent to separation without rabbinical support. Most of the nurses were Catholic, and they refused to be involved unless a priest assured them it was morally acceptable. Koop, among other things, feared potential homicide charges, and he would not perform the separation unless a court granted him prospective legal immunity from criminal prosecution.

What differentiates this case from the anencephalic baby, the Tay-Sachs baby, or the trisomy-13 baby is that there is a possible (albeit highly experimental and so-far unsuccessful) intervention that has the potential to permit one of the two children to live. Thus it is not simply a question of killing one child or letting it die because it cannot survive long in any event. The case is more analogous to attempted selective feticide when amniocentesis discloses that one of two fetuses is affected with a severely handicapping condition, and the mother would definitely abort both if not given the option to try to abort only the affected twin. It is only the current status of the abortion laws that permit a selective abortion decision to be made by the woman prior to viability. After birth, selective infanticide is not a legal option. But should it be if the twins are physically connected and can be thought of as literally, although innocently, killing each other?

The rabbinical scholars involved in the 1977 case reportedly relied primarily on two analogies.[3] In the first, two men jump out of a burning airplane. The parachute of the second man does not open, and as he falls past the first man, he grabs his legs. If the parachute cannot support both of them, is the first man morally justified in kicking the second man away to save himself? Yes, said the rabbis, since the man whose parachute didn't open was "designated for death."

The second analogy involves a caravan surrounded by bandits. The bandits demand a particular member of the caravan be given up for execution and the rest will go free. Assuming that the named individual has been "designated for death," the rabbis conclude it was acceptable to surrender him to save everyone else. Accordingly, they concluded that if twin A was "designated for death," and could not survive in any event, but twin B could, surgery that would kill twin A to help improve the chances of twin B was acceptable.

The Catholic justification, which employed the principle of the double effect, was even more strained. That principle states generally that if an action has two effects, one good and one bad, it can still be acceptable if the good effect does not come about because of the bad effect, and there is a proportionate reason for permitting the bad effect. Here the bad effect is the death of twin A and the good effect is the possibility of preserving the life of twin B. When the carotid artery feeding blood to the brain of twin A is tied off, this causes the death of twin A. It was argued that this action, however, was not done to terminate twin A's life, but to preserve the life of twin B by protecting it from the poisons that would build up in twin A's blood after its death.[4]

Application of the principle of the double effect, however, seems to fail because it is precisely the bad effect that permits the good effect: killing twin A permits twin B to have a chance to live (twin A's blood becomes poisoned and threatens twin B only after it is dead). One might respond that it is nonetheless better that twin B have a chance to live than that both twins die, but this does not address the fact that twin A has been killed to try to save twin B. The good end has been used to justify the evil means. One must argue further that twin A is a threat to twin B merely because its body requires more support than their shared heart can provide. Then it could be argued that one is relieving the pressure on twin B's heart by tying off the carotid artery, and twin A's death becomes an inevitable, but unintended, result of a good act.

A three-judge panel of the family court heard the hospital lawyers make two additional arguments on behalf of Koop. The first was that because the two twins had only one heart between them, there was only one person. This argument was rejected, primarily because the concept of brain death was already well established. On the other hand, if the child had only one body and two heads, the court might well have concluded that it was just one child, and that removing one of the heads would be similar to removing an extra arm or leg. Their second argument was an analogy similar to the rabbinical one. Two mountain climbers are attached together by a rope. One falls from his perch, but is saved from instant death by the rope attached to his partner. His partner has a more secure hold, but not so secure that he can hold both of them. In this circumstance (like the parachute case) the lawyers argued that it was acceptable for the mountain climber with the more secure hold to cut the rope to save himself.[5] After deliberating for a few minutes, the court authorized Koop to perform the surgery. It was done the next day. The separation was successful, but the surviving twin died three months later.

Three things should be noted about the 1977 case. First, the analogies are weak. In all of them adults are consciously and voluntarily engaged in known, risky behaviors, and one adult always puts the other's life in peril by his own actions. Neither voluntary assumption of the risk nor any personal act on the part of the twins can justify treating them like mountain climbers or parachuters. Second, there was great consternation and ethical and legal debate about this case, which was seen as problematic by almost everyone involved. Third, homicide charges were considered such a real possibility that the surgeon demanded a court order before he would proceed.

In a similar case in Little Rock, Arkansas, that same month, surgery was not performed until both the state attorney general and the county prosecutor agreed that no criminal prosecution would be pursued. The Arkansas case was described by the physicians involved as an "amputation" (of the right twin from the left twin). Even though it was recognized that the surgical result was very suboptimal, the physicians thought "it seemed unwise in view of the prolonged survivals of some dicephalus twins not to attempt separation."[6](!)

Ten years later, in early 1987, the same basic case was again presented to the physicians at Philadelphia Children's Hospital. In the meantime, there had been a number of versions of the Baby Doe regulations, and the first (and still only) attempted criminal prosecution of a physician for nontreatment of a newborn—the Danville, Illinois, Siamese twins case.[7] Nonetheless, the legal aspects of the case were handled more calmly. The surgeon, James A. O'Neill, Jr., did not demand or expect prospective legal immunity from a court. The hospital's lawyers, however, did ask the district attorney's office to sign a letter saying the surgeons would not be prosecuted for homicide. The D.A.'s office complied, but thought the entire exercise unnecessary and a simple "CYA" bid by the hospital attorneys.

Instead of going to court, the surgeon sought concurrence from a group not available in 1977: the hospital ethics committee. The committee talked the matter over for an hour and a half and agreed with the surgeon's plan. He was pleased with both the process and the outcome. The surgery was performed, but neither twin survived.

THE POTENTIAL TO SURVIVE

There are two ways in which these cases can appear easy. The first is to assume that there is some "objective medical criteria" that can determine which one of the twins has a significantly better chance to survive. In this case, the decision is not which twin will survive (their own condition has determined this), but whether the separation should be carried out at all. Also, since the separation procedure remains experimental, and survival is unprecedented, there is no question that the parents have a right to refuse to have the separation performed. The second is the "monster" approach, which concludes that the twins are so grotesque that they are not really human. Therefore, we are justified in doing anything medically reasonable to make at least one of them "human," even if it is highly probable that it will result in both of their deaths.

The case is much more difficult if there is no significant difference in the survival potential of the two twins, and thus neither is "designated for death." Rather, one must be chosen to die for the sake of the other. How should this decision be made? The more apt (though equally unlikely) analogy is now clear. A man jumps out of a burning plane with two infant children in his arms. His parachute opens. As he descends, he begins to lose his grip on both of them. Which one does he drop to save the other?

If this is the case with Siamese twins, the fairest way to determine which survives is random, by the flip of a coin. Besides having the advantage of eliminating human prejudices, it also has a potential advantage for the surviving twin (assuming that one will survive) who doesn't have to live with the knowledge that his life was paid for by a conscious decision to kill his identical twin. A decision to kill one to save the other in this circumstance would be homicide (as Koop knew), but the relevant legal issue is whether it would be justifiable homicide.

The closest legal cases deal with necessity, actions taken in response to natural disasters and acts of God. In a lifeboat, for example, it has been thought to be acceptable to cast lots to see which individuals get thrown overboard if some must die to keep the boat afloat. But having the stronger simply throw the weaker overboard is not justified by the circumstances. What really seems to be at issue in this case is the more modern notion of the "choice of evils" defense, which now serves to exculpate justified conduct no matter what the source of the threat.[8]

Restated, does society regard it as justified to kill one twin to attempt to save the other? As long as the rescue attempt is medically reasonable and the choice of which twin to kill is made fairly, the answer is almost unquestionably "yes." Although flipping coins is the fairest, society would likely find it too callous and arbitrary. That is why we continue to look for "objective medical criteria" to decide, for example, who gets the next heart for transplant. In this case we would also probably let the physician decide which twin was most likely to survive to maintain the fiction that the decision was an "act of God." Likewise, our parachutist with his two children would likely instinctively drop the one he held in the weakest grasp, to try to make sure that he could rescue at least one child.

A more formal best interests analysis "works" only if we make some strained assumptions. Having twin A separated from twin B is in twin B's best interests if it enhances his chances to survive. It cannot, however, be said to be in twin A's best interests objectively (unless one accepts the monster analysis and concludes that the life of such a twin is so degrading to it that it is better off dead) since twin A is experiencing life and is not suffering, and its life will be cut short by the procedure.

If we want to fantasize a substituted judgment scenario, we can ask twin A if he will consent to being killed, understanding that he will die soon in any event, and unless he undergoes this sacrifice his twin brother will also die. Since his twin brother carries his identical genes, the only way his genes have any chance to survive is if he makes the supreme sacrifice. Using this wildly speculative scenario, one might conclude that twin A might consent to die for his twin or at least that the scenario is plausible enough that the parents of twins A and B should be permitted to make this terribly difficult decision under these unique and tragic circumstances.

We can also complicate the matter further by unequivocally declaring that there really are two patients here, not just one. Thus separate representation in some form should be considered. For example, prior cases have all assumed that one child must die for the other to have a chance to live, and this may indeed be true. But unless each child has its own advocate, alternatives that might permit them both to have some chance at survival might not be vigorously pursued. At some point in the future, for example, it seems likely that it will be possible for the twin who will not have its circulation maintained to be a candidate for a heart transplant. Although this will present a logistical nightmare, it may at least be possible to put the "doomed" twin on a heart transplant list, and if a heart becomes available (and if it cannot be used by a more "medically suitable" candidate) before separation surgery must be performed, to try to preserve the lives of both children.

This approach "solves" the problem of choosing between the two twins, but brings us back to a question that underlies our entire discussion: When is it reasonable to perform an experimental intervention on a human being that has little chance of success? In terms of separating Siamese twins with conjoined hearts, it seems likely that most people would agree with the fictional physician in *Attachments*, who concluded "the condition is enough reason to attempt the cure." Stated somewhat differently, it is better to intervene to try to save one life than to passively observe two lives end. Both law and ethics support reasonable medical attempts to separate Siamese twins with conjoined hearts. Nonetheless, defining a rationale better than human instinct is perplexing, and developing a fair and useful procedure to apply it remains an unmet challenge.

19
Killing Machines

The adoption of military metaphors by the medical profession is well known.[1] Physicians aggressively combat disease on the front lines, using their armamentarium to destroy invaders of the body. The military also adopts medical metaphors, ranging from surgical strikes to antiseptic operations. Less commented on is the adoption of modern technology by both the military and medicine, and what insights we might gain about medicine by examining military technology. In the wake of operation Desert Storm, however, it is difficult to ignore the striking similarities. In both cases, for example, we will pay double or triple for a small increase in efficacy. As retired Admiral Eugene Carroll put it: "The military always stresses performance at all cost." For a 10 percent increase in performance, the military will pay twice as much, and the new technology will be twice as difficult to operate and maintain.

One of the most intriguing parallels between military technology and medical technology is that some technologies, often the most efficient and effective, are considered either unethical or unfair. Western civilization, at least until 1500 A.D., seems to have considered weapons that allowed their users to kill "from a distance and behind cover" unfair, because "such weapons obscured the vital distinction between war and plain murder."[2] Thus, for example, both the long bow and the cross bow were regarded as "cowardly" and unfair. More recently, chemical and biological weapons have entered the unfair category, apparently because they are so feared and effective, but also perhaps because they have the capability to indiscriminately kill both civilian populations and military personnel.

Two days before American war planes attacked Iraq, the Public Broadcasting System aired a *Nova* program entitled "The Killing Machines." The program focused on the new technology of war. It ultimately concluded that technology is only useful against technology, that the increased information available to commanders, and their decreased time for decisionmak-

240

ing, increases the risk of human error. Whatever one thinks about these observations regarding war machines, their applicability to medicine seems beyond dispute.

Desert Shield was converted into Desert Storm six months later. Much of the country, probably the vast majority, felt themselves simply spectators in an event, sometimes described by administration officials and military experts as a "game," that they were totally helpless to influence. Although much of the discussion was certainly coincidental, it seemed that at least some of the heightened and sharpened debate about the "right to die" during the Gulf war period was an attempt by a passive populace to assert at least some measure of control over their own lives and over the medical machines that might be employed to prolong their dying.

Historically, for example, the Karen Ann Quinlan case (see Chapter 8) is often portrayed as a question of "turning off the machine." And the case that has occasioned the most heated debate has not focused on either a doctor or a patient, but on a machine itself: Jack Kevorkian's "suicide machine," first used in the death of Janet Adkins. Kevorkian was hardly the first U.S. physician to assist in a patient's suicide. The difference is that previously deaths involved patients taking prescription drugs; this was the first case of a physician using a "killing machine" to produce death. Is it too far a stretch to think that what upset most ethicists was more the machine than the act itself? Is the machine seen as an "unfair" or unethical weapon that makes the distinction between murder and the practice of medicine difficult or impossible?

THE MICHIGAN SUICIDE CASES

Kevorkian, whose business card reads "Bioethics and Obituary, Special Death Counseling, by Appointment Only," reportedly picked Michigan to showcase his suicide machine because he believed that assisted suicide was legal in Michigan. He apparently based this belief on his own reading of two Michigan cases. The first, *People v. Roberts*,[3] was decided by the Michigan Supreme Court in 1920. In that case Frank C. Roberts plead guilty to the charge of murder in the first degree for killing his wife, Katie. Katie Roberts was terminally ill, practically helpless, and suffering from multiple sclerosis. At his wife's request, Roberts mixed a quantity of paris green (which contains arsenic) in a drink. Mrs. Roberts drank the potion with the intention of taking her own life and died a few hours later. After being sentenced to life imprisonment on the basis of his confession, Roberts appealed. The primary argument was that since there was no crime of suicide in Michigan, there could be no crime of being an accessory before the fact of suicide—that is, since Mrs. Roberts committed no crime in killing herself, Mr. Roberts could have committed no crime in helping her.

The Michigan Supreme Court rejected this argument on the basis that the charge was murder "by means of poison." The Michigan homicide statute provided in part that "All murder which shall be perpetrated by means of poison, or lying in wait . . . shall be deemed murder of the first degree." The court agreed that, if there is no crime of suicide, there can be no crime of being an accessory to suicide, but continued: "The real criminal *act* charged here is not suicide, but the *administering of poison*." (emphasis added) The sentence for using a chemical weapon was accordingly affirmed.

In 1983 the Michigan Court of Appeals[4] dismissed the indictment of Steven Paul Campbell on the charge of murder in connection with the suicide death of Kevin Basnaw. On the night of his suicide, Basnaw had been drinking heavily with Campbell. Just two weeks before this, Campbell had caught Basnaw in bed with his wife. Basnaw began to talk about suicide, but said he didn't have a gun. They drove to the home of Campbell's parents to get a gun. Upon returning with the gun and five shells, Basnaw told his girlfriend to go home because he was going to kill himself. The next morning Basnaw was found dead with a self-inflicted wound to the temple.

The prosecutor relied on *Roberts* to justify the first-degree murder charge. The appeals court agreed that the case could not be distinguished from *Roberts*, but ruled that *Roberts* was no longer good law. The court found: "The term suicide excludes by definition a homicide. Simply put, the defendant here did not kill another person." The court invited the legislature to pass a statute against this type of conduct, which the court found "morally reprehensible" but not "criminal under the present state of the law."

KEVORKIAN AND ADKINS

Kevorkian's original suicide machine consisted of three hanging bottles connected to an IV. Once the IV is in place, it delivers saline. The "patient" can switch the saline to a second bottle containing thiopental. The third bottle, containing potassium chloride, is activated automatically by a timer and is fatal within minutes. Janet Adkins, a 54-year-old Oregon schoolteacher who was suffering from early Alzheimer disease, flew to Michigan with her husband to use Kevorkian's machine. Unable to obtain a motel room or space at a funeral parlor, they eventually wound up in a public park in the back of his Volkswagen bus. There Kevorkian, assisted by his two sisters, inserted the IV into Mrs. Adkins' arm, after which she switched the IV to thiopental and eventually died.

Two days later the story was on the front page of the *New York Times*, and Kevorkian appeared on most of the national talk shows during the following week. Although he is admittedly a very strange person, what really caught the public's imagination was his machine, which he was pictured with on the front page of the *Times* and in national magazines. Headlines varied, but almost all mentioned the machine, including "Dr.

Death's Suicide Machine" (*Time*), "Doctor Tells of First Death Using His Suicide Device" (*New York Times*), and "Ban Sought on Doctor's 'Suicide Machine'" (*USA Today*).

The following day the *New York Times*, focusing on the similarities between the machine and devices used to execute condemned prisoners by lethal injection, noted that to some his actions "seemed a lot more like an execution" than a dignified death:

> True, Mrs. Adkins was in Michigan and not, say, in the death house in Texas; and lying on a cot in a rusting van rather than on a gurney in a windowed execution chamber. One might also say that Mrs. Adkins had a choice whereas the condemned do not. . . . Here comes a Dr. Jack Kevorkian to publicize himself, his "Rube Goldberg apparatus" and his willingness to make a martyr of himself. "They'll be after me for this," he says. They should be.[5]

In early December 1990, Kevorkian was charged with first-degree murder in the death of Janet Adkins. Less than two weeks later, after a two-day preliminary hearing, Judge Gerald McNally dismissed all charges against Kevorkian. The judge relied on *Campbell*, ruling that Adkins had caused her own death and that Michigan had no specific law against assisting suicide. Another judge ruled similarly in July 1992 after Kevorkian was charged with murder in the deaths of two more middle-aged women.

In a related civil case, a temporary injunction was issued restraining Kevorkian from using his machine again. A two-week hearing took place in January 1991 on a request to make the injunction permanent. Kevorkian had by this time said he was not planning to use the machine again: "I would now like to work cooperatively with the legislative and medical communities to see if we can rationally solve this terrible problem [assisted suicide]. I'm not out to make Michigan a suicide capital."[6] Nonetheless, Judge Alice Gilbert granted the permanent injunction in February 1991, saying, "his goal is self-service rather than patient service."

WHY THE METHOD MATTERS

From a purely logical perspective, one might imagine that the intent to produce death and the death itself, rather than the means, would be determinative in judging the act. From this perspective, there should be no distinction between discontinuing a mechanical ventilator and discontinuing tube feeding, if the intention in both cases is to end the patient's life, and that is the result. Nonetheless, many still feel a major emotional distinction between discontinuing these two medical interventions. Likewise, although warfare ethics is an oxymoron, military professionals view chemical and biological weapons as unethical and different in kind from "conventional" weaponry, even though both are designed to do precisely the same thing: frighten, maim, and kill. In the realm of suicide and assisted suicide, it seems fair to conclude that the means will matter, and may even be determinative in the debate.

We expect physicians, for example, to use "medical procedures," but not to end life in ways that do not require a doctor's skill. For example, physicians participate in the execution of condemned prisoners primarily when the skills of a trained medical expert are needed. The French physician Joseph-Ignace Guillotin encouraged the National Assembly to pass a law in 1789 that required the death sentence to be carried out painlessly and "by means of a machine," and he later developed the guillotine for this purpose. In the United States, physicians have historically been present at executions to declare death, and sometimes they pin targets over the hearts of prisoners for firing squads. But physicians have never been thought to be appropriate to act as the hangman, a firing squad member, or the electrocutioner. With the advent of lethal injection as the preferred method of execution, however, physicians have become prominent in the execution itself, since it is often seen as the physician's role to prescribe the drugs needed to insure death, to insert the IV, and to supervise the administration of the drugs.

Had Kevorkian made a noose for Janet Adkins to hang herself with, or helped her point a gun at her head and indicated when to pull the trigger, there seems little doubt that he would have been charged with and convicted of manslaughter (the reckless endangerment of another's life), if not murder. Had he simply prescribed medication for her, and informed her that taking a certain number of the pills was likely to cause death, it is unlikely he would have been charged with anything. But he took an intermediate position: devising his own machine, which has no medical use, but, because of the IV and drugs involved, seems to be a medical machine. The suicide machine stands as a hybrid between medical and nonmedical technology. Judge McNally ultimately saw this machine as medical in nature, and the act of using it one that a physician did for a patient. That is why Kevorkian was treated much kinder than a man who later came to Michigan to help his wife commit suicide and was charged with murder for, among other things, tying a plastic bag over her head.

Similarly, it will be viewed as militarily appropriate for soldiers to kill or maim enemy soldiers by shooting them, stabbing them, or simply blowing them up, but it would be seen as wrong for the military to use chemical weapons, biological weapons, or even to inject enemy soldiers with a deadly drug in hand-to-hand combat. If the method does matter, it must be because the methods used are limited by the role (and thus the authority) society assigns to professionals. Professional soldiers are to obey "the rules of war," and physicians are to obey "the rules of medical practice."

In this respect personal responsibility seems central. Machines have a tendency to depersonalize death and to make us seem less responsible for it. B-52 pilots, for example, cannot see the devastation their bombs cause on other humans; nor can missile technicians or users of many other high-tech military weapons. Like the use of the bow in the middle ages, use of these weapons seems unfair to many. This may, nonetheless, be acceptable in the modern military. It is not in medicine. We still expect physicians to be responsible for what they do to their patients. Thus when a physician develops a "suicide machine" that seems to remove accountability and responsibility from the physician, we are faced with a new reality that is destabilizing, to use the military-political term, and we are not sure how to react.

One possibility is to try to keep suicide out of medicine. In one of the original *Star Trek* programs, Robert Hammer's 1967 "A Taste of Armageddon" the Enterprise encounters two planets at war. Their 500 year long war is different: it is played entirely by computers, which determine the casualties on each side. But the casualties are real; real citizens are required to voluntarily walk into a "disintegration chamber," which instantly vaporizes them. Kurt Vonnegut in his 1960 short story "Welcome to the Monkey House," had earlier envisioned "ethical suicide parlors" being set up around the country to encourage people to painlessly end it all. Everything was voluntary. The parlors were tended by beautiful young women who talked with you, brought you your last meal, played your favorite music, and, upon your request, induced death by lethal injection.

The function of the ethical suicide parlor was to make death seem desirable, at least more desirable than continued life. One could as well argue that the purpose of war is to make life seem more desirable than death. But this lets it incorporate the metaphors of medicine (and life) into an activity that primarily deals in death. In this regard Paul Fussell is entirely persuasive when he argues that the reason infantry men seldom talk about their experiences is that no one wants to hear the real details of death and mutilation: "What listener wants to be torn and shaken when he doesn't have to be? We have made unspeakable mean indescribable: it really means nasty."[7]

The use of military metaphors in medicine tends to obliterate the patient, just as the use of medical metaphors by the military tends to obliterate the horrors of war. In both cases, we prefer to concentrate on the technology because, unlike death, it seems clean and controllable.

20

Health Law and Bioethics at the Millennium: Concluding Thoughts and a Proposal

The evolution of stars is inexorable. From the form in which we currently view our own sun, it and similar stars eventually expand as their exterior cools to become red giants. When a red giant runs out of fuel, its exposed core will collapse to form first a degenerate white dwarf and eventually a dead black dwarf. Health law and bioethics as disciplines seem to be on an opposite trajectory: from black dwarfs to white dwarfs, they are on their way to becoming red giants. What is health law, how is it related to bio-ethics, and why is the influence of both fields expanding exponentially? The search for an answer to these questions ends in our nation's law schools.[1]

HEALTH LAW IN LAW SCHOOLS

In the 1950s and 1960s the field of "Law and Medicine" was defined by courses in law schools that were almost exclusively concerned with issues of forensic psychiatry and forensic pathology and were properly considered advanced courses in criminal law. In the late 1960s some law and medicine courses began concentrating on broader medicolegal issues in the court-room, including disability evaluation and medical malpractice. These courses were properly considered as either advanced torts or trial practice courses.

In the 1970s, the concerns of at least some law and medicine courses expanded to include public policy, including issues of access to health care and the quality of that care. At the same time, advances in medical technol-ogy created new legal issues to explore: from brian death to organ donation, and from abortion to *in vitro* fertilization. These issues were increasingly incorporated into law and medicine courses, which were themselves becoming known by the broader rubric of "Health Law."

Teachers of health law in law schools, medical schools, schools of public health, and schools of management began meeting together on a regular basis in 1976 when the first national health law teachers meeting took place at Boston University.[2] It took more than a decade, but in 1987, the American Association of Law Schools sponsored its first teaching workshop on health law.[3] Although this more narrow group convened late, its program and proceedings offer a useful insight into the current state of health law in law schools. As the organizers of the workshop saw it, law and medicine (a field having primarily to do with medical malpractice, forensic medicine, and psychiatric commitment) had become a subdivision of the new field of health law.[4] Health law itself can be said to have three additional subdivisions, currently denoted Economics of Health Care Delivery; Public Policy and Health Care Regulation; and Bioethics. As one of the participants reasonably argued, these three subdivisions are actually three different approaches to the same subject matter: the health care industry.[5] All participants seemed either to admit or to tacitly assume that health law is *applied* law, much the way astronomy and physics are to a large extent applied mathematics.[6] As one participant persuasively argued: "It quickly appears that the common denominator that best unifies the study of health care law is the health care industry itself."[7]

As applied law, health law has immediate relevance to students in medical schools and schools of public health.[8] It has become increasingly apparent to even the most traditional medical school dean that physicians will be at a distinct disadvantage in their practices, and thus will be both less effective and more frightened than necessary, if they do not have a basic understanding of the law as it relates to medical practice. Accordingly, most medical schools now have formal courses in either law and medicine or medical law.[9] Although the realization that public health measures almost always have a major legal component came late to schools of public health, it has arrived, and virtually all such schools now have health law courses. Boston University's School of Public Health, for example, has both a health law concentration and a health law course that is required of all graduates. But where does a course in applied law fit in the law school curriculum?

Obviously it must be a second or third year course, since the students need to know something about law, especially torts, contracts, constitutional law, criminal law, and administrative law, the main types of law they will be applying to the health care field. The more interesting question, however, is what distinguishes law and medicine and health law courses from other "law and" courses. These courses are sometimes referred to generically as "law and a banana" courses (in an attempt to distinguish them from the basic or "real" law courses). Such courses are often viewed as luxuries that professors generally teach not because the course is particularly relevant to a legal career but because the professor is personally interested in the subject matter.

In commenting on "law and" courses today, one law professor worried that the proliferation of such courses might lead to the neglect of legal practice skills and make law school education even less relevant to legal practice and the legal profession than it already is.[10] He said these courses made him think of the ironic line in the movie *Dr. Strangelove*: "There will be no fighting in the war room." In his words: "Now some people say there will be no law in the law schools." Others have concurred, noting that the trend in law school courses that question the underpinnings and legitimacy of current law and legal structures, including the critical legal studies movement, has the potential to turn law schools into academic graduate schools and to deflect them from their traditional role of training lawyers for legal practice.[11]

There is much truth to all of these comments, but even if they can be aptly applied to such courses as sports law, education law, energy law, transportation law, entertainment law, or space law (to name just a few), I do not think they have much to say about health law. That is because health law is worth studying on its own merits for at least five reasons:

1. No other field can match the "magnitude, complexity, and universality of health care."[12]
2. Health law introduces lawyers to the problems confronted by the other great profession in the United States, medicine.
3. Changes in medicine can directly affect not only what humans can do but also how humans think about being human itself (and therefore what rights and obligations humans should have).
4. As issues of public health and safety capture center stage in American culture, the importance of prudent use of law to protect health and safety becomes central.
5. Issues of social justice and resource allocation are presented more starkly in the medical care context than in any other context.

Other reasons could, of course, be added to this list. Health care accounts for almost 15 percent of the gross national product and cost increases continue out of control. Most important constitutional law questions are now focusing on medical issues such as abortion, the "right to die," and free speech in the doctor–patient relationship. Legal jobs in health care exist in a wide variety of settings—including local, state, and federal regulatory agencies; private health care facilities; insurance companies; and law firms, to name just the major employers. And, perhaps as important to most who teach health law, there is no more intrinsically fascinating area of law than law applied to the health care field. In fact, whole courses in law schools have been taught around just one medical development, such as organ transplantation, and around one specialized medical activity, such as human experimentation.

Not only does health law provide a uniquely critical and intrinsically fascinating field to which to apply law, but it is also a field that can be fruitfully approached from a wide variety of perspectives. Rand Rosenblatt, for example, has suggested that health law can be approached not only from the traditional law and medicine avenue, but also from three more modern perspectives: a law and economics approach, a social justice approach, and a bioethics approach. A fourth approach would be a public health approach, and a fifth approach, of course, would try to integrate (or at least expose) all of these approaches.[13] Each approach deserves comment.

The Law and Economics Approach

In ransacking the rest of the university to find relevant disciplines to teach in law schools, economics has become the first to take ascendancy and actually become a method of legal analysis. Based primarily on the work of the Chicago School, and especially that of Judge Richard Posner, the "law and economics" approach postulates that most legal problems can be best analyzed or solved by applying the principles of economic theory based on the private market rather than immediate resort to governmental regulation or other value systems.[14] To oversimplify, the basic viewpoint from which health law is approached is that private property regimes presumptively serve to maximize social welfare; that in a many-seller market, goods will be available at marginal cost; that private contracts should be enforced; that relationships among noncontracting parties must be governed by explicit legal rule; and that income distribution is and should be primarily a function of productive capabilities. Even some of its harshest critics concede that the law and economics movement "provides the most coherent and intelligible realization of the liberal social theoretical agenda."[15]

My own view is that it is extremely strained to try to apply private market principles to the medical field, since none of the classic market assumptions apply in medical care. Specifically, unlike Adam Smith's market model, in medical care individuals do not have perfect knowledge about alternatives, do not shop for the best bargains, and do not (in most cases) pay for their medical care directly (but rather through insurance); most of the means of production (physicians, medical schools, nursing schools, and hospitals) are directly or indirectly subsidized by the government; and barriers to entry create governmentally enforced monopolies in many sectors of the health care industry. Perhaps most critically, the goal of health care should be prevention that decreases the need for medical care rather than attempts to get the public to consume more and more drugs, medical procedures, visits to the doctor, and days in the hospital. (See Chapter 16) Nonetheless, if these market imperfections are recognized, a reasonable course could be taught from this perspective, and certainly a very worthwhile course in antitrust law can be taught by using the health care industry as the only example.

The Critical Legal Studies (CLS) Approach

Like the law and economics rubric, the CLS rubric is used here as oversimplified shorthand for a course that is approached from an ideological perspective which dominates the discussion. Unlike the law and economics school, with its market model, CLS has no single, coherent set of principles to apply to any given industry. Nonetheless, those who describe the approach as a "social justice" one imply that it will be concerned with questioning the assumptions of capitalism (or at least looking "critically" at those assumptions).[16] It will employ what Duncan Kennedy has described as "fancy theory," by which he means "a mélange of critical Marxism, structuralism, and phenomenology."[17] Such an approach to the health law industry will not ignore how we got to where we are and will not assume that traditional race, class, and gender power relationships are proper and deserve to be privileged and given presumptive validity.

Rather than concentrating on economic efficiency as the primary goal of the health care system, there is likely to be primary commitment to social justice attained by equal access to care and equality of treatment. Cost and quality issues will certainly be considered, but it will be taken for granted that if individuals cannot afford the health care they need, income should be redistributed in a way that insures that they can. Nor will the health care industry be seen as an inherently private domain. Instead, it is likely that much class time will be devoted to considering how the system can be made more responsive to the needs of the public, with both national health insurance and the nationalization of the health care industry examined as reasonable policy alternatives.

The Bioethics Approach

Adherents of both the law and economics and the CLS schools are at home on the theoretical and macroeconomic levels. When it comes to dealing with the real problems of real physicians and patients, however, they each have much less to say. Perhaps that is why members of both of these politically hostile camps agree on at least one thing: issues of medical decisionmaking, such as autonomy and the doctor–patient relationship (the natural focus, for example, of a medical school course) should be relegated to a separate course called bioethics.

The term "bioethics" itself is extremely unsatisfactory when used in the context of a law course in either law school or medical school because it seems to denote the old style, 1970s, law and medicine course that concentrated on medical malpractice, with the recognition that new technologies have expanded the scope of medicine, and thus the scope of relevant legal topics. Sylvia Law, for example, sees this area as including termination of treatment, new reproductive technologies, organ transplantation, and definition of death.[18] Alexander Capron, rightly I think, sees the utility of a bioethics approach in combining factual knowledge about scientific developments (for example, clinical issues in the neonatal ICU or how genetic engineering is actually done) with a discussion of the most useful and constructive approaches the law can take to the social problems posed by new technologies. As Capron notes in espousing a case-based approach:

Social policy does not exist solely at the level of abstraction; it merges also from the resolution of cases. . . . One of the attractions to the field of law and medicine is that it ultimately involves not only basic values of justice, autonomy, and beneficence but actual minute-to-minute life-and-death decisions in a way most legal decisions do not.[19]

The Public Health Approach

This approach has yet to receive much attention in law schools and is currently used primarily in schools of public health. Nonetheless, as issues of public health continue to dominate the news and public policy development—issues such as teenage pregnancy, drug abuse, drunk driving, smoking, AIDS, nuclear energy, the quality of the environment, worker health and safety—such courses will naturally find a home in the law school. When they do, the pioneering work that has been done in the school of public health context will find a ready home in the development of courses that take a public health approach.[20]

THE FUTURE

A decade ago it would have been difficult to predict the state of health law today. What will it be in the year 2000? Prediction in this field is fraught with danger and uncertainty. Nonetheless, with the aid of futurists, and extending current trends, reasonable guesses can be hazarded and a proposal developed. First the reasonable guesses. French futurist Bertrand de Jouvenel postulated three ages of history: those ruled by priests, by lawyers, and by scientists.[21] The politics of the first age are derived from sacred scripture and the ignorance of the people. The politics of the second are derived from human scripture and the presumption that "we the people" can judge matters of common concern. The politics of the third are anomalous: the people retain the responsibility for judging technology, but lose the capacity to judge it. Technological experts, such as scientists and physicians, cannot run society directly, but can do so indirectly as experts and pressure groups. This reduces the state to the role of the sorcerer's apprentice.

Is this our future? One in which we equate the good with the new? One in which we assume that we can live forever and pretend that science and technology can grant us replaceable body parts and, ultimately, a replaceable body into which the information stored in our brains can be "dumped"? Can we have it all—economic growth and clean air and water? massive military expenditures and social justice? extreme and expensive rescue medicine and adequate disease prevention programs? human dignity and ruthless human experimentation?

A decade ago, before the reconstitution of the U.S. Supreme Court, before the Chernobyl and Challenger disasters, before Barney Clark and

Baby Fae, before the hole in the ozone layer, before the AIDS epidemic and the crack epidemic, most Americans would probably have answered a resounding yes. Today only those who live in caves could be so optimistic. We still claim to have the "best" technological health care system in the world, but we also know that 40 million Americans have no health care insurance at all and about the same number have inadequate coverage. We still want to live forever, but we also recognize that "miracles" like effective artificial hearts and gene therapy are years, if not decades, in the future. And when that future comes, society will not be able to afford to provide all its members with all of the extreme and expensive interventions medicine will be able to produce. How will we decide what technologies to pursue, which to utilize, and which to make available to all? (See, e.g., Chapter 17)

Bioethicist Daniel Callahan has persuasively argued that medical technology is uniquely powerful in that it not only changes what we can do, it also changes the way human life itself can be lived and thus can change our very concept of human life itself. The legal consequences of medical advances are seldom directly acknowledged, although they are profound. A few examples at the beginning and end of life illustrate the power of medicine to change the way we think about ourselves. The first concerns human reproduction. Oral contraception made sex without reproduction consistently possible for the first time in human history, and thus changed the role of women in society by making childbirth plannable. The new reproductive technologies, such as in vitro fertilization (IVF), have now closed the circle by making reproduction without sex possible for the human race. This process has generally been greeted with great fanfare, but we have only just begun to realize the impact this new technology has upon our views of children, gestation, motherhood, and human reproduction. As discussed in Chapters 5 and 6, when the embryo created in the petri dish in IVF is transferred for gestation to a woman other than the woman who contributed the ovum, we have an entirely novel legal question: As between the child's genetic mother and the woman who gestates and gives birth to the child, which woman should the law consider the child's legal mother with rearing rights and responsibilities?

Perhaps the most spectacular example of medical technology changing how we think about ourselves at the end of life is heart transplantation. This procedure, discussed in Chapter 15, requires taking the heart of a dead person and transplanting it into a dying person, after the dying person's own heart has been removed. Prior to the advent of this dramatic procedure, the law had always considered a person dead when their heart stopped beating. A strict application of this traditional definition of death would make a human heart transplant a double homicide. To permit transplantation, a new definition of death that takes full account of the technological ability to maintain respiration artificially after death of the brain had to be formulated. The death of the brain thus became the basis for human death. It was the combination of the technology of mechanical ventilators and heart transplantation that forced our society to reexamine what it means to die and to determine that the death of the entire brain is the equivalent of the death of the person for all purposes.[22] This "new" definition of death permitted the "harvesting" of heart and other vital organs from persons who, although dead (by brain death criteria), had their circulation and respiration artificially maintained by a mechanical ventilator. Obviously, an individual who is dead ceases to have legal rights. Prior to redefining death, a person with a dead brain, but whose circulation and respiration was nonetheless being maintained artificially, was a person under the constitution and retained the legal rights of citizenship. Upon legal acceptance of brain death, however, that same individual, in identical circumstances, is a corpse, with no human or constitutional rights, and can be used as a source of spare parts for others.

HEALTH LAW AS A LITERARY MOVEMENT

It has become increasingly popular to use literature in two different senses in law schools. The first is to actually teach courses in law by using literary works that deal with legal themes for the course readings. The second, and somewhat more interesting, is to use literary theory to analyze judicial decisions and other legal texts. It is through this approach, for example, that the concepts of structuralism have become commonplace in legal discourse, especially notions that language (and thus court decisions) is indeterminant. The structuralist view of literature "coincides with that of the twentieth-century physicists who posit a world model of indeterminacy, relativity, and uncertainty."[23] Instead of positing a rational order in which legal opinions can be logically deduced, "structuralists depict a self-reflexive world of language which is attached only arbitrarily and conventionally to things out there." A third approach, one I have used in my own course, Law, Medicine, and Literature, is to combine these two methods by using both literature about bioethical issues and literary theory to analyze contemporary issues in health law and bioethics.[24]

Because of the ability of new medical technologies to change the way we think about ourselves and our place in the world, the subject matter of health law is especially well suited for explicating structural literary (and legal) theories. It is also by reviewing contemporary literature itself, especially contemporary science fiction literature, that we can gain more of an insight into the potential uses of health law and bioethics instruction in the modern law school.

Like traditional law school courses, traditional science fiction writing has slipped into familiar plots and patterns, with little left to the imagination and almost no creativity and little relevance to our immediate futures. One reaction against this traditional view is the so-called cyberpunk movement.

This movement is probably best represented by William S. Burroughs (although William Gibson is usually portrayed as its prophet). Cyberpunk blends high tech with an aggressive outlaw culture and underclass to paint visions of our near future by extrapolating trends in our society, such as global communications networks, increasingly large corporations and bureaucracies, and use of advanced medical technologies, more to warn us than to entertain us.[25]

One of Burroughs's lesser known works, for example, is a movie treatment of Alan E. Nourse's 1974 novel, *The Bladerunner*.[26] Nourse, a practicing physician, concentrated his energies in the novel on exploring the dark side of our health care delivery system. In Nourse's story, increasing costs and decreasing access to health care eventually lead to the national health riots of 1994. Two years later, a system of universal health insurance is adopted, and care is provided free to all citizens at public hospitals and outpatient facilities. There is, however, a catch: free care is limited to those who have not been treated more than three times. For treatment after the third time, sterilization is required. These laws are enforced by the health control police. The overall thesis is that our health care system carries within it the seeds of its own destruction: the more sophisticated the medical technology, the better it works at keeping those with serious diseases alive to reproduce, the more it costs, and the more people it keeps alive to spend more money. Medicine thus continues to do more and more for fewer and fewer people at higher and higher costs. The sickest members of society swallow all the money we can spend on social welfare, and America is in danger of becoming one giant hospital.

Burroughs is faithful to the basic story, but he adds his own distinctive touches. He presents an especially compelling view of an underclass served by outlawed underground medicine, whose physicians are supplied with equipment and surgical instruments by couriers known as "bladerunners." In his treatment, an especially virulent flu virus (which could be taken as a precursor or prediction of the AIDS virus) sweeps the population. It can only be stopped if the underground doctors persuade their patients to be immunized, and this can only happen if the eugenic laws are suspended.

Burroughs himself began medical school in Vienna but soon dropped out. In *The Western Lands* (1987) his hero, Joe the Dead (a natural outlaw "dedicated to breaking the so-called natural laws of the universe foisted upon us by physicists, chemists, mathematicians [and] biologists") says of medical school: "By the time a student gets through medical school his brain is so crammed with undigested, often misleading, data that there is no room left to think in. In addition to misinformation, the student has also absorbed a battery of crippling prejudices." Like the best of the modern science fiction writers, Burroughs often comes back to transplantation as a theme. Joe the Dead becomes a transplant surgeon for a while. "Joe is able to hide his potentials and act like any idiot surgeon, addicted to his operations and the adulation of patients, nurses and colleagues." Transplant surgeons have gained enormous celebrity, and the aspects of their personality that Burroughs finds problematic are equally applicable to academicians.

Bruce Sterling, science fiction writer and cyberpunk promoter, notes that certain basic themes recur in cyberpunk, especially "the theme of body invasion: prosthetic limbs, implanted circuitry, cosmetic surgery, genetic alteration and the even more powerful theme of mind invasion: brain-computer interfaces, artificial intelligence, neurochemistry—techniques radically redefining the nature of humanity, the nature of self."[27] Genetic engineering and organ transplants are medical techniques whose implications are often explored in this writing. Literary critic Larry McCaffery contends that, "Issues such as these which are so massive, troubling, and profoundly disruptive cannot be dealt with by mainstream writers, in part because these issues challenge the normative bed rocks upon which the fantasies of 'realism' are grounded."[28] He goes on to assert that "most contemporary American authors continue to write novels as if these enormous shifts in our world had never occurred."

It is probably fair to say that the vast majority of law school courses as well continue to be taught "as if these enormous shifts in our world had never occurred" and that traditional courses cannot take reasonable account of these shifts. What shifts are we likely to see in the 90s?

The first shift will of necessity involve a strategy to deal with the AIDS epidemic, discussed in part in Chapters 10 and 11. We will either use it to expose the underlying inequities and inefficiencies in our current health care system, and take the epidemic as an opportunity to radically restructure it and provide equal access to it, or we will use it to reinforce and "legitimize" the notion of an underclass that "deserves" to be sick and die. The AIDS epidemic also provides an almost unique opportunity for lawyers and physicians to work together cooperatively since, as others have noted, the AIDS epidemic is the first modern epidemic where lawyers can be more helpful to most patients than physicians.[29] This is because medicine has been all but helpless in the face of AIDS, and lawyers can at least help prevent discrimination in housing, education, employment, and insurance.

The second shift, as outlined in Chapters 17 and 18, will involve coming to grips with the proper goals of medicine itself. We have seemed to believe that its proper goal is to keep people alive as long as possible and at any cost. This view, never a realistic one, is no longer economically or socially tenable. We will have to confront such boogymen as the "quality of life," the "right to die," and meaningless political slogans such as the "right to life" and the injunction to always "err on the side of life." Death is central to human life, and our mortality is not confronted so directly in any other law school course.

The third shift, a focus of Chapters 2 and 7, will involve the increasing use of the state's police powers to force its citizens to live healthy lives. How far should the law go in requiring its citizens to eat healthy foods? to take safety precautions, such as using seat belts? to refrain from using mind-altering drugs and intoxicating beverages? to refrain from performing certain unhealthy acts, such as smoking, in public? We have already seen food transformed into medicine, with advertisements and labeling touting the absence of fat or cholesterol in various products. Fitness is a fetish, and weight control books regularly appear on best seller lists. Fields traditionally dominated by other discourses have been preempted by public health. For example, nuclear energy, once seen as the cornerstone of any coherent energy policy (and of any course in energy law), is now seen primarily as a public health and safety problem. Highway safety is no longer seen exclusively as a police problem or a transportation problem, but as a public health and safety problem. Drunk drivers are a particularly focused public health problem. Alcoholism, once a crime, is now a medical and public health problem. Drug addiction is still viewed primarily as a law enforcement problem, but the trend is to see it as a public health problem. The safety of our food supply is increasingly viewed as a public health problem. Safety in the workplace, stress on the job, and the quality of environment are increasingly seen as public health issues. Of course, on a global level, disruption of the ozone layer, the fouling of the ocean, toxic chemicals in the air, as well as nuclear fallout and the AIDS epidemic, are all seen as primary public health problems.

The fourth major shift will occur in the cyberpunk issues of changing medical technology, discussed in Chapters 6, 12, 13, and 16. How will we deal with new methods of human reproduction, new transplantation techniques, genetic engineering, and man-machine hybrids? How will we judge what new developments are "good" and can be counted as progress, and which will create more problems for us than they solve? Is it possible, for example, to develop a "social impact statement" (analogous to an environmental impact statement) to give us some advance warning of where we are going, and to help temper our most self-destructive tendencies?

There will undoubtedly be major transformations in each of these four areas during the remainder of the 1990s. It is in this sense that the fields of health law and bioethics, whose subject matter these developments comprise, will grow from their current white dwarf state into red giants. This book has suggested ways in which society can meet the new challenges to its existence and norms by using health law and bioethics. Since bioethics has been primarily driven and shaped by law in the United States, and since most of the chapters in this book have focused on judges and legislators, it seems reasonable to conclude this book with a proposal aimed at our nation's law schools.

A PROPOSAL

It is no secret to most law students and faculty that the final semester of the third year is often a lost semester. It is also no secret that law school curriculum is becoming increasingly detached from the real world, that lawyers are becoming increasingly alienated from their work, and that their fellow citizens are becoming increasingly alienated from them.[30] One way to bring meaning to the final semester of law school, and at the same time help equip tradition-bound lawyers for the real world of the 21st century, is to devote the entire final semester (perhaps even the entire final year) of law school to an intensive study of health law. As already stressed, health law is applied law, and giving students the opportunity to apply what they have learned in law school to a particular field of human endeavor gives them an opportunity to try to synthesize their knowledge and approach the world in a encompassing rather than a reductive mode. Of course, experts in other types of applied law might argue for their own fields to be the focus, but health law has unique attributes that especially suit it for this role in revitalizing law school education. As Dean George Schatzki of the University of Connecticut Law School stressed in opening a 1989 health law symposium: "Law is concerned with making the world a better place to live in."[31] Dean Schatzki went on to list the four areas that are central to our lives, but which are seldom dealt with in law school: family, work, recreation, and health. Health law is the only field that can cover all of these areas, and in this way can play a key role in humanizing the law school curriculum and in encouraging lawyers and law students to get involved in and help solve critical human problems.

In addition, the health care industry has undergone tremendous change in the recent past, and changes are likely to be even more dramatic during the Clinton administration. The model of professional dominance is rapidly giving way to multiple influences. As such, it provides a real-world laboratory for examining the influences of law — from the courtroom (especially medical malpractice and termination of treatment) to constitutional litigation (especially the right of privacy) to legislation (various proposals of Medicare reform and national health insurance) and regulations (from the FDA and revising drug safety rules to state rules on licensing physicians and facilities). New medical technologies present new legal challenges, and these are of the type that are so intrinsically fascinating that they routinely appear on the front pages of newspapers and news magazines, and they will have no trouble keeping the attention of even hardened third-year law students.

The cases of Karen Ann Quinlan, Nancy Cruzan, and Mary Beth Whitehead are only a few examples of the health law dramas played out in the courts. *Roe v. Wade*, the premier health law case, continues to be contested and contracted, and the right of privacy, so central to medicine and the doctor–patient relationship, continues to play the key role in the politics of judicial appointments. Issues of organ transplants and implants, including the case of Barney Clark, also present particularly compelling case studies that lead naturally to broader policy discussions. Public health issues are of direct importance to the day-to-day lives of students, including drugs, alcohol, tobacco, food consumption, the quality of the environment, exercise, and use of seat belts and motorcycle helmets. And, perhaps as important, health law permits direct study of (and possibly joint courses with) the other major profession in the United States, the medical profession. Relationships between the two professions have become increasingly adversarial, and increased knowledge may help restore a more reasonable and socially constructive relationship. Finally, the advice lawyers give their clients in the health law field often has a direct impact on the lives and the manner of deaths of real people. Professional responsibility has an immediacy in this legal field that is lacking in most others.

There are a variety of curriculum options. One would be to have all students take a basic overview course on health law in the fall of the third year, with special emphasis on developing an understanding of the health care industry itself. The second semester would then consist of three or four courses, each approaching the industry from a different perspective (such as law and economics, social justice, bioethics, technology, public health, environmental law, occupational health and safety law, and law and medicine). Students would then each participate in a writing seminar, and/or a clinical project, preferably with one or more medical students.[32] Health law presents an opportunity to apply law, and its rules and procedures, to the most intrinsically fascinating and substantively influential industry in the United States. As the subject matter of health law—the fields of medicine, public health, and bioethics—continue to expand, so does the field of health law itself. Of course, once our health care system is under control, the final semester could concentrate on other real world problems such as the criminal justice system, education, energy, transportation, and the environment.

Mythologist Joseph Campbell has noted that most cultures are held together by mythology that is handed down from one generation to another: "But in America we have people from all kinds of backgrounds, all in a cluster, together, and consequently law has become very important in this country. Lawyers and law are what hold us together. There is no ethos."[33] This is a difficult role for the law to perform, and an impossible one if we insist on acting as if the world is not changing and on teaching law the way we have always taught it. An intense study of health law is not a magic cureall for alienation, but it provides a way for law students to work on real life problems that both they and society must confront, and to do so in a constructive and humanistic manner that has the potential to benefit both them and the society at large.

Notes

INTRODUCTION

1. *Roe v. Wade,* 410 U.S. 113 (1973). *Roe v. Wade* is discussed in Chapter 4.

2. *Webster v. Reproductive Health Services,* 492 U.S. 490 (1989). *Webster* is discussed in Chapter 4.

3. The brief is partially reprinted in *Am. J. Law & Med.* 15:169–177; 1989.

4. *Cruzan v. Director, Missouri Dept. of Health,* 497 U.S. 261 (1990). *Cruzan* is discussed in Chapter 7.

5. Annas, G. J., Arnold, B., Aroskar, M., *et. al.,* Bioethicists' Statement on the U.S. Supreme Court's *Cruzan* Decision, *New Engl. J. Med.* 323:686–687; 1990.

6. Annas, G. J., In re Quinlan: Legal Comfort for Doctors, *Hastings Center Report* 6(3):29–31; July 1976. This portion of the introduction is adopted from my last regular column, Annas, G. J., Ethics Committees: From Ethical Comfort to Ethical Cover, *Hastings Center Report* 21(3):18–20; May 1991.

7. *In re Quinlan,* 355 A.2d 647 (N.J. 1976). *Quinlan* is discussed in Chapter 7.

8. *Doe v. Bolton,* 410 U.S. 179 (1973).

9. For a detailed discussion of the Baby Doe regulations see Elias, S. & Annas, G. J., *Reproductive Genetics and the Law,* St. Louis: Mosby-Yearbook, 1987.

10. *See generally* Glantz, L. H., What Lessons Ethics Committees Can Learn from IRBs (in) Cranford, R. & Dondera, E., eds., *Institutional Ethics Committees,* Ann Arbor, MI: Health Research Press, 1982.

11. *See, e.g.,* Dubler, N., *Ethics on Call,* New York: Harmony Books, 1992.

12. Ethics Committee of the American Fertility Society, Ethical Considerations of the New Reproductive Technologies, *Fertility and Sterility* 53(6)(Supp. 2):34S; 1990.

13. Ethics Committee of the American College of Obstetricians and Gynecologists, Multifetal Pregnancy Reduction and Selective Fetal Termination, No. 94, April 1991.

14. Solzhenitsyn, A., The Exhausted West, *Harvard Magazine,* July/Aug. 1978, p. 22.

15. *Rust v. Sullivan,* 111 S.Ct. 1759 (1991).

16. Campbell, J. (with Bill Moyers), *The Power of Myth,* New York: Doubleday, 1988, p. 9.

CHAPTER 1

1. This chapter is based on Annas, G. J., Restricting Doctor–Patient Conversations in Federally Funded Clinics, *New Engl. J. Med.* 325:362–365; 1991.

2. Statutory prohibition on use of appropriate funds in programs where abortion is a method of family planning, Standard of compliance for family planning services projects, Final rule. DHHS, Public Health Service, *Federal Register* 53:2921–2946; 1988.

3. *Massachusetts v. Sullivan,* 899 F.2d 53 (1st Cir. 1990) and *Planned Parenthood Federation of America v. Sullivan,* 913 F.2d 1492 (10th Cir. 1990).

4. *New York v. Bowen,* 889 F.2d 401 (2nd Cir. 1989).

5. *Rust v. Sullivan,* 111 S.Ct. 1759 (1991).

6. *Maher v. Roe,* 432 U.S. 464 (1977).

7. Entralgo, P. L., *Doctor and Patient,* New York: McGraw-Hill, 1969, p. 32.

8. *United States v. Krass,* 409 U.S. 434, 460 (1973) (dissenting opinion).

9. Annas, G. J., Glantz, L. H. & Mariner, W. K., The Right of Privacy Protects the Doctor–Patient Relationship, *JAMA* 263:858–861; 1990.

10. Shawn, W., *The Fever,* New York: Farrar, Straus, Giroux, 1991, p. 54.

11. President George Bush, Veto message on H.R. 2707, Nov. 19, 1991.

12. *National Family Planning & Reproductive Health Services Assoc. v. Sullivan,* 1992 U.S. App. LEXIS 28469 (D.C. Cir. Nov. 3, 1992).

CHAPTER 2

1. *See, e.g.,* Butterfield, F., U.S. Expands Its Lead in the Rate of Imprisonment, *New York Times,* Feb. 11, 1992, p. C18.

2. *Ibid.* and Langan, P. A., America's Soaring Prison Population, *Science* 251: 1568–1573; 1991.

3. This portion of the chapter is based on Annas, G. J., Crack, Symbolism and the Constitution, *Hastings Center Report* 19(3):35–37; May 1989.

4. *Skinner v. Railway Labor Executives' Association,* 489 U.S. 656 (1989).

5. *National Treasury Employees Union v. Von Raab,* 489 U.S. 656 (1989).

6. Shabecoff, P., Captain of Tanker Had Been Drinking, Blood Tests Show, *New York Times,* March 31, 1989, p. 1.

7. This portion of the chapter is based on Annas, G. J., One Flew Over the Supreme Court, *Hastings Center Report* 20(3):28–30; May 1990.

8. *Washington v. Harper,* 494 U.S. 210 (1990).

9. *Harper v. State,* 759 P.2d 358 (Wash. 1988).

10. *See, e.g.,* Annas, G. J., *Judging Medicine,* Totowa, NJ: Humana, 1988, pp. 238–243, and cases discussed therein.

11. Oral remarks, Conference on Nazi Doctors and the Nuremberg Code, Dec. 1989, Boston University, Boston, Mass.

12. Treaster, J., Some Think the 'War on Drugs' is being Waged on Wrong Front, *New York Times,* July 28, 1992, p. 1. *And see Political Pharmacology: Thinking about Drugs, Daedalus,* Summer, 1992.

CHAPTER 3

1. William Carlos Williams, The Use of Force (in) *The Doctor Stories,* New York: New Directions, 1984, pp. 56–60.

2. *Jefferson v. Griffin Spalding Co. Hospital Authority,* 247 Ga. 86, 274 S.E.2d 457 (1981).

3. This chapter is based on two articles, Annas, G. J., She's Going To Die: The Case of Angela C, *Hastings Center Report* 18(1):23-25; Feb. 1988, and Annas, G. J., Foreclosing the Use of Force: A.C. Reversed, *Hastings Center Report* 20(4): 27-29; July 1990.

4. Quotations from the hearing are taken from the transcript.

5. *In re: A.C.,* 533 A.2d 611 (D.C. 1987).

6. *In re: A.C.,* 539 A.2d 203 (D.C. 1988).

7. *In re: A.C.,* 573 A.2d 1235 (D.C. 1990).

8. *See supra* note 2.

9. *In re Mayden,* 114 Daily Wash. L. Rptr. 2233 (D.C. Super. Ct. July 26, 1986).

10. William Carlos Williams, Danse Pseudomacabre in *supra* note 1, p. 88.

11. A malpractice and civil rights suit by the estate of Ms. Carder against the hospital, *Stoner v. G.W.U.,* was settled in November 1990, with the hospital agreeing to set up procedures to insure that hospitalized pregnant women have the right to make their own medical decisions in the future.

CHAPTER 4

1. This chapter is based on Annas, G. J., The Supreme Court, Liberty, and Abortion, *New Engl. J. Med.* 327:651-654; 1992; Annas, G. J., The Supreme Court, Privacy, and Abortion, *New Engl. J. Med.* 321:1200-1203; 1989; Annas, G. J., Webster and the Politics of Abortion, *Hastings Center Report* 19(2):36-38; March 1989; and Annas, G. J., Four-One-Four, *Hastings Center Report* 19(5):27-29; 1989.

2. Lamanna, M. A., Social Science and Ethical Issues: The Policy Implications of Poll Data on Abortion (in) Callahan, S. & Callahan, D., eds., *Abortion: Understanding Differences,* New York: Plenum Press, 1984. *See also* Dionne, E. J., Poll Finds Ambivalence on Abortion Persists in U.S., *New York Times,* Aug. 3, 1989, p. A18.

3. Elias, S. & Annas, G. J., *Reproductive Genetics and the Law,* St. Louis: Mosby-Yearbook, 1987.

4. President's News Conference, *New York Times,* Jan. 28, 1989, p. 7.

5. Attorney General "Guesses" at Shift in Abortion Law, *Boston Globe,* Jan. 23, 1989, p. 1.

6. *Roe v. Wade,* 410 U.S. 113 (1973).

7. Woodward, B. & Armstrong, S., *The Brethren: The Inside Story of the Supreme Court,* New York: Simon & Shuster, 1979.

8. Hunter, N. D., Time Limits on Abortion (in) Cohen, S. & Taub, N., eds., *Reproductive Laws for the 1990s,* Totowa, NJ: Humana Press, 1989.

9. *Planned Parenthood of Central Missouri v. Danforth,* 428 U.S. 52 (1976).

10. Quoted in Elias, S. & Annas, G. J., *Reproductive Genetics and the Law, supra,* note 3, pp. 160-161.

11. Glantz, L. H., Abortion: A Decade of Decisions (in) Milunsky, A. & Annas, G. J., eds., *Genetics and the Law III,* New York: Plenum Press, 1985, p. 305.

12. *Reproductive Health Services v. Webster,* 662 F. Supp. 407 (W.D. Mo. 1987).

13. *Reproductive Health Services v. Webster,* 851 F.2d 1071 (8th Cir. 1988).

14. *Webster v. Reproductive Health Services,* 492 U.S. 490 (1989).

15. *Akron v. Center for Reproductive Health,* 462 U.S. 416 (1983) (O'Connor, dissenting).

16. Dworkin, R., The Great Abortion Case, *N.Y. Review of Books,* June 29, 1989, p. 51.

17. *Planned Parenthood of Southeastern Pennsylvania v. Casey,* 112 S.Ct. 2791 (1992).

18. Hall, M., Activists Aside, Justices' Ruling Pleases Many, *USA Today,* July 1, 1992, p. 3A, and Shribman, D., Abortion Issue Could Benefit Clinton's Bid, *Wall Street J.,* July 10, 1992, p. A14.

19. *See* Tribe, L., Write *Roe* Into Law, *New York Times,* July 27, 1992, p. A17, and Tribe, L., *Abortion: The Clash of Absolutes,* New York: Norton, 1992 ed., pp. 251–256.

CHAPTER 5

1. This chapter is based on Annas, G. J., Fairy Tales Surrogate Mothers Tell, *Law, Med. & Health Care* 16:27–33; 1988.

2. Ephron, D., In This Year's Movies Baby Knows Best, *New York Times,* March 13, 1988, p. 1 (A&L).

3. Keane, N. & Breo, D., *The Surrogate Mother,* New York: Everest House, 1981, p. 27. Quotations in this section are all from this book.

4. Kane, E., *Birthmother,* New York: Harcourt Brace Jovanovich, 1988, p. 275. *And see* Chesler, P., What Is a Mother?, *Ms.,* May 1988, pp. 26–39.

5. Barron, J., Views on Surrogacy Harden after Baby M Ruling, *New York Times,* April 2, 1987, pp. 1, B2.

6. *Matter of Baby M,* 537 A.2d 1227, 1234 (N.J. 1988).

7. Harlow, H. F., The Nature of Love, *Am. Psychol.* 13:673; 1958, and Harlow, H. F., Blazek, N. C., & McClearn, G. E., Manipulative Motivation in the Infant Rhesus Monkey, *J. Comp. Physiol. & Psychol.* 14:44; 1956.

8. Peterson, I., Feminists See Unfair Maternal Norm in Baby M Case, *New York Times,* March 20, 1987, p. 13.

9. *Planned Parenthood of Central Missouri v. Danforth,* 428 U.S. 52 (1976).

10. *Murray v. Vandevander,* 522 P.2d 302, 304 (Okla. App. 1974).

11. *In the Matter of Baby M,* 217 N.J. Super. Ct. 313, 525 A.2d 1128 (1987).

12. McPherson, J. M., *Battle Cry of Freedom: The Civil War Era,* New York: Oxford U. Press, 1988, p. 38.

13. *Ibid.,* pp. 38–39. For a modern retrospective on the family-destruction aspects of slavery, *see* Toni Morrison's Pulitzer Prize–winning *Beloved,* New York: Alfred A. Knopf, 1987.

14. Radin, M. J., Market-Inalienability, *Harv. L. Rev.* 100:1849; 1987.

15. Ms. Kane has since repudiated her role. See Kane, *Birthmother, supra* note 4.

16. *Geraldo,* The Happy Surrogates, aired Sept. 29, 1987.

17. *Ibid.*

18. Kolder, V. E. B., Gallagher, J. & Parson, M. T., Court-Ordered Obstetrical Interventions, *New Engl. J. Med.* 316:1192; 1987. *And see* Note, Maternal Rights and Fetal Wrongs: The Case against the Criminalization of 'Fetal Abuse,'" *Harv.*

L. Rev. 101:994; 1988, and Annas, G. J., Protecting the Liberty of Pregnant Patients, *New Engl. J. Med.* 316:1213; 1987.

19. *See, e.g.,* Robertson, J., Embryos, Families, and Procreative Liberty: The Legal Structure of the New Reproduction, *So. Cal. L. Rev.* 59:939,995–1000; 1986.

20. Elias, S. & Annas, G. J., *Reproductive Genetics and the Law,* St. Louis: Mosby-Yearbook, 1987.

21. Annas, G. J., Making Babies without Sex: The Law and the Profits, *Am. J. Public Health* 74:1415,1417; 1987.

22. By mid-1992, 18 states had acted to outlaw or sharply curtail the role of brokers in commercial surrogacy. Belkin, L., Childless Couples Hang on to Last Hope, Despite Law, *New York Times,* July 28, 1992, p. 1.

CHAPTER 6

1. This chapter is adapted from Annas, G. J., A French Homunculus in a Tennessee Court, *Hastings Center Report* 19(6):20–22; Nov. 1989; Annas, G. J., Crazy Making: Embryos and Gestational Mothers, *Hastings Center Report* 21(1):35–37; Jan. 1991; and Annas, G. J., Using Genes To Define Motherhood: The California Solution, *New Engl. J. Med.* 326:417–420; 1992.

2. Gillers, S., Taking L.A. Law More Seriously, *Yale L. J.* 98:1607–1623; 1989.

3. Rosenberg, C. B., An L.A. Lawyer Replies, *Yale L. J.* 98:1625–1629 (arguing that *L.A. Law* is not primarily about law and lawyers, but about "interesting people, some of whom happen to be lawyers").

4. *Davis v. Davis v. King,* Fifth Jud. Ct., Tennessee, E-14496, Sept. 21, 1989 (Young, J.).

5. *Scopes v. State,* 289 S.W. 362 (Tenn. 1927).

6. All of these statements are taken from the judge's own summary of the testimony. The words in quotation marks are Dr. Lejeune's.

7. Trial on Couple's Frozen Embryos Left to Judge, *St. Cloud (Minnesota) Times,* Aug. 11, 1989, p. 4A.

8. Fitzgerald, M., Embryo Trial Goes to Judge, *USA Today,* Aug. 11, 1989, p. 3A.

9. Goodman, E., A Ruling in the Realm of Scientific Fantasy, *Boston Globe,* Sept. 26, 1989, p. 16.

10. *Davis v. Davis,* 1989 Tenn. App. LEXIS 641 (Sept. 21, 1989), *aff'd* 1992 Tenn. LEXIS 400 (June 1, 1992).

11. *Johnson v. Calvert,* Cal. Super. Ct., Orange Co., Dept. 11, No. X633190 (Oct. 22, 1990).

12. Bouchard, T. J., Lykken, D. T., McGue, M., Segal, N. & Tellegen, A., Sources of Human Psychological Differences: The Minnesota Study of Twins Reared Apart, *Science* 250:223,228; 1990.

13. *Anna J. v. Mark C.,* 286 Cal. Rptr. 369 (Ct. App., 4th Dist. 1991).

14. *Michael H. v. Gerald D.,* 491 U.S. 110 (1989).

15. Balkin, J. M., Tradition, Betrayal, and the Politics of Deconstruction, *Cardozo L. Rev.* 1990; 11:1613, 1618–1621.

16. Levran, D., Dor, J., Rudak, E., *et al.,* Pregnancy Potential of Human Oocytes—the Effect of Cryopreservation, *New Engl. J. Med.* 323:1153–1156; 1990. Sauer, M. V., Paulson, R. J. & Lobo, R. A., A Preliminary Report on Oocyte

Donation Extending Reproductive Potential to Women over 40, *New Engl. J. Med.* 323:1157–1160; 1990. Angell, M., New Ways To Get Pregnant, *New Engl. J. Med.* 323:1200–1202; 1990.

17. Kolata, G., Young Women Offer To Sell Their Eggs to Infertile Couples, *New York Times,* Nov. 10, 1991; p. 1.

18. Harrison, M., The Baby with Two Mothers. *Wall St. J.,* Oct. 24, 1990, p. A12.

19. American College of Obstetricians and Gynecologists Committee on Ethics, Ethical Issues in Surrogate Motherhood, No. 88, Nov. 1990.

CHAPTER 7

1. The chapter is adapted from Annas, G. J., The Long Dying of Nancy Cruzan, *Law, Med. & Health Care* 19:52–59; 1991.

2. *Cruzan v. Director, Missouri Dept. of Health,* 497 U.S. 261 (1990).

3. *Estate of Nancy Beth Cruzan v. Harmon,* Estate No. CV384-98, Cir. Ct., Jasper Co., Mo. July 27, 1988. Portions of this section are adapted from Annas, G. J., The Insane Root Takes Reason Prisoner, *Hastings Center Report* 19(1):29–31; 1989.

4. *Cruzan v. Harmon,* 760 S.W.2d 408 (Mo. 1988) (en banc).

5. *In re Quinlan,* 70 N.J. 10, 355 A.2d 647, cert. den. sub. nom. *Garger v. New Jersey,* 429 U.S. 922 (1976).

6. *In re Jobes,* 108 N.J. 394, 529 A.2d 434 (1987), and *In re Conroy,* 98 N.J. 321, 486 A.2d 1209 (1985). The *Jobes* case is discussed in Chapter 8.

7. *In re Storar,* 52 N.Y.2d 363, 420 N.E.2d 64, cert. den. 454 U.S. 858 (1981).

8. Portions of this section are adapted from Annas, G. J., Nancy Cruzan and the Right To Die, *New Engl. J. Med.* 323:670–673; 1990. And see note 2 *supra* for case citation.

9. *Storar, supra* note 8.

10. *In re Westchester Co. Medical Center on behalf of O'Connor,* 581 N.E.2d 607 (N.Y. 1988).

11. For a more complete discussion of the fluids and nutrition issue, *see* Cantor, N., The Permanently Unconscious Patient, Non-Feeding and Euthanasia, *Am. J. Law & Med.* 15:381–438; 1989.

12. Marzen, T., 'Insane Roots and Serpent's Teeth': Death and the Law (in) Andrusko, D., ed., *The Triumph of Hope: A Pro-Life Review of 1988 and a Look to the Future,* Washington, D.C.: National Right to Life Committee, 1989, pp. 159–170.

13. A photo of Ms. Busalacchi from the videotape ran in the *New York Times* (State Makes Public Videotape in Right-to-Die Case, *New York Times,* Feb. 5, 1991, p. B6.) *See, e.g., Berthiaume v. Pratt,* 365 A.2d 762 (Me. 1976).

14. Marzen, *supra* note 12, p. 166.

15. The history of the Baby Doe rules is chronicled in Elias, S. & Annas, G. J., *Reproductive Genetics and the Law,* St. Louis: Mosby-Yearbook, 1987, pp. 168–194.

16. *Ohio v. Akron Center for Reproductive Health,* (1990).

17. In one survey prior to the U.S. Supreme Court's decision, 88 percent of the public thought the family should decide on treatment, 8 percent thought the doctors

should decide, 1 percent the courts, and no one selected the state. (Coyle, How Americans View the High Court, *National L. J.,* Feb. 26, 1990, pp. 1, 36.)

18. Sabatino, C. P., *Health Care Powers of Attorney,* Chicago: American Bar Association, 1990.

19. *In re Guardianship of Browning,* 568 So.2d 4 (Fla. 1990).

20. Rosenthal, Filling the Gap Where a Living Will Won't Do, *New York Times,* Jan. 17, 1991, p. B9.

21. Foucault, M., *The History of Sexuality: An Introduction,* Vol. 1, New York: Random House, 1990, pp. 135–159.

22. Moral Sentiments, 4, ii, as quoted in Wills, G. *Inventing America: Jefferson's Declaration of Independence*, New York: Vintage Books, 1978, p. 254.

CHAPTER 8

1. This chapter is based on Annas, G. J., Precatory Prediction and Mindless Mimicry: The Case of Mary O'Connor, *Hastings Center Report* 18(6):31–33; Dec. 1988, and Annas, G. J., In Thunder, Lightning or in Rain: What Three Doctors Can Do, *Hastings Center Report* 17(5):28–30; Oct. 1987.

2. *In the Matter of Mary O'Connor,* 581 N.E.2d 607 (N.Y. 1988).

3. *Matter of Storar, Matter of Eichner,* 52 N.Y.2d 363 (1981).

4. *In the Matter of Claire Conroy,* 486 A.2d 1209 (N.J. 1985).

5. Annas, G. J., *Judging Medicine,* Totowa, NJ: Humana Press, 1988, pp. 244–324.

6. 529 A.2d 404 (N.J. 1987).

7. *In re Quinlan,* 70 N.J. 10, 355 A.2d 647, cert. den. sub. nom. *Garger v. New Jersey,* 429 U.S. 922 (1976).

8. *Doe v. Bolton,* 410 U.S. 179 (1973).

9. 42 U.S.C. 1395(a)(1) et. seq. (as amended Nov. 1990).

10. The remainder of this chapter is adapted from Annas, G. J., The Health Care Proxy and the Living Will, *New Engl. J. Med.* 324:1210–1212; 1991.

11. Kutner, L., Due Process of Euthanasia: The Living Will—a Proposal, *Indiana L. Rev.* 44:539; 1969.

12. Annas, G. J., *The Rights of Patients,* 2d ed., Carbondale, IL: So. Ill. U. Press, 1989, pp. 196–255.

13. Legal Advisers to Concern for Dying, The Right To Refuse Treatment: A Model Act, *Am. J. Public Health* 73:918–922; 1983. *See also* Veatch, R., *Dying and the Biological Revolution,* New Haven, CT: Yale U. Press, 1976, pp. 184–186, and Relman, A. S., Michigan's Sensible "Living Will," *New Engl. J. Med.* 300: 1270–1272; 1979.

14. Sabatino, C. P., *Health Care Powers of Attorney,* Chicago: American Bar Association, 1990.

15. Davis, M., Sutherland, L. I., Garrett, J. M., *et. al.,* A Prospective Study of Advance Directives for Life-sustaining Care, *New Engl. J. Med.* 324:882–888; 1991.

16. Emanuel, L. L. & Emanuel, E. J., The Medical Directive: A New Comprehensive Advance Care Document, *JAMA* 261:3290; 1989. *See also* Emanuel, L. L., Barry, M. J., Stoeckle, J. D., Ettelson, L. M. & Emanuel, E. J., Advance Directives for Medical Care: A Case for Greater Use, *New Engl. J. Med.* 324:889–895; 1991.

17. New York State Task Force on Life and the Law, *Life-Sustaining Treatment:*

Making Decisions and Appointing a Health Care Agent, New York: New York State Task Force on Life and the Law, 1990.

18. Mass. G.L. c. 201D.

19. Copies are available from the Office of Elder Affairs, Commonwealth of Massachusetts, 38 Chauncy Street, Boston, MA 02111; bulk orders from Massachusetts Health Decisions, P. O. Box 417, Sharon, MA 02067.

20. Task Force on Organ Transplantation, *Organ Transplantation,* Washington, D.C.: Department of Health and Human Services, 1986, p. 38.

21. *New York Times,* Feb. 4, 1991, p. B1.

CHAPTER 9

1. This chapter is based on Annas, G. J., Not Saints but Healers: The Legal Duties of Health Care Professionals in the AIDS Epidemic, *Am. J. Public Health* 78:844–849; 1988.

2. Winner, L., *The Whale and the Reactor,* Chicago: U. Chicago Press, 1986, p. 51.

3. Tienstra, J. D., Letter to the Editor, *JAMA* 259:517; 1988.

4. *E.g.,* Annas, G. J., Legal Risks and Responsibilities of Physicians in the AIDS Epidemic, *Hastings Center Report* April/May 1988. *See also* Boffey, P. M., Doctors Who Shun AIDS Patients Are Assailed by Surgeon General, *New York Times,* Sept. 10, 1987, p. 1, and Editorial, When Doctors Refuse To Treat AIDS, *New York Times,* Aug. 3, 1987, p. A16.

5. Oral remarks, AIDS Conference, Boston, Mass., Dec. 1, 1988. *See also* Breo, D. L., Dr. Koop Calls for AIDS Tests before Surgery, *Am. Med. News,* June 26, 1987, p. 1.

6. Goodman, E., For Doctors, an AIDS Dilemma that's Spreading with the Disease, *Boston Globe,* Feb. 25, 1988, p. 21.

7. *See* Barnes, M., Rango, N. A., Burke, G. R., & Chiarello, L., The HIV-Infected Health Care Professional: Employment Policies and Public Health, *Law, Med. & Health Care* 18:311–330; 1990.

8. Banks, T. L., The Right to Medical Treatment (in) Dalton, H. & Burris, S., eds., *AIDS and the Law,* New Haven, CT: Yale U. Press, 1987.

9. Annas, G. J., *The Rights of Patients,* 2d ed., Carbondale, IL: So. Ill. U. Press, 1989.

10. Annas, G. J., Your Money or Your Life: "Dumping" Uninsured Patients from Hospital Emergency Wards, *Am. J. Public Health* 76:74–77; 1986.

11. OSHA, Dept. of Labor, Occupational Exposure to Hepatitis B Virus and Human Immunodeficiency Virus; Advance Notice of Proposed Rulemaking, 52 *Fed. Reg.* 45438 (1987); Final Rule, 56 *Fed. Reg.* 64004 (1991); and Centers for Disease Control, Public Health Service, U.S. Department of Health and Human Services, Recommendations for Prevention of HIV Transmission in Health-Care Settings, *Morbidity and Mortality Weekly Report,* Aug. 21, 1987; 36:3S–18S. *And see* AIDS and HIV Update: Acquired Immunodeficiency Syndrome and Human Immunodeficiency Virus Infection among Health Workers, *Mortality Weekly,* 37: 229; 1988.

12. Tokarz, W., Odyssey of AIDS Victim Ends in Death, *Am. Med. News,* Nov. 4, 1983. *And see* other cases cited in Annas, *supra* note 9.

13. *Doe v. Shasta General Hospital,* Shasta Co. Super. Ct., 92336 (*AIDS Policy & Law,* Jan. 27, 1988, pp. 9–10).

14. Mass. Bd. of Registration in Medicine, 243 CMR 2.06 (10). The genesis of the regulation is discussed in Annas, G. J., *Judging Medicine,* Totowa, NJ: Humana Press, 1988, pp. 42–45.

15. *See, e.g.,* Fein, R., *Medical Care, Medical Costs,* Cambridge, MA: Harvard U. Press, 1986, and Relman, A., Universal Health Insurance: Its Time Has Come, *New Engl. J. Med.* 320:117; 1989.

16. Annas, G. J., *The Rights of Hospital Patients,* New York: Avon, 1975, p. 95.

17. *Lyons v. Grether,* 239 S.E.2d 103 (Va. 1977).

18. *School Board of Nassau Co. v. Arline,* 481 U.S. 1024 (1987). Parmet, W. E., AIDS and the Limits of Discrimination Law, *Law, Med. & Health Care* 15:61; 1987. The statute defines as handicapped one who "(i) has a physical or mental impairment which substantially limits one or more of such person's major life activities, (ii) has a record of such impairment, or (iii) is regarded as having such an impairment."

19. Parmet, W. E., Discrimination and Disability: The Challenge of the ADA, *Law, Med. & Health Care* 18:331–344; 1990.

20. Leonard, A. S., AIDS in the Workplace (in) Dalton, H. & Burris, S., eds., *AIDS and the Law,* New Haven: Yale U. Press, 1987.

21. *See supra* note 11.

22. *Gateway Coal Co. v. United Mine Workers of America,* 414 U.S. 368 (1974), and Leonard, *supra* note 20.

23. Hagan, M. D., Klemens, K. B., & Pauker, S. G., Routine Preoperative Screening for HIV, *JAMA* 259:1357–1359; 1988.

24. *Ibid.,* p. 1359. *Compare* Emanuel, E. J., Do Physicians Have an Obligation to Treat Patients with AIDS?, *New Engl. J. Med.* 318:1686; 1988.

25. For an in-depth discussion of this issue see Glantz, L. H., Mariner, W. K. & Annas, G. J., Risky Business: Screening Health Care Professionals for HIV Infection, *Milbank Q.* 70:43–79; 1992.

26. Position Paper, Acquired Immunodeficiency Syndrome, *Ann. Int. Med.* 104: 575–581; 1986.

27. The Doctor's Duty toward AIDS Patients, *Lancet,* May 30, 1987, p. 1274.

28. Council on Ethical and Judicial Affairs, Ethical Issues Involved in the Growing AIDS Crisis, *JAMA* 259:1360–1361; 1988.

29. Unethical To Refuse To Treat HIV-infected Patients, AMA Says, *Am. Med. News,* Nov. 20, 1987, p. 1.

30. Refusing Care of AIDS Patients: New Policies and Admissions Emerge, *Hospital Ethics,* Jan./Feb. 1988, p. 5. *And see* Pear, R., What Would Hippocrates have said about AIDS? *New York Times,* Jan. 3, 1988, p. E7.

31. AMA Delegates Vote on AIDS Care Ethics, *Med. World News,* Dec. 28, 1987, p. 16.

32. TMA Policy Lets MDs Refuse AIDS Patients if They Refer, *Am. Med. News,* Dec. 4, 1987, p. 3.

33. *Ibid.*

34. Annas, G. J., Glantz, L. H. & Katz, B. F., *The Rights of Doctors, Nurses and Allied Health Professionals,* Cambridge, MA: Ballinger, 1981.

35. Copies available from the Massachusetts Board of Registration in Medicine, 10 West Street, Boston, MA 02111.

36. Zuger, A., AIDS on the Wards: A Residency in Medical Ethics, *Hastings Center Report,* June 1987, pp. 16–20.

37. Shenson, D., When Fear Conquers, *New York Times Magazine,* Feb. 28, 1988, p. 35.

38. Sullivan, R., 13 Medical Colleges Say Staffs Must Treat AIDS, *New York Times,* Dec. 9, 1987, p. B3.

39. *E.g.,* Pinkey, D. S., AIDS Increases Strain on N.Y. Hospitals' Finances, Manpower, *Am. Med. News,* March 11, 1988, p. 1, and *supra* note 15.

CHAPTER 10

1. This chapter is based on Annas, G. J., Faith (Healing), Hope and Charity at the FDA: The Politics of AIDS Drug Trials, *Villanova L. Rev.* 34:771-797; 1989, which should be consulted for full text of notes.

2. Katz, J., *The Silent World of Doctor and Patient,* New York: Free Press, 1984, p. 151.

3. *Trials of War Criminals before the Nuremberg Military Tribunals under Control Council Law No. 10, The Medical Case,* Vols. I and II, Washington, D.C.: U.S. Gov. Print. Office, 1950.

4. Annas, G. J., Glantz, L. H. & Katz, B. F., *Informed Consent to Human Experimentation,* Cambridge, MA: Ballinger, 1977. Surprisingly, when the U.S. Supreme Court had a chance to adopt and endorse the principles of the Nuremberg Code in 1987, it failed to recognize the code as a basis to award damages in the United States military by a 5 to 4 vote. *U.S. v. Stanley,* 483 U.S. 669 (1987).

5. Ingelfinger, F., Informed (but Uneducated) Consent, *New Engl. J. Med.* 287: 465-466; 1972.

6. *Ibid. And see* Reinhold, R., Infected but Not Ill, Many Try Unproved Drugs To Stave Off AIDS, *New York Times,* May 20, 1987, p. B12.

7. For example, a French AIDS researcher experimenting with HPA-23 said of AIDS patients in 1984: "What do these people have to lose?" (Quoted in Shilts, R., *And the Band Played On,* New York: St. Martin's Press, 1987, p. 496.)

8. Fletcher, J., The Evolution of the Ethics of Informed Consent (in) Berg, K. & Treanoy, K., eds., *Research Ethics,* New York: A. R. Liss, 1983, p. 211.

9. *New York Times,* Sept. 26, 1988, p. A16 (transcript of the presidential debate).

10. *U.S. v. Rutherford,* 442 U.S. 544, 1979. See Culbert, M., *The Fight for Laetrile Vitamin B17,* New Rochelle, NY: Arlington House, 1974, and Kittler, G. D., *Laetrile: Control for Cancer,* New York: Warner Books, 1963.

11. *Rutherford,* at p. 549. Laetrile's advocates, on the other hand, accused the government of suppressing a "cure" for cancer.

12. FDA, HHS, Investigational New Drug, Antibiotic, and Biological Drug Product Regulations; Treatment Use and Sale, 52 *Fed. Reg.* 19,465-77 (1987). *See* Young, F., Norris, J., Levitt, N., & Nightingale, S., The FDA's New Procedures for the Use of Investigational New Drugs, *JAMA* 259:2267; 1988.

13. Pear, R., U.S. To Allow Use of Trial Drugs for AIDS and Other Terminal Ills, *New York Times,* May 21, 1987, p. 1. A year later these new rules were termed a "failure" by the President's AIDS Commission. Report of the Presidential Commission on AIDS, 50 (1988).

14. Boffey, P., FDA Will Allow Patients To Import AIDS Medicines, *New York Times,* July 25, 1988, p. A15. Up to three months supply can be imported and a physician's name must be given.

15. Booth, P., An Underground Drug for AIDS, *Science,* Sept. 9, 1988, p. 1279.

16. Shilts, *supra* note 16, p. 562. "About 100 Americans were part of the AIDS

exile community in Paris, making long daily treks to Percy Hospital on the edge of the city for their shots of HPA-23" (*Ibid.,* p. 563).

17. Eckholm, R., Should the Rules be Bent in an Epidemic?, *New York Times,* July 13, 1987, p. 30E.

18. Clark, M., Lerner, M. & Stadtman, N., AIDS: A Breakthrough?, *Newsweek,* Nov. 11, 1985, p. 88.

19. Brooke, J., In Zaire, AIDS Awareness vs. Prevention, *New York Times,* Oct. 10, 1988, p. B4.

20. *See, e.g.,* Kolata, G., Recruiting Problems in New York Hinder U.S. Trials of AIDS Drug, *New York Times,* Dec. 18, 1988, p. 1.

21. 53 *Fed. Reg.* 41515-24 (1988). *See also* Waldholz, M., Drug Firms Hope FDA Broadens Plan To Speed Approval of Some Medicines, *Wall St. J.,* Oct. 21, 1988, p. B3.

22. Silver, L., FDA Offers Plan To Speed Process of Drug Approval, *Boston Globe,* Oct. 20, 1988, p. 3.

23. Altman, L., At AIDS Talks Reality Weighs Down Hope, *New York Times,* July 26, 1992, p. 1.

24. McKinlay, J., From "Promising Report" to "Standard Procedure": Seven States in the Career of a Medical Innovation, *Milbank Mem. Fund Q.* 59:374; 1981, and sources cited therein. In an RCT trial a new drug is compared with a placebo or other drug, each being assigned at random to comparable patients. In a double blind study, neither the physician nor the patient know who is getting the new drug and who is getting the placebo.

25. New Ideas for New Drugs, *Wall St. J.,* Dec. 28, 1988, p. A6. *See also* Waldholz, M., Drug Firms Hope FDA Broadens Plan To Speed Approval of Some Medicines, *Wall St. J.,* Oct. 21, 1988, p. B3.

26. *See, e.g.,* Editorial, Forcing Poverty on AIDS Patients, *New York Times,* Aug. 30, 1988, p. A18, stating in part, "A drug company should not unusually have to justify its profit, but AZT is a special case." *And see* Arno, P. & Feiden, K., *Against the Odds: The Story of AIDS Drug Development, Politics and Profits,* New York: HarperCollins, 1992.

27. O'Reilly, Drug Makers Under Attack, *Fortune* 124(3):48-63, July 29, 1991.

28. *But see* Edgar, H. & Rothman, D. J., New Rules for New Drugs: The Challenge of AIDS to the Regulatory Process, *Milbank Mem. Fund Q.* 68:111–141; 1990.

29. Brauer, R., The Promise that Failed, *New York Times Magazine,* Aug. 28, 1988, pp. 46, 76.

CHAPTER 11

1. This chapter is based on Annas, G. J., Mapping the Human Genome and the Meaning of Monster Mythology, *Emory L. J.* 39:629–664; 1990, which should be consulted for more detailed references.

2. Langbaum, R., Introduction, Shakespeare, W., *The Tempest,* New York: New American Library ed., 1964 (first published in 1611), p. 9.

3. Bloom, H., Afterword, *Frankenstein,* New York: New American Library ed., 1963 (first published in 1817), p. 56.

4. Charyn, I., Afterword: Who Is Hyde? (in) *Dr. Jekyll and Mr. Hyde,* New York: Bantam, 1981 (first published in 1886).

5. Aldiss, B., Afterword, *The Island of Dr. Moreau,* New York: New American Library, 1988 (first published in 1896). *See also,* Ringel, Genetic Experimentation: Mad Scientists and the Beast, *J. Fantastic in the Arts* 2(1):64; 1989.

6. *See, e.g.,* U.S. Congress, Office of Technology Assessment, *Mapping Our Genes: Genome Projects, How Big, How Fast?,* Washington, D.C.: U.S. Gov. Print. Office, 1988, pp. 21–24.

7. Quoted in Hall, James Watson and the Search for Biology's "Holy Grail," *Smithsonian,* Feb. 1990, pp. 41, 47.

8. *Mapping Our Genes, supra* note 6, p. 57.

9. Quoted in Breo, D., DNA Discoverer James Watson Now Dreams of Curing Genetic Diseases, *JAMA* 262:3340,3343; 1989.

10. Elias, S. & Annas, G. J., *Reproductive Genetics and the Law,* St. Louis: Mosby-Yearbook, 1987, p. 29.

11. National Academy of Sciences, *Genetic Screening: Programs, Principles and Research,* Washington, D.C.: National Academy of Sciences, 1975.

12. Holtzman, N. A., *Newborn Screening for Genetic-Metabolic Diseases: Progress, Principles and Recommendations,* Washington, D.C.: National Academy of Sciences, 1977.

13. Rothstein, M., *Medical Screening and the Employee Health Cost Crisis,* Washington, D.C.: Bureau of National Affairs, 1989, p. 221.

14. Koshland, D., The Molecule of the Year, *Science,* 246:1541; 1989.

15. *Buck v. Bell,* 274 U.S. 200, 207 (1927).

16. *Mapping Our Genes, supra* note 6, p. 84.

17. Quoted in Jaroff, L., The Gene Hunt, *Time,* March 20, 1989, p. 62.

18. Snow, C. P., *The Two Cultures,* New York: Cambridge U. Press, 1964, p. 5.

19. Roszak, T., *The Making of a Counter-Culture,* Garden City, NY: Doubleday, 1969, p. 273.

20. Quoted in *Science* 199:33; 1978.

21. Swazey, J., Sorenson, J. & Wong, P., Risks and Benefits, Rights and Responsibilities: A History of the Recombinant DNA Research Controversy, *So. Cal. L. Rev.* 51:1019; 1978.

22. Roberts, L., Carving Up the Human Genome, *Science* 246:1244; 1989.

23. Department of Health and Human Services, National Institutes of Health, Guidelines for Research Involving Recombinant DNA Molecules, 48 *Fed. Reg.* 24556 (1983).

24. Quoted in President's Commission for the Study of Ethical Problems in Medicine and Biomedical and Behavioral Research, *Splicing Life: The Social and Ethical Issues of Genetic Engineering with Human Beings,* Washington, D.C.: U.S. Gov. Print. Office, 1982, p. 23.

25. *Ibid.,* p. 24.

26. Areen, J., King, P., Goldberg, S. & Capron, A., *Law, Science and Medicine,* Mineola, NY: Foundation Press, 1984, p. 65.

27. *Splicing Life, supra* note 24, p. 4.

28. Anderson, F. & Fletcher, J., Gene Therapy in Human Beings: When Is It Ethical To Begin?, *New Engl. J. Med.* 303:1293; 1980. *And see generally* Nichols, E., *Human Gene Therapy,* Washington, D.C.: National Academy of Sciences, 1988.

29. Rogers, M., *Biohazard,* New York: Knopf, 1977, pp. 92–93. *And see* Dworkin, R., Science, Society, and the Expert Town Meeting: Some Comments on Asilomar, *So. Cal. L. Rev.* 51:1471; 1978.

30. Quoted in Rhodes, R., *The Making of the Atomic Bomb,* New York: Simon & Shuster, 1986, p. 761.

31. Havel, V., *Living in Truth,* London: Faber & Faber, 1989, pp. 136, 138, 144, 149–150. (J. Vladislavrd, Tr. 1989).

32. Excerpts from Czech Chief's Address to Congress, *New York Times,* Feb. 22, 1990, p. A14.

33. Havel, V., The End of the Modern Era, *New York Times,* March 1, 1992, p. E17.

34. *Ibid.*

35. Fitzgerald, F. Scott, *The Great Gatsby,* New York: Scribners, 1925, p. 182.

CHAPTER 12

1. This chapter is based on Annas, G. J., Whose Waste Is It Anyway? The Case of John Moore, *Hastings Center Report* 18(5):37–39; 1988, and Annas, G. J., Outrageous Fortune: Selling Other Peoples's Cells, *Hastings Center Report* 20(6): 36–38; 1990.

2. Stone, J., Cells for Sale, *Discover,* August 1988, pp. 34–35.

3. *Moore v. Regents of the U. of California,* 88 Daily Journal D.A.R. 9520 (Cal. Ct. App., 2d Dist., Div. 4, 1988).

4. *Browning v. Norton Children's Hospital,* 54 S.W.2d 713 (Ky. 1974).

5. American Medical Association, Office of General Counsel, *Medicolegal Forms,* Chicago: American Medical Association, 1973, p. 58.

6. Judge Rothman attributes the analogy to Rori Sherman, The Selling of Body Parts, *National L. J.,* Dec. 7, 1987, p. 1. And *see generally* Note, Toward the Right of Commerciality: Recognizing Property Rights in the Commercial Value of Human Tissue, *UCLA L. Rev.* 34:207–264; 1986.

7. Congress of the United States, Office of Technology Assessment, *New Development in Biotechnology: Ownership of Human Tissues and Cells,* Washington, D.C.: U.S. Gov. Print. Off., 1987, pp. 83–85.

8. *Ibid.*

9. *Moore v. Regents of the University of California,* 793 P.2d 479, 271 Cal. Rptr. 146 (1990).

10. *Cobbs v. Grant,* 502 P.2d 1, 104 Cal. Rptr. 505 (1972).

11. Relying on Mary Taylor Danforth's recommendations in Cells, Sales, and Royalties: The Patient's Right to a Portion of the Profits, *Yale Law & Policy Rev.* 6:179–202; 1988.

CHAPTER 13

1. This chapter is adapted from an article which was coauthored with Sherman Elias, who is the source of the medical information contained herein. Annas, G. J. & Elias, S., The Politics of Transplantation of Human Fetal Tissue, *New Engl. J. Med.* 320:1079–1082; 1989.

2. *Roe v. Wade,* 410 U.S. 113 (1973), discussed in Chapter 4.

3. Robertson, J. A., Fetal Tissue Transplants, *Washington U. L. Q.* 66:443–498; 1988.

4. *Ibid.* The states that prohibit such research are Arizona, Arkansas, Illinois, Indiana, Louisiana, New Mexico, Ohio, and Oklahoma.

5. Consultants of the Advisory Committee to the Director of the National Insti-

tutes of Health, *Report of the Human Fetal Tissue Transplant Panel,* Washington, D.C.: National Institutes of Health, 1988.

6. Butchaell, J. T., University Policy on Experimental Use of Aborted Fetal Tissue, *IRB* 10(4):7–11; 1988.

7. Bopp, J., Use of Fetal Tissue Will Increase the Number of Abortions, *National Right to Life News,* Nov. 17, 1988, p. 4. *See also* Under Secretary of HHS James Mason on *60 Minutes* ("Life, Death and Politics"), Feb. 23, 1992 (arguing that using fetal tissue for "humanitarian purposes" could tilt the woman's decision in favor of abortion).

8. Nolan, K., *Genug ist Genug:* A Fetus Is Not a Kidney, *Hastings Center Report* 18(6):13–19; 1988.

9. Freedman, B., The Ethics of Using Human Fetal Tissue, *IRB* 10(6):1–4; 1988.

10. *Strachan v. John F. Kennedy Memorial Hospital,* 538 A.2d 346 (N.J. 1988).

11. Greely, H. T., Hamm, T., Johnson, R., *et. al.,* The Ethical Use of Human Fetal Tissue in Medicine, *New Engl. J. Med.* 320:1093–1096; 1989.

12. Warburton, D., Stein, Z., Kline, J., & Susser, M., Chromosome Abnormalities in Spontaneous Abortion (in) Porter, I. H. & Hook, B., eds., *Human Embryonic and Fetal Death,* New York: Academic Press, 1980, pp. 261–287.

13. Sever, J. L., Infectious Cause of Human Reproductive Loss (in) Porter, I. H., Hook, B., eds., *Human Embryonic and Fetal Death,* New York: Academic Press, 1980, pp. 169–175.

14. Hilts, P., Fetal-Tissue Bank Not Viable Option Agency Memo Says, *New York Times,* July 27, 1992, p. 1.

15. Mason, J. O., Should the Fetal Tissue Research Ban Be Lifted? *J. NIH Res.* 2:17–18; Jan. 1990.

16. Lewin, R., Cloud over Parkinson's Therapy, *Science* 240:390; 1988.

17. Editorial, Embryos and Parkinson's Disease, *Lancet* 1:1087; 1988. *See also* Goetz, C. G., *et. al.,* Multicenter Study of Autologous Adrenal Medullary Transplantation to the Corpus Striatum in Patients with Advanced Parkinson's Disease, *New Engl. J. Med.* 320:337; 1989.

18. Lindvall, *et al.,* Fetal Dopamine-rich Mesencephalic Grafts in Parkinson's Disease, *Lancet* 2:1483; 1988.

19. Lewin, R., Caution Continues Over Transplants, *Science* 242:1379; 1988.

20. Reports of their work, with editorial comments, appear in *New Engl. J. Med.* 327:1541–1555; 1589–1595 (Nov. 26, 1992).

21. Sladek, J. R. & Shoulson, I., Neural Transplantation: A Call for Patience Rather Than Patients, *Science* 240:1386–1388; 1988.

CHAPTER 14

1. This chapter is based on Annas, G. J., Brain Death and Organ Transplantation: You Can Have One without the Other, *Hastings Center Report* 18(3):28–30; May 1988, and Annas, G. J., From Canada with Love: Using Anencephalics for Organ Transplants, *Hastings Center Report* 17(6):36–38; Dec. 1987.

2. *Strachan v. John F. Kennedy Memorial Hospital,* 507 A.2d 718 (N.J. Super. A.D. 1986). All quotations not otherwise referenced and other facts regarding this case are from this opinion or the one in note 3.

3. *Strachan v. John F. Kennedy Memorial Hospital,* 538 A.2d 346 (N.J. 1988).

4. A good example is the suffering endured by the family of Paul Brophy when New England Sinai Hospital refused to terminate his artificial feeding upon the request of the family.

5. This is because the most that either the court or a committee could do would be to ask the neurologist who had previously determined the patient to be dead, if the patient was in fact dead. An additional neurologist might reasonably be called in to consult in a difficult case, but courts and committees add nothing to this factual determination.

6. For a more detailed discussion, *see* Martyn, S., Wright, R. & Clark, L., Required Request of Organ Donation: Moral, Clinical, and Legal Problems, *Hastings Center Report* 18(2):27–34, April 1988.

7. Task Force on Organ Transplantation, *Organ Transplantation Issues and Recommendations,* Washington, D.C.: U.S. DHHS, 1986, p. 38.

8. Kantrowitz, A., *et al.,* Transplantation of the Heart in an Infant and an Adult, *Am. J. Cardiol.* 22:782; 1968.

9. Capron, A., Anencephalic Donors: Separate the Dead from the Dying, *Hastings Center Report* 17(1):5, Jan. 1987.

10. Caplan, A., Should Fetuses or Infants Be Utilized as Organ Donors?, *Bioethics* 1:119; 1987.

11. President's Commission for the Study of Ethical Issues in Medicine, *Defining Death,* Washington, D.C.: U.S. Gov. Print. Off., 1981, p. 3.

12. Task Force for the Determination of Brain Death in Children, Guidelines for the Determination of Brain Death in Children, *Ann. Neurol.* 21:616–617; 1987.

13. Peabody, J. L., Emery, J. R. & Ashwal, S., Experience with Anencephalic Infants as Prospective Organ Donors, *New Engl. J. Med.* 321:344–350; 1989; *and see,* Committee on Bioethics, American Academy of Pediatrics, Infants with Anencephaly as Organ Sources: Ethical Considerations, *Pediatrics* 89:1116–1119; 1992.

14. *In Re: T.A.C.P.,* 1992 Fla. LEXIS 1932 (Nov. 12, 1992).

CHAPTER 15

1. This chapter is based on Annas, G. J., Death and the Magic Machine: Informed Consent to the Artificial Heart, *Western New Engl. L. Rev.* 9:89–112; 1987, which should be consulted for more detailed references and notes.

2. Solzhenitsyn, A. I., *The Cancer Ward,* 1968, quoted in Katz, J., *The Silent World of Doctor and Patient,* New York: Free Press, 1984, p. xv.

3. Fletcher, J., The Evolution of the Ethics of Informed Consent (in) Berg, K., & Teanoy, K., eds., *Research Ethics,* New York: A. R. Liss, 1983, p. 211.

4. Barnard, C. & Pepper, C. B., *One Life,* New York: Macmillan, 1969, p. 348.

5. Quoted in Thompson, T., *Hearts,* New York: McCall Pub. Co., 1971, p. 216.

6. Quoted in Thorwald, J., *The Patients,* New York: Harcourt Brace Javonovich, 1971, p. 402. *And see Karp v. Cooley,* 493 F.2d 408, 423 (5th Cir. 1974) affirming *Karp v. Cooley,* 349 F. Supp. 827 (S.D. Tex. 1972).

7. Artificial Heart, NOVA, Transcript, Time-Life Video, p. 3 (1984). The other major problem was and remains the incompatibility of human blood and the device's surface that leads to clotting.

8. For a fuller discussion of this form, *see* Annas, G. J., Consent to the Artificial Heart: The Lion and the Crocodiles, *Hastings Center Report* 13(2):20–22; April 1983.

9. Altman, L., The Ordeal of a "Human Experiment," *New York Times,* May 14, 1985, p. C3.

10. *Newsweek,* Dec. 13, 1982, pp. 35–36.

11. Altman, L., Recipient of Artificial Heart Calls Ordeal Worthwhile, *New York Times,* March 3, 1983, p. A1.

12. *See* Williams, R., Why IRBs Falter in Reviewing Risks and Benefits, *IRB* May/June 1984, pp. 1–5. On December 20, 1985, the FDA held a hearing to determine if DeVries should be permitted to complete his "series of seven" permanent implants that had originally been approved, or whether such research should be suspended in view of the devastating effects it had had on the first four recipients. The FDA decided to permit DeVries to continue, but only if additional information was supplied to the FDA and if future implants were reviewed on a case-by-case basis. *See* Boffey, P., More Implants of Artificial Hearts Are Urged by U.S. Health Panel, *New York Times,* Dec. 22, 1985, p. 34. *See also* Clark, Stiffer Rules for the Heart, *Newsweek,* Dec. 30, 1985, p. 68. No major problems were seen by the agency in the consent form or process, although DeVries reported to a U.S. Congressional committee on February 5, 1986, that modifications were planned for both. In retrospect we can see that experimentation with the Jarvik-7 as a permanent device ended with the death of William Schroeder in August 1985.

13. Cooley, Liotta & Hallman, Orthotopic Cardiac Prosthesis for Two-staged Cardiac Replacement, *Am. J. Cardiol.* 24:723; 1969. *See also* Cooley, D., Staged Cardiac Transplantation: Report of Three Cases, *Heart Transplant* 1:145; 1982.

14. Annas, G. J., No Cheers for Artificial Hearts, *Hastings Center Report* 15(5): 27–28; Oct. 1985. *Contra,* Hill, *et al.,* Use of a Prosthetic Ventricle as a Bridge to Cardiac Transplantation for Postinfarction Cardiogenic Shock, *New Engl. J. Med.* 314:626; 1986.

15. Following Barnard's initial human-to-human heart transplant, about 150 human heart transplants were done at sixty hospitals around the world in the next two years. There were almost no long-term survivors in the unseemly rush to join the "me-too" club of heart transplant surgeons, and this episode stands as one of the blackest marks in the history of surgery. *See* Jennett, B., *High Technology Medicine,* London: Nuffield Provincial Hospital Trust, 1984, pp. 84–85.

16. The case of Thomas Creighton is described in more detail in Annas, G. J., The Phoenix Heart: What We Have to Lose, *Hastings Center Report* 15(3):15–16; June 1985. *See also* Copeland, J., *et al.,* The Total Artificial Heart as a Bridge to Transplantation: A Report of Two Cases, *JAMA* 256:2991; 1986.

17. Altman, L., Anguish, Hope, a Moment of Fame: A Heart's Story Is Told, *New York Times,* March 19, 1985, pp. C1–2. *See also* Hubert & Ring, Tucsonian Gets Mechanical Heart at UMC, *Arizona Daily Star,* March 7, 1985, pp. 1–2. Blakeslee, S., Arizona Surgeon Defends Heart Implant, *New York Times,* March 12, 1985, p. C2. Kuhn & Pesce, Heartmaker: A Dentist with a Dream, *USA Today,* March 8, 1985, p. 1A. The Man with the Illegal Heart, *New York Times,* March 9, 1985, p. 22. *Time,* March 18, 1985, p. 63. *Newsweek,* March 18, 1985, pp. 86–88. Altman, L., Learning To Live with the Artificial Heart, *New York Times,* March 17, 1985, p. D7.

18. Hubert & Rothenberg, Patient Has a Long Shot, *Arizona Daily Star,* March 8, 1985, pp. 1–2.

19. Copeland, J., We Can't Sacrifice Lives to Risks, *USA Today,* March 11, 1985, p. 10A.

20. FDA, HHS, Guidance for Emergency Use of Unapproved Medical Devices: Availability, 50 *Fed. Reg.* 42866 (1985).

21. The original four hospitals to obtain FDA approval were the University of Arizona at Tucson, Pennsylvania State University at Hershey, Abbott-Northwestern, Hospital, Minneapolis, and Presbyterian-University Hospital, Pittsburgh.

22. The implant was done at the West Berlin Charlottenburg University Clinic by Emil Buecheri. *See New York Times,* March 10, 1986, p. A17.

23. Hubert, Chayrez Dies, *Arizona Star,* Oct. 12, 1986, pp. 1, 5.

24. All quotations in this paragraph are from Epstein, Heart Patient's Death: Sorrow, Lessons Endure, *Am. Med. News,* Nov. 7, 1986, p. 3.

25. I presented a proposal to this effect to the Subcommittee on Investigations and Oversight of the Committee on Science and Technology, U.S. House of Representatives, on February 5, 1986. (Annas, G. J., Legal and Ethical Issues in Artificial Heart Experimentation, *Status of the Artificial Heart Program, Hearings,* pp. 163–209.) The two committee members present were not supportive, nor was the FDA. The hearing itself took place one week after the explosion of the space shuttle Challenger, and this disaster was commented on by almost all of the witnesses. Their point was that we should not let the disaster stop the space program. Of course no one had suggested that it should, any more than anyone would seriously suggest the disasters suffered by Barney Clark, William Schroeder, Murray Hayden, and Jack Burcham should end the quest for an effective, efficient, and totally implantable artificial heart. But just as reality has caught up with the private hope and public hype of the space program, so it has caught up with the hype of the artificial heart. Our reactions to disappointment should be basically the same in both programs: to reassess; to move forward with more knowledge and more caution; and "to liberate the space program [artificial hearts] and technology in general from the mystique that we have placed on it. . . . Our technology is imperfect, because we are imperfect, so either worshipping or despising our technological age is just a neat shifting of blame." (Walter McDougal, quoted by Wilford, J., After the Challenger: America's Future in Space, *New York Times Magazine,* March 16, 1986, pp. 38, 106.)

In 1991 an Institute of Medicine panel reviewing the artificial heart gave it its first only lukewarm endorsement saying:

> The committee recommends that NHLBI continue to support TAH [total artificial heart] development for an interim period . . . NHLBI's commitment to TAHs could be reexamined in 1994 or 1995 . . . aided by another cost-effectiveness analysis that reflects updated estimates about projected TAH clinical effectiveness, complications, and costs. (Institute of Medicine, *The Artificial Heart: Prototypes, Policies and Patients,* Washington, D.C.: National Academy Press, 1991, p. 12.)

CHAPTER 16

1. Klein, R., *The Politics of the NHS,* 2d ed. London: Longman, 1989, pp. 67–68.

2. Callahan, D., *What Kind of Life: The Limits of Medical Progress,* New York: Simon & Schuster, 1990.

3. Havinghurst, C., Prospective Self-Denial: Can Consumers Contract Today to Accept Health Care Rationing Tomorrow?, *U. Penn. L. Rev.* 140:1755, 1807; 1992.

4. Illich, I., *Medical Nemesis*, London: Calder & Boyars, 1975, p. 149.

5. Lubitz, J. & Prihoda, R., The Use and Costs of Medicare Services in the Last 2 Years of Life, *Health Care Financing Rev.* 5:117; 1984.

6. *See, e.g.,* Moravec, H., *Mind Children: The Future of Robot and Human Intelligence,* Cambridge, MA: Harvard U. Press, 1988.

7. Quoted in Farney, D., Novelist Updike sees a Nation Frustrated by its own Dreams, *Wall St. J.,* September 16, 1992, p. A8.

CHAPTER 18

1. This chapter is based on Annas, G. J., Siamese Twins: Killing One To Save the Other, *Hastings Center Report* 17(2):27–29; 1987.

2. Marin-Padilla, M., Chin, A. J. & Marin-Padilla, T. M., Cardiovascular Abnormalities in Thoracopagus Twins, *Teratology* 23:101–113; 1981.

3. Drake, D. C., The Twins Decision: One Must Die So One Can Live, *Philadelphia Inquirer,* Oct. 16, 1977.

4. Meehan, F., The Siamese Twin Operation and Contemporary Catholic Medical Ethics, *Linacre Q.* 45:157–162; 1978.

5. Drake, *supra* note 3.

6. Golladay, E. S., Williams, G. D., Seibert, J. J., *et al.,* Dicephalus Dipus Conjoined Twins: A Surgical Separation and Review of Previously Reported Cases, *J. Pediatric Surgery* 17:259–264; 1982.

7. *See generally* The Treatment of Handicapped Newborns (in) Elias, S. & Annas, G. J., *Reproductive Genetics and the Law,* St. Louis: Mosby-Yearbook, 1987.

8. Robinson, P. H., Criminal Law Defenses: A Systemic Analysis, *Columbia L. Rev.* 82:199, 234–235; 1982.

CHAPTER 19

1. This chapter is based on Annas, G. J., Killing Machines, *Hastings Center Report* 21(2):33–35; March 1991.

2. Van Creveld, M., *Technology and War,* New York: Free Press, 1989, p. 71.

3. *People v. Roberts,* 211 Mich. 187, 178 N.W. 690 (1920).

4. *People v. Campbell,* 335 N.W.2d 27 (Mich. App. 1983).

5. Editorial, Dying, Dr. Kevorkian's Way, *New York Times,* June 7, 1989, p. A22.

6. Lewin, T., Doctor Cleared of Murdering Woman with Suicide Machine, *New York Times,* Dec. 14, 1990, p. B8.

7. Fussell, P., *The Great War and Modern Memory,* New York: Oxford U. Press, 1975, p. 170.

CHAPTER 20

1. This chapter is adopted from Annas, G. J., Health Law at the Turn of the Century: From White Dwarf to Red Giant, *Conn. L. Rev.* 21:551–569; 1989.

2. I chaired the first national health law teachers conference, which was sponsored by Boston University's Center for Law and Health Sciences. Since 1976 the

Health Law Teacher's Meeting has been held a dozen times, biannually until 1985, and annually since.

3. *See* Teaching Health Law: A Symposium, *J. Legal Educ.* 38:485–576; 1988.

4. Law, S., Teaching Health Law: A Symposium: Introduction, *J. Legal Educ.* 38:485,486; 1988. *See also* Curran, W. J., Titles in the Medicolegal Field: A Proposal for Reform, *Am. J. Law & Med.* 1:10; 1975. The basic text for the standard law and medicine course is Curran, W. J., Shapiro, E. D. & Hall, M., *Law, Medicine and Forensic Science,* 4th ed., Boston: Little, Brown, 1991.

5. Rosenblatt, R., Conceptualizing Health Law for Teaching Purposes: The Social Justice Perspective, *J. Legal Educ.* 38:489; 1988.

6. This is the approach I suggested at the first health law teachers conference, noting that "just as astronomy and physics can be viewed as applied mathematics, health law can be viewed as applied law, concerned with a particular area of human endeavor." (Quoted in Christoffel, T., *Health and the Law,* New York: Free Press, 1982, p. 7.)

7. Havighurst, C., Health Care as a Laboratory for the Study of Law and Policy, *J. Legal Educ.* 38:499; 1988.

8. *See, e.g.,* Annas, G. J., Law and Medicine: Myths and Realities in the Medical School Classroom, *Am. J. Law & Med.* 1:195; 1975.

9. Grumet, B., Legal Medicine in Medical Schools: A Survey of the State of the Art, *J. Med. Educ.* 54:755; 1979.

10. Martin Redish of Northwestern University Law School, quoted in Rothfeld, What Do Law Schools Teach? Almost Anything, *New York Times,* Dec. 23, 1988, p. B8.

11. *E.g.,* Mark Tushnet of Georgetown Law Center, noting that the law school "is more an academic department than a professional school." Quoted in Middleton, Legal Scholarship: Is It Irrelevant?, *National L. J.,* Jan. 9, 1989, p. 1.

12. Havighurst, *supra* note 7.

13. An introductory course that exposes all three approaches can be taught from Annas, G. J., Law, S., Rosenblatt, R. & Wing, K., *American Health Law,* Boston: Little, Brown, 1990.

14. *See, e.g.,* Posner, R., *Economic Analysis of Law,* 3rd ed., Cambridge, MA: Harvard U. Press, 1986; and Posner, R., Utilitarianism, Economics, and Legal Theory, *J. Legal Studies* 8:103; 1979.

15. *Ibid., and see* Kelman, M., *A Guide to Critical Legal Studies,* Cambridge, MA: Harvard U. Press, 1987, p. 186.

16. Rosenblatt, *supra* note 5.

17. Kennedy, D., Distributive and Paternalist Motives in Contract and Tort Law, with Special Reference to Compulsory Terms and Unequal Bargaining Power, *Maryland L. Rev.* 41:563,564; 1982.

18. Law, *supra* note 4, p. 486.

19. Capron, A., A 'Bioethics' Approach to Teaching Health Law, *J. Legal Educ.* 38:505,509; 1988. A casebook he coauthored also takes this approach. (Areen, J., King, P., Goldberg, S. & Capron, A., *Law, Science and Medicine,* Mineola, NY: Foundation Press, 1984.)

20. *See, e.g.,* Wing, K., *The Law and the Public's Health,* 3rd ed., Ann Arbor, MI: Health Administration Press, 1985. *See also* Christoffel, *supra* note 6.

21. Quoted in McDougall, W., *The Heavens Themselves: A Political History of the Space Age,* New York: Basic Books, 1985, p. 441.

22. President's Commission for the Study of Ethical Problems in Medicine and Biomedical and Behavioral Research, *Defining Death,* Washington, D.C.: U.S. Gov. Print. Off., 1981.

23. Staton, S. F., ed., *Literary Theories in Praxis,* Philadelphia, Pa.: U. Pennsylvania Press, 1987, p. 4.

24. Some of the novels used are *Frankenstein, The Plague, Cider House Rules, The Fifth Child, White Noise, Brave New World, 1984,* and *The Handmaid's Tale.*

25. *See, e.g.,* Farrell, J., The Cyberpunk Controversy, *Boston Globe Magazine,* Feb. 19, 1989, p. 18.

26. The Burroughs' movie "script" *The Bladerunner* (1979) and the Nourse novel are not to be confused with the 1982 Warner Brothers movie of the same name. The movie *Blade Runner* takes place in 2019. Blade runners are special police whose job it is to kill "replicants," or robots, which have become just as intelligent as human beings, but are much stronger. They are designed for work off earth, but following a mutiny, some have returned "home." The movie explores issues of control, power, mortality, and identity. Based on the novel by Philip Dick (*Do Androids Dream of Electric Sheep?*), the only thing it has in common with the Nourse and Burroughs works is its title.

27. Sterling, B., ed., *Mirrorshades: The Cyberpunk Anthology,* New York: Ace Books, 1986, p. xiii.

28. Quoted by Farrell, *supra* note 36, p. 56.

29. *See, e.g.,* Fox, D., Physicians versus Lawyers: A Conflict of Cultures (in) Dalton, H. L., *et al.,* eds., *AIDS and the Law: A Guide for the Public,* New Haven, CT: Yale U. Press, 1987, p. 217.

30. *See, e.g.,* Bok, D., A Flawed System of Law Practice and Teaching, *J. Legal Educ.* 33:570; 1983. *See also* Wellington, H., Challenges to Legal Education: The 'Two Cultures' Phenomenon, *J. Legal Educ.* 37:327; 1987, and White, J., Doctrine in a Vacuum: Reflections on What a Law School Ought (and Ought Not) To Be, *J. Legal Educ.* 36:155; 1986.

31. Welcoming Remarks, Conference on Law and Medicine: Unresolved Issues for the 1990s, University of Connecticut School of Law, March 29, 1989. When the Dean Robert Clark of Harvard Law School was asked what he considered the "leading issues in the study of law today" he listed "health care regulation" first. (*New York Times,* March 31, 1989, p. B6.)

32. This approach should not be confused with the "clinical studies movement" that views medical education as the proper model for legal education, a model properly criticized in Carrington, P., The Dangers of the Graduate School Model, *J. Legal Educ.* 36:11; 1986.

33. Campbell, J. (with Bill Moyers), *The Power of Myth,* New York: Doubleday, 1988, p. 9.

Index